BIOCHEMICAL SOCIETY SYMPOSIA

No. 63

MAMMARY DEVELOPMENT AND CANCER

BIOCHEMICAL SOCIETY SYMPOSIUM No. 63
held at The University of Liverpool, Spring 1996

Mammary Development and Cancer

ORGANIZED AND EDITED BY

P.S. RUDLAND, D.G. FERNIG, S. LEINSTER AND G.G. LUNT

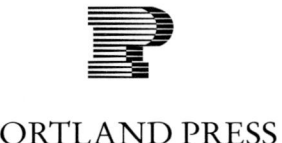

PORTLAND PRESS

Published by Portland Press, 59 Portland Place, London W I N 3AJ, U.K.
on behalf of The Biochemical Society
In North America orders should be sent to Ashgate Publishing Co.,
Old Post Road, Brookfield, VT 05036-9704, U.S.A.

ISBN I 85578 087 9   ISSN 0067-8964

British Library Cataloguing in Publication Data
A catalogue record for this book is available from the British Library

Typeset by Portland Press Ltd
Printed in Great Britain by Information Press Ltd, Eynsham, UK

Contents

Preface

This book on Mammary Development and Cancer arose from the Annual Symposium of The Biochemical Society of Great Britain, held at the University of Liverpool on 16–18 April 1996. It was organized as part of The Biochemical Society's 658th Meeting, held under the auspices of Professor B.E.H. Maden, Dr. A.G. McLennan, Professor H.H. Rees and the Department of Biochemistry of the University of Liverpool. Each speaker kindly agreed to provide a chapter based on their lecture, and since they are all internationally recognized in their areas, the book provides an authoritative and up-to-date review of what is a particularly fast-moving field. The cost of bringing the speakers together was provided, in part, by sponsorship from a local charity, The Cancer and Polio Research Fund, and from a local pharmaceutical company, Zeneca, both based in the North West of England, as well as by The Biochemical Society itself.

The Symposium, and now this book, have been designed to appeal to a wide audience of biochemists/molecular biologists, making use of the fact that the mammary gland is probably the most intensively studied mammalian developmental system in use today. There are five quite separate reasons for this intensive research into mammary development, as follows. (1) The mammary gland is one of the few organs that develops after birth, so making many experiments more tractable than in those organs that develop prior to birth. (2) The hormones that control breast development are well known and are important in a major commercial product, i.e. milk. (3) Genetic engineering of the mammary glands of small mammals and of suitable farm animals for industrial use is more advanced than for other mammalian tissues. (4) The major disease of the human mammary gland, breast cancer, is one of the most common forms of cancer in the Western world. (5) Breast cancer is virtually incurable when it has disseminated to other organs of the body.

The resulting intensive research into the mammary gland has led to discoveries and models that are applicable not only to the mammary gland itself but also to many other biological systems. Thus the mammary gland has served as a prototype for mammalian development in many areas of biology in the past, and in the areas of biochemistry and molecular biology today, and will continue to do so in the foreseeable future.

The individual sections of the book reflect the five reasons for intensive research into the mammary gland, and are particularly topical at the present time because of the rapid advances in the molecular understanding of the various developmental processes underpinning each of these areas. The sections consist of chapters on the control of mammary development, on the regulation of milk production, on mammary transgenics, on genetic changes in mammary cancer and on mammary metastasis.

In Section 1, the Control of Mammary Development, the evidence for a cellular model for development of the normal mammary gland is reviewed. This model is based on the existence of stem cells that are capable of differentiating in a stepwise fashion into the major cell types, i.e. the ductal epithelial, smooth-muscle-like myoepithelial and casein-secretory alveolar cells seen in the mammary gland. The formation of mammary cancer in rats and of breast cancer in humans is then viewed as a gradual truncation of the differentiation pathways towards myoepithelial and alveolar cells, and the vestiges of these pathways allow the ectopic expression of proteins that may assist in the formation of the malignant state (Rudland et al.). The genes that can induce morphogenesis in transfected mammary glands of mice include those encoding the short-range signalling molecule Wnt-4, which induces ductal branching; the overactive mutant ErbB-1/epidermal growth factor (EGF) receptor, which induces ductal enlargement; and the overactive mutant of the growth factor receptor ErbB-2, which causes local development of alveoli. These findings suggest that it may be possible to relate oncogenic effects to normal growth controls (Edwards).

The normal hormones that control the early development of the mammary gland *in vivo* are the oestrogens. However, they probably do not work directly to stimulate cell growth. The oestrogens themselves can modulate the responsiveness of breast epithelial cells in culture to insulin-like growth factors (IGFs) at several points in the IGF signal transduction pathway, and this may, in part, be an explanation for their growth-promoting effects *in vivo* (Westley et al.). Modulation of the EGF signal transduction pathway may also play a role in oestrogen action. IGF-l and EGF-related proteins can also regulate the transcriptional activity of the oestrogen receptor itself via a common N-terminal domain of this receptor. Once the oestrogen has bound, a second region of the receptor can interact with co-activators of transcription of oestrogen-responsive genes (Parker); these genes presumably include those for IGF-1 and the EGF-related growth factor, transforming growth factor α (TGFα). Hence there is a complex network of interactions between the oestrogens, the IGFs and the EGFs. There are also other hormonally regulated, locally produced, growth stimulators and inhibitors of mammary development. These include the stimulator pleiotrophin, a heparin-binding protein of the midkine family that is involved in early developmental processes, and a mammary-derived growth inhibitor related to intracellular fatty acid binding proteins; the latter can also induce alveolar cell development and milk protein synthesis *in vitro* (Kürtz et al.). Thus there appear to be several locally produced, hormonally regulatable candidates for mediating/amplifying the effects of the mammatrophic hormones.

In Section 2, the Regulation of Milk Production, the end-point of mammary gland development is viewed as the production of milk. Milk production is largely controlled by peptide hormones based on prolactin, assisted by the synergistic action of the glucocorticoids. However, as with the earlier developmental stages of the gland, there is considerable evidence for local control of alveolar cell function and hence milk production. A feedback inhibitor of lactation accumulates during milk storage within the mammary gland and may thus regulate the local rate of milk secretion (Peaker et al.). This inhibitor is a small acidic glycoprotein that can inhibit the production of aqueous milk constituents *in vitro* and *in vivo*, primarily by blocking the early calcium-independent stages of the mammary secretory pathway (Wilde et al.). The later stages of the secretion of casein are partially dependent on intracellular calcium ions, and intra-organelle calcium is required for casein phosphorylation in freshly isolated lactating mouse acini (Burgoyne et al.).

At the molecular level, prolactin and cortisol 'turn on' the synthesis of milk proteins such as β-casein and whey acidic protein in rodents via composite response elements in the promoters of the genes. These composite response elements contain multiple binding sites for several transcription factors, including Stat5 (where Stat denotes signal transducers and activators of transcription) and, in the case of the β-casein gene, a leucine zipper class of DNA binding proteins, CCAAT/enhancer binding protein (C/EBP). The C/EBP family may play a pivotal role in maintaining a balance between cell proliferation and terminal (apoptotic) differentiation (Rosen et al.). In addition to hormones and locally produced growth factors, cellular confluence and matrix deposition are also required for milk protein synthesis in cultured cells. These cellular interactions exert their effect, in part, through regulatory elements; for example in the β-casein gene promoter by conferring transcriptional competence to the lactogenic hormones. One such regulatory element contains overlapping sites for DNA binding factors with both positive and negative regulatory activities. A single-stranded DNA repressor can be sequestered by binding to the 5′ untranslated region of β-casein mRNA after hormonal stimulation, and this allows the binding of a single-stranded DNA activator whose activity is enhanced by cell confluence *in vitro* and by suckling *in vivo* (Altiok and Groner). It is quite possible that the balance of transcription factors may be shifted away from processes involving terminal differentiation and apoptotic death, and towards cell proliferation, in breast cancers.

In Section 3, Mammary Transgenics, it is shown how a knowledge of the promoters activated during milk production has enabled transgenes to be expressed in the lactating glands of rodents and farm animals, both for experimental purposes and for potential commercial production. Thus some of the discrete promoter elements of the sheep milk protein gene for β-lactoglobulin have been used to target the expression of foreign genes to the mammary glands of transgenic mice for the production of therapeutic proteins in their milk. In such circumstances the promoter rarely functions optimally, but strategies have been developed to overcome this problem (Clark). When similar elements of this promoter are used to express foreign proteins in transgenic sheep, the transgenic protein can comprise over 50% of the milk protein, at least in the case of α_1-antitrypsin. However, expression from the endogenous promoter may interfere with that from the transgene, since knockout mice in which both endogenous α-lactalbumin genes have been deleted produce much more human α-lactalbumin (Colman).

Transgenic mice can also be used to overexpress genes in order to study their effects on abnormal development *in vivo*. Such is the case for the gene for the tyrosine kinase receptor, c-erbB-2/neu, which occurs in some human breast cancers. When a transmembrane point-mutated or activated form of neu is coupled downstream of a lactation-inducible promoter derived from the mouse mammary tumour virus (MMTV), its expression in the lactating glands of the resultant transgenic mice causes the appearance of adenocarcinomatous nodules with varying degrees of latency and frequency (Muller et al. and Jolicoeur et al.). When the non-mutated form of c-erbB-2 is similarly introduced into transgenic mice, there is only a stochastic appearance of focal tumours, and these arise because of in-frame deletions adjacent to the transmembrane domain producing another form of activated c-erbB-2 different from neu (Muller et al.). Moreover, re-examination of a transgenic mouse strain expressing the original activated neu gene, but producing only focal tumours after a long latent period, suggests that such tumours are clonal in origin and that other genetic events are additionally required to produce the adenocarcinomas (Jolicoeur et al.). These conclusions have been broadly confirmed by MMTV-induced overexpression of the non-activated human genes for the EGF-related growth factor TGFα and the ErbB-2 receptor in the rat. Overexpression of the TGFα gene produces only severe hyperplasia and focal tumours after long latency, whereas c-erbB-2 produces both benign tumours and malignant forms of adenocarcinoma in a stochastic manner after a long latent period (Davies et al.).

In Section 4, Genetic Changes in Mammary Cancer, some of the principles elucidated in normal mammary development are applied to the formation of breast cancer. The view from the clinic stresses the importance of accurate diagnosis, prognosis and effective treatment of this disease. The present clinico-pathological parameters are useful for grouping patients into broad prognostic categories, but they are not precise enough for use in individual treatment decisions. The hope is that the identification of molecular events actually involved in the progression of breast cancer may ultimately be more reliable for prognosis and as targets for treatment than existing regimes (Leinster). Overexpression of the type 1 family of growth factor receptors, i.e. the EGF receptor, ErbB-2 and ErbB-3, has been commonly found in solid human tumours, including those of the breast. ErbB-4 has not yet been examined in breast tumour cells. Changes such as these appear to be one of the causes of malignant transformation. They may also provide information regarding the course of the disease, response to current treatments and targets for new forms of treatment (Gullick). These receptors can be activated by many different ligands, resulting in the formation of a spectrum of heterodimer complexes and biological outcomes. This system has been dissected out in clones of mouse fibroblasts, demonstrating that transformation in vitro and tumour formation in vivo occur only in cells expressing two different ErbB family members. Furthermore, for a breast carcinoma cell line containing multiple ErbB family members, activation of ErbB-3 results in cellular differentiation but activation of ErbB-4 is mitogenic (Cohen et al.).

In addition to alterations in dominantly acting genes that affect cell growth, there are also genes that encode products that are believed to be involved in the normal suppression of cellular proliferation during development. Deletion of these genes or inactivation of the gene products leads either directly or indirectly to uncontrolled growth in cancer cells; the mutant p53 is the most widely occurring example in breast cancer (Leinster). One method believed to probe for genetic alterations indicative of inactivated tumour suppressor genes is loss of heterozygosity. So far, 12 arms of chromosomes have been found to be so affected in breast tumours. Another method relies on identifying the relevant genes that are deactivated by MMTV integration and which contribute to specific stages of mouse mammary tumorigenesis. Using this approach two new loci, *INT3/NOTCH4* and *INT6*, have been identified; the former encodes a receptor protein involved in determination of the fate of cells during the development of *Drosophila*, and the latter is novel (Callahan). At present there appear to be two inherited genes that predispose humans to breast cancer, but these occur in high-risk families and not in the common sporadic forms of breast cancer. One of these, *BRCA1*, appears to be hormonally regulated in normal mammary glands, and acts as a tumour suppressor gene. Mutations towards the N-terminus of the molecule are correlated with breast cancers, and those towards the C-terminus with ovarian cancers. The other, *BRCA2*, is another suppressor gene with mutations that are commonly found in male breast cancers (Ponder). Thus the uncontrolled growth of breast cancers appears to arise from alterations in the normal genes that control various aspects of mammary development.

Section 5, the final section, is concerned with Mechanisms of Mammary Metastasis. In addition to the loss of growth control that allows the primary tumour to expand, breast cancers possess the additional and important property of being able to invade the local tissue and disseminate to other parts of the body. This process of tumour progression and metastasis involves the tumour cells surmounting various biological hurdles, presumably with the aid of a series of different genetic products, in a stepwise manner. Oncogenes such as the mutant *ras*, when transfected into benign mammary epithelial cells, can induce rapid rates of phenotypic change and cellular diversity, concomitant with the acquisition of the metastatic phenotype, perhaps by disruption of gap-junction communications. This may allow genes involved in motility, such as the *MTA1* gene, and cell surface mucin-like glycoproteins that may be involved in cell adhesion, to be expressed at the appropriate times (Nicolson). Similar conclusions are drawn in the next chapter. One of the adhesion molecules of the integrin family, integrin α2β1, which mediates interactions with the extracellular matrix (particularly collagen I), and the E-cadherins, which maintain cell junctions and hence the amount of mammary tissue architecture and cell polarity, are reduced in breast cancers. The decreases in these molecules can be simulated by transfection and expression in normal human mammary epithelial cell lines of oncogenes, including the breast cancer-related c-*erbB-2*. This results in a decrease in branching morphogenesis in a collagen I matrix *in vitro* (Alford et al.). Another gene, *nm23*, is underexpressed in highly metastatic carcinoma cell lines and in human carcinomas *in vivo*, including those of the breast. Transfection of this gene into experimental systems also seems to reduce cellular motility, local invasion of artificial matrices and the metastatic, but not tumorigenic, potential of metastatic cell lines. Moreover, Nm23 increases the ability of certain breast cancer cell lines to acquire more characteristics of normal differentiated epithelial cells, including branching morphogenesis in collagen gels. Homologues of Nm23 have been found to be required for the normal development of *Drosophila*, and Nm23 also seems to be developmentally regulated in mammals, pointing to a role in cellular signalling pathways, perhaps for apoptosis (Freije et al.).

The integrins $\alpha 2\beta 1$, E-cadherin and Nm23 are all suppressors of human tumour progression and metastasis. There are also dominantly acting inducers, and these fall into the cellular motility, adhesion and destruction categories outlined already. Direct transfection of genes and genetic DNA fragments into benign mammary cells has identified two genes encoding calcium binding proteins, S100A4 (p9Ka) and osteopontin, that can induce metastasis in a syngeneic rat system. The former targets the cytoskeleton and increases cellular motility, while the latter probably targets the vitronectin receptor ($\alpha v\beta 3$ integrin) and affects cell adhesion. In the former case S100A works in conjunction with oncogenes such as c-*erbB-2* in producing the metastatic phenotype in transgenic mice, and in the latter case the expression of osteopontin can be induced by different regulatory regions of DNA specifically found in breast cancer cell lines (Barraclough et al.). Finally, transfection of a mouse mammary carcinoma cell line by the gene for the matrix metalloproteinase gelatinase A, but not with the genes for collagenase or stromelysin, causes an increase in the cells' ability to invade Matrigel *in vitro* and to demonstrate lung colonization *in vivo* after injection into the tail vein of immuno-incompetent mice. This malignant/metastatic phenotype can be reversed by a gelatinase inhibitor but also, surprisingly, by peptides to its non-catalytic C-terminal domain. The latter result suggests that specific interactions of the proteinase with the surface of the cancer cell may be required for its anti-cancer effects (Docherty et al.). Molecules such as S100A4, osteopontin and gelatinase A are normally produced by differentiated cells within the mammary gland and not by ductal epithelial cells, but all these appear to be produced in human breast carcinomas, despite the lack of fully differentiated mammary cell types. These results suggest that the normal pathways of mammary differentiation are subverted in different ways (perhaps by truncation as outlined earlier) which can, under suitable circumstances, lead to breast cancer. Thus breast cancer may be viewed as aberrant development which still utilizes some of the normal developmental processes while adapting others to its own ends, through processes of natural selection at a cellular level. The end result is to generate cellular systems that are able to survive and even prosper in apparently alien environments of the body.

In conclusion our grateful thanks are extended to The Cancer and Polio Research Fund, Zeneca Pharmaceuticals and The Biochemical Society for sponsoring the Symposium, without which this book would not have been possible, and to the Officers of The Biochemical Society and Portland Press for adding a touch of professionalism to the production of this volume.

Philip S. Rudland
David G. Fernig
Sam J. Leinster

Abbreviations

AB	alveolar bud
AF	activation function
α_1AT	α_1-antitrypsin
BAPTA	bis-(o-aminophenoxy)ethane-$N,N,N'N'$-tetra-acetic acid
$[Ca^{2+}]_i$	intracellular free calcium concentration
CAT	chloramphenicol acetyltransferase
C/EBP	CCAAT/enhancer binding protein
DCIS	ductal carcinoma *in situ*
DMBA	dimethylbenzanthracene
DTT	dithiothreitol
EGF	epidermal growth factor
EGFR	EGF receptor
EHS matrix	reconstituted basement membrane derived from the Engelbreth–Holm–Swarm tumour
eIF4E	eukaryotic translation initiation factor 4E
ER	endoplasmic reticulum
ERK	extracellular-signal-related kinase
ES cells	embryonic stem cells
(h-)FABP	(heart-type) fatty acid binding protein
(b)FGF	(basic) fibroblast growth factor
FGFR	FGF receptor
FIL	feedback inhibitor of lactation
GR	glucocorticoid receptor
HER	human EGF-like receptor
HGF	hepatocyte growth factor
HOG	hyperplastic outgrowth line
HSPG	heparan sulphate proteoglycan
IDC	invasive ductal carcinoma
IGF	insulin-like growth factor
IGFBP	IGF binding protein
ir-	immunoreactive
IRS-1	insulin receptor substrate-1
JAK	Janus kinase
LAP	liver-enriched activating protein
LIP	liver-enriched inhibitory protein
LOH	loss of heterozygosity
LTR	long terminal repeat
MAP kinase	mitogen-activated protein kinase

MDGI	mammary-derived growth inhibitor
MetaDNA	metastasis-inducing DNA sequences
MGF	mammary-gland-specific factor
MMP	matrix metalloproteinase
MMTV	mouse mammary tumour virus
MPBF	milk protein binding factor
MT-MMP	membrane-type MMP
NDPK	nucleotide diphosphate kinase
NF	nuclear factor
OR	oestrogen receptor
P.I.	Prognostic Index
PMGF	pituitary-derived mammary growth factor
Rb	retinoblastoma protein
RIP	receptor-interacting protein
RTK	receptor tyrosine kinase
RT-PCR	reverse transcription-PCR
SARP	sequence-specific single-stranded DNA activator region binding protein
Shc	Src-homology/collagen
Stat	signal transducers and activators of transcription
STR	sequence-specific single-stranded DNA binding transcriptional repressor
tBHQ	2,5-di-(t-butyl)-1,4-benzohydroquinone
TEB	terminal end bud
TGF	transforming growth factor
TIMP	tissue inhibitor of metalloproteinases
UTR	untranslated region
WAP	whey acidic protein
YY	Yin Yang

Biochem. Soc. Symp. **63**, 1–20
Printed in Great Britain

Growth and differentiation of the normal mammary gland and its tumours

P.S. Rudland*, R. Barraclough, D.G. Fernig and J.A. Smith

Cancer and Polio Research Fund Laboratories, Department of Biochemistry, University of Liverpool, Liverpool L69 3BX, U.K.

Abstract

The mammary glands of non-pregnant rodents and humans consist of epithelial, intermediate stem and myoepithelial cells, and these have been isolated as cell lines *in vitro*. Growth factors produced by the myoepithelial cells, e.g. transforming growth factor α (TGFα) and basic fibroblast growth factor (bFGF), can stimulate the growth of the intermediate stem cells *in vitro*. One protein, p9Ka, a calcium binding regulatory protein, arises at an early stage of the differentiation of epithelial into myoepithelial cells *in vitro* and is associated with the cytoskeleton; another, cathepsin D, is a protease associated with this pathway *in vivo*. Unlike normal glands and benign lesions, malignant mammary carcinomas of rats and humans do not contain fully differentiated myoepithelial cells, and the resultant cell lines fail to differentiate completely into myoepithelial cells. Loss of the myoepithelial cells in some human invasive carcinomas may account, in part, for compensatory changes in the malignant cells. For example, overexpression of TGFα/ErbB-2 receptors may compensate for a decrease in TGFα, whereas ectopic production of bFGF and its receptors, and of p9Ka and cathepsin D, may help in tumorigenesis and in metastasis respectively. Thus compensation for, or retention of, molecules potentially involved in growth and/or differentiation by some human invasive carcinomas may be a mechanism by which a malignancy progresses.

Introduction

The normal mammary glands of rodents and humans consist of a branching network of ducts terminating in end buds prior to puberty, thereafter in increasing numbers of alveolar lobules, and finally in secretory alveoli during pregnancy and lactation (Fig. 1) [1]. These developmental changes are con-

---

*To whom correspondence should be addressed.

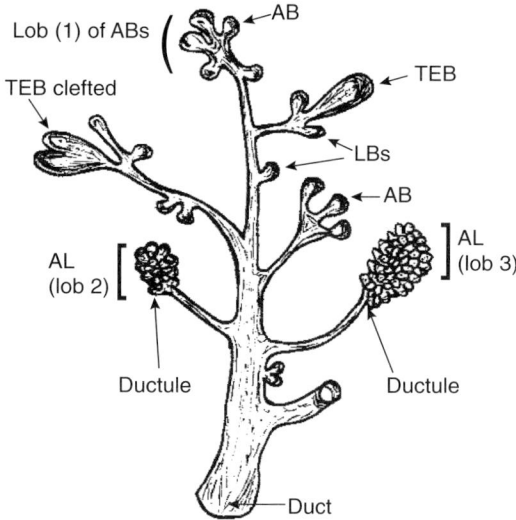

Fig. 1. Diagrammatic representation of the structures in the developing breast. Abbreviations: TEB clefted, TEB subdivided by a cleavage furrow at its tip (further cleavage results in alveolar buds); LBs, lateral buds; AB, alveolar bud; AL, alveolar lobule. The lobules have been classified previously as type 1 (lob 1), synonymous with lobule of ABs, and types 2 and 3, which correspond to ALs containing smaller numbers of larger ductules (lob 2) and ALs containing larger numbers of smaller ductules (lob 3) respectively. Modified from Russo and Russo [78] and Rudland [8].

trolled by the circulating levels of mammatrophic hormones; in particular, oestrogen produces ductal growth, progesterone produces alveolar lobules and prolactin produces the alveoli that secrete milk products, including casein. Other circulating hormones such as cortisol and insulin are required to promote mammary development *in vivo*, probably by synergizing with the primary mammatrophic hormones (Fig. 2) [2]. In addition, local trophic agents produced in the vicinity of the mammary glands are also involved in growth control, since rodent mammary tissues and cells will grow when transplanted into the mammary fat pad, but not when transplanted subcutaneously [3].

For a spectrum of increasingly malignant mammary tumours, there is a gradual loss of the requirement for circulating hormones for growth. Thus benign tumours most closely akin to the normal gland require the majority of the mammatrophic hormones to grow, e.g. the carcinogen-induced tumours of rats [4] and the spontaneously arising benign tumours of humans [5]. Some (low-grade) malignant tumours of rats [6] and humans still require the mammatrophic hormones to enable them to grow. These are the so-called hormone-dependent tumours, and comprise 25–30% of all human carcinomas [7]. The remaining 70–75% of human malignant tumours no longer require normal circulating levels of the mammatrophic hormones, and are said to be hormone-independent for growth. Moreover, hyperplastic rodent lesions require the fat-

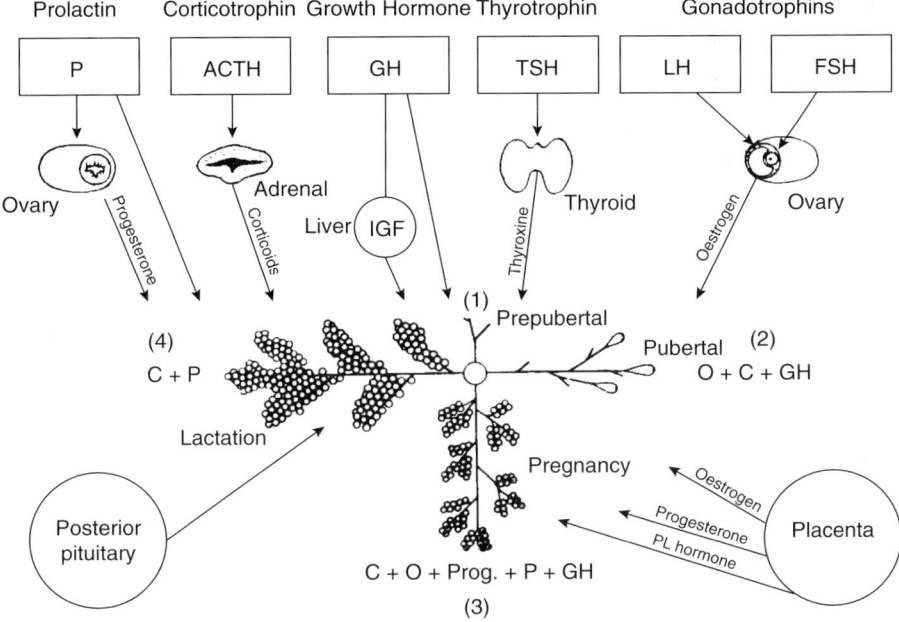

**Fig. 2. Diagrammatic representation of hormones involved at differ-
ent stages of breast development.** (1) Prepubertal gland; (2) pubertal
gland; (3) gland in pregnancy; (4) lactating gland. Abbreviations: LH, luteinizing
hormone; FSH, follicle-stimulating hormone; C, corticoids; O, oestrogen; Prog,
progesterone; PL hormone, placental lactogen; IGF, insulin-like growth factor.
Modified from Lyons et al. [79].

pad environment for growth, but neoplastic lesions often no longer require this
tissue for sustained development [3]. Thus changes in both systemic and local
growth control can be observed in the development of a breast carcinoma.

Cellular organization in normal and neoplastic mammary glands

The normal mammary gland consists of two cellular compartments: the
mesenchymal compartment of fatty stroma, which is permeated by blood vessels and nerves, and the epithelial compartment of ducts and lobules. These two
cellular compartments are separated by a basement membrane of type IV collagen, laminin and glycosaminoglycans [8]. During the development of
malignant tumours, the fatty environment may be lost, the density of blood
vessels is increased [9], and the basement membrane is reduced or lost completely in high-grade, more malignant carcinomas [10].

The normal epithelial compartment consists of three cell types: the
epithelial cells which line ducts, the alveolar cells which line alveoli, and the
myoepithelial cells sandwiched between the epithelial/alveolar cells and the

basement membrane (Fig. 3) [11]. Benign hyperplastic and benign neoplastic lesions of the mammary glands, termed benign breast disease and (fibro)adenomas respectively, contain both epithelial and myoepithelial cells and, if the animal or patient is pregnant, milk-secreting alveolar cells as well. In contrast,

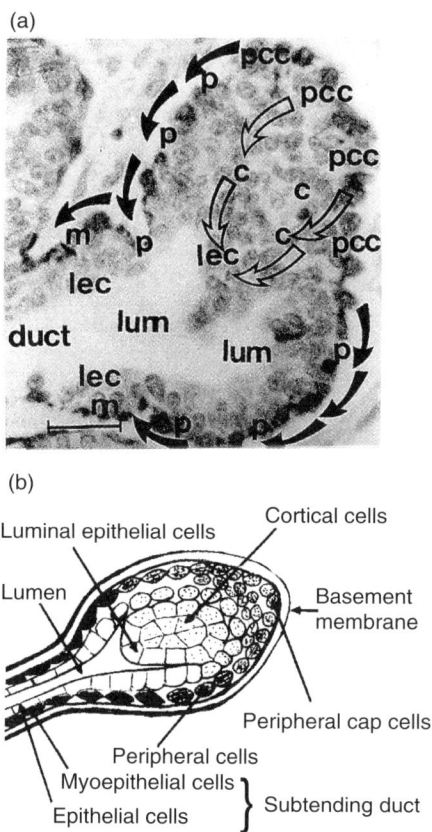

Fig. 3. Myoepithelial markers in growing terminal ducts and TEBs.
(a) Section of human TEB incubated with a monoclonal antibody to smooth muscle actin. The peripheral cap cells (pcc) stain moderately; this staining increases gradually the further such cells are positioned from the distal tip (solid arrows). The staining decreases for the central cells (c) and is lost completely from the luminal epithelial cells (lec) (outlined arrows) which line the lumen (lum). p, peripheral cells; m, myoepithelial cells. Scale bar = 20 μm. (b) Diagrammatic representation of staining patterns. The peripheral cap cells are stained moderately for actin/myosin (dotted circles), and their staining increases through peripheral cells, closer to the subtending duct, where they eventually merge with the myoepithelial cells of the duct (black ovoids). The central epithelial cells show usually only a weaker staining for actin/myosin (dotted squares). Staining for the basement membrane proteins laminin and type IV collagen encircles the TEB completely, producing a thin band at its distal tip which increases gradually in thickness in the neck regions of the TEB, where it merges with that of the subtending duct. Modified from Rudland [8].

malignant carcinomas of rodents and humans contain only epithelial cells; they have lost both the myoepithelial cell and, even when pregnant, the secretory alveolar cell (Fig. 4) [8,12].

Single-cell-cloned epithelial cell lines have been isolated from normal and benign lesions of rat and human glands that can give rise, in a stepwise manner, to myoepithelial-like and secretory alveolar-like cells in culture. Some of the intermediate cells along the myoepithelial pathway can be isolated as cell lines [8,12]. Similar cellular stages of differentiation are observed *in vivo* in growing terminal end buds (TEBs) (Fig. 3) and certain alveolar lobules [8,13]. However, single-cell-cloned epithelial cell lines from rat and human breast carcinomas largely fail to differentiate into either myoepithelial or alveolar cells in culture (Fig. 4). The environment produced by the myoepithelial cell is additional to that provided by the mesenchymal compartment, and as such represents a further loss experienced by the developing mammary carcinoma. With these changes in mind, the detailed requirements for growth and differentiation at a cellular level can now be investigated. The cell lines used for this purpose are shown in Table 1.

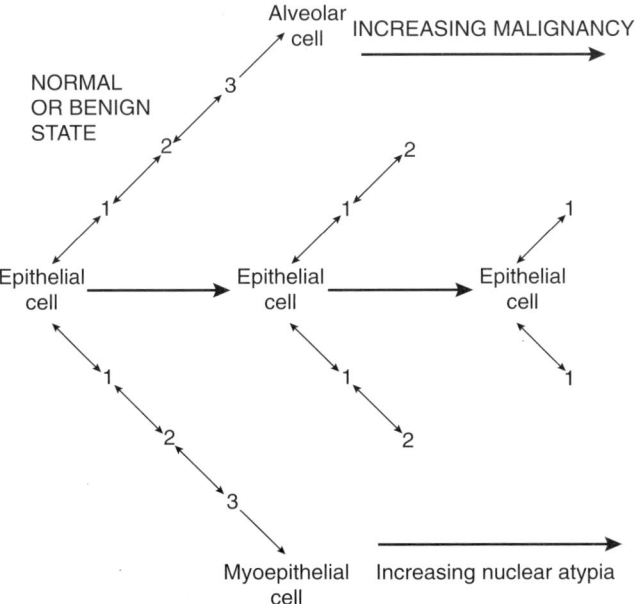

Fig. 4. Cellular model for the development of the normal breast and breast cancer. Normal epithelial cells in terminal ductal structures can differentiate into myoepithelial cells and into secretory alveolar cells via a series of cellular intermediates (here represented by numerals) [12]. It is suggested that many benign hyperplastic and neoplastic lesions arise directly from such epithelial and closely related intermediate cells, which still retain much of their ability to differentiate into myoepithelial and alveolar cells. Insults leading to malignant changes produce epithelial and related intermediate cells with a decreasing ability to differentiate into either cell type [8].

Table 1. Summary of breast cell lines. These cell lines have been reviewed in detail previously [8,12]. Abbreviation: SV40, simian virus 40.

Mammary tissue	Cell line	Identity	Differentiate
Normal rat	Rama 704	Epithelial	Yes
	Rama 401	Myoepithelial-like	No
Benign DMBA	Rama 25	Epithelial	Yes
rat tumour	Rama 25-I1, I2, I4	Intermediate	Yes
	Rama 29	Myoepithelial-like	No
	Rama 37	Epithelial	Yes
Weakly metastasizing rat tumour TR2CL	Rama 600	Epithelial	Very incompletely
Moderately metastasizing rat tumour TMT-081	Rama 800	Anaplastic epithelial	No
Strongly metastasizing rat tumour SMT-2A	Rama 900	Anaplastic epithelial	No
Normal human immortalized by SV40	SVE3, Huma 7	Epithelial	Yes
	Huma 25, 62	Myoepithelial-like	No
Benign breast disease, parent HMT 3522	Huma 121, 123	Epithelial	Yes
	Huma 101, 109	Myoepithelial-like	No
Human ductal carcinoma	Ca2-83	Malignant epithelial	No
Metastatic pleural effusion	MCF-7, ZR-75	Malignant epithelial	No

Hormonal agents and micronutrients

Despite results obtained *in vivo*, the established mammatrophic hormones are much less effective than might be anticipated in promoting cell growth *in vitro* [14–17]. Thus attempts have been made to identify those agents that stimulate DNA synthesis and cell division directly in mammary cells in culture, and then to relate them back to possible growth-controlling processes *in vivo*. One type of growth factor identified using this approach in defined media may be characterized as essential micronutrients.

The most important micronutrient is probably iron, and the iron-binding protein transferrin is essential for the growth of many cultured cells in defined media [18], including our mammary epithelial cell lines [17]. Since addition of haemoglobin and ferritin also promotes growth of our Rama 37 epithelial cells

Table 2. Binding of transferrin to breast cell lines. The K_d values and numbers of receptors were calculated from the data pooled from at least two independent binding experiments and are presented as means $\pm$ S.E.M. The binding of ^{125}I-labelled diferric transferrin was performed and analysed as described previously [29,42].

Cell line	K_d (nM)	$10^{-3} \times$ No. of receptors per cell
SVE3 normal epithelial	44 ± 28	41 ± 14
MCF-7 malignant epithelial; oestrogen-free	120 ± 70	350 ± 120
MCF-7 malignant epithelial; plus oestrogen	200 ± 120	810 ± 160

[19], the iron requirement may be an artefact of the culture system. However, a high number of transferrin receptors has been reported in rapidly proliferating cells, including those in mammary glands in pregnancy and lactation [20]. Transferrin and its mRNA are also found within the developing rat mammary gland; transferrin itself constitutes 2% of cytosolic protein in late pregnancy and lactation [21]. Thus transferrin may be acting like a growth factor, either in an autocrine/paracrine manner if produced locally and/or in an endocrine manner if its levels in blood vary appreciably.

With the MCF-7 breast carcinoma cell line, transferrin is secreted into the culture medium; its secretion is stimulated by oestrogen and reduced by tamoxifen [22]. Moreover, the numbers of transferrin receptors are greater in malignant as opposed to non-malignant breast cell lines (Table 2). Their numbers are also higher for the MCF-7 breast cancer cell line in medium containing oestrogen than in medium antagonistic to the action of oestrogen. Transferrin receptors are also overexpressed in the majority of cells in 71% of invasive breast carcinomas, and in some cells of all breast carcinomas [20]. Thus the possibility exists of a hormonally controlled autocrine loop involving transferrin and its overexpression in breast carcinomas.

Pituitary-derived activity

Although prolactin has little growth-promoting effect *in vitro*, pituitary extracts are mitogenic for mammary cells [16]. The pituitary-derived mammary growth factor (PMGF) that promotes the growth of our rat mammary epithelial-like, but not myoepithelial-like, cell lines has still only been partially purified. Nonetheless, it is separable from bovine prolactin, growth hormone and known growth factors found in the pituitary gland [17,19]. PMGF is also implicated in the process of mammary development *in vivo*, since the activity of PMGF from pituitary glands of early lactating or perphenazine-treated rats, when the mammary glands are growing rapidly, is 4–10 times greater than the activity found in untreated virgin females [17]. Pure rat or bovine prolactin, however, stimulates production of casein-secreting, alveolar-like cells in confluent epithelial cultures [23]. Thus, although prolactin and PMGF may be under similar hypothalamic control in the pituitary gland, prolactin acts on the epithelial cells of the mammary gland to induce differentiation, whereas PMGF may serve to promote the proliferation of the epithelial cells in glandular growth.

PMGF fails to stimulate the growth of highly malignant, metastatic carcinoma cell lines of rat (Rama 800, Rama 900) or human (Ca2-83) origin. This result is consistent with results *in vivo*, whereby hypophysectomy of rats or humans bearing such advanced tumours largely fails to cause regression [7,24]. In contrast, benign tumours of rats and humans largely regress after the systemic use of anti-pituitary agents [5,25], and epithelial cells from such tumours are still responsive to the growth-promoting effects of PMGF in culture [17]. Therefore the malignant cells are refractory to the growth-promoting effects of PMGF. The loss of differentiating ability and failure to respond to pituitary-related growth factor(s), however, are changes that may not occur simultaneously in the malignant cell, since weakly metastasizing rat cell lines are responsive to PMGF in culture (Rama 600) [17], and about 25% of all human breast cancers, when first diagnosed, are responsive to hormone (including pituitary-ablative) therapy [7]. Thus initiation of the loss of the differentiating ability of the neoplastic epithelial cell may occur at an earlier stage in the malignant process than does the loss of response to pituitary (possibly PMGF) control of cell growth.

Epidermal growth factors (EGFs)

The most abundant growth factor of the EGF family in the mammary gland is transforming growth factor α (TGFα). Both epithelial (Rama 25) cells and, particularly, myoepithelial (Rama 29) cells in culture have been shown to secrete mature, bioactive TGFα, and it is found also in the rat mammary gland *in vivo* (Figs. 5A and 5B) [26].

The activity of rat TGFα [26], like that of EGF [17], is not specific for a particular cell type; it stimulates the growth of fibroblastic, myoepithelial-like and epithelial cell lines from normal mammary glands and from benign tumours. The amounts of TGFα secreted from the Rama 29 myoepithelial-like cells in culture are sufficient to stimulate the growth of the myoepithelial-like cells themselves, or of epithelial or stromal cell lines. On the face of it, this suggests a paracrine or autocrine role for TGFα in the mammary gland *in vivo*. Apparent confirmation of a pattern in which differentiation from the epithelial to the myoepithelial phenotype is accompanied by an increase in TGFα production came from immunofluorescent and immunocytochemical studies [27]. Again, immunofluorescence with anti-TGFα serum is greater in Rama 29 myoepithelial cells than Rama 25 epithelial cells, while immunocytochemical staining of the rat mammary gland shows the presence of immunoreactive TGFα (ir-TGFα) primarily in the myoepithelial cells and to a lesser extent in the epithelial cells during development. The intermediate cells in growing TEBs are stained at an intermediate level (Figs. 5A and 5B). In lactating glands, alveolar secretions are also stained strongly.

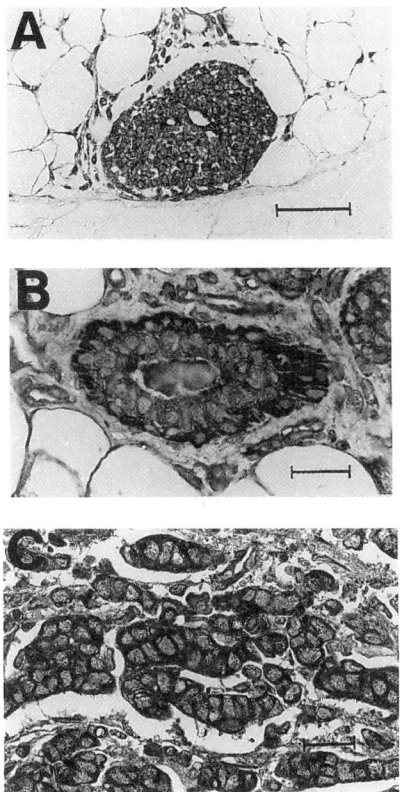

Fig. 5. Immunocytochemical staining of mammary tissues by anti-TGFα. (A) TEB from 50-day-old rat in cross-section, showing moderate to strong staining of all growing parenchymal cells. (B) Duct from 50-day-old rat showing strong staining of outer myoepithelial cells of the duct and little or no staining of the inner epithelial cell layer. (C) Human invasive ductal carcinoma showing intense staining of the carcinoma cells. Scale bars: (A) 75 μm, (B) 20 μm and (C) 25 μm.

However, Western blotting of ir-TGFα in extracts of rat mammary glands and cell lines shows that ir-TGFα consists mainly of a 50 kDa protein, and the amounts of ir-TGFα are considerably in excess of the amounts of bioactive TGFα observed in the same extracts. Moreover, ir-TGFα is also found in rat mammary fibroblasts *in vivo*, and ir-TGFα and mRNA for TGFα are found in the equivalent Rama 27 cell line *in vitro* [28], which does not secrete bioactive TGFα into the culture medium [26]. These results warn against too simplistic interpretations in relation to growth control.

TGFα normally binds to the EGF receptor (EGFR) in many different cell types. All of our rat mammary cell lines possess high-affinity receptors for EGF, with dissociation constants ranging from 0.4 nM to 1.3 nM [26,29]. Furthermore, there is no alteration in the EGFRs when epithelial cells differentiate along the myoepithelial-like pathway *in vitro* [29]. Hence locally produced TGFα may stimulate the growth of epithelial, intermediate and myoepithelial cell types *in vivo*.

The overexpression of TGFα and of its cognate receptor, EGFR, has been implicated in the abnormal growth of the malignant breast [30,31]. In support of an autocrine model involving TGFα/EGFR *in vivo* [32,33], ir-TGFα has been detected in 30–70% of human breast carcinomas (Fig. 5C), and its presence correlates with the tumour burden [27,34,35]. As in normal epithelial cells, the major component of ir-TGFα appears to be a 50 kDa protein, and the relationship of this to mature, bioactive TGFα is unknown [27]. Moreover, the expected outcome of an uncontrolled TGFα/EGFR autocrine loop would be a rapidly growing tumour, such as is found in squamous carcinomas of the head and neck, in which the EGFR is invariably overexpressed [36]. In contrast, breast carcinomas, at least in the early stages, tend to be slow growing, and frequently still under a degree of hormonal control. Thus a more gradual evolution to an oestrogen-refractory state is required in which changes in TGFα/EGFR may well contribute, but other changes may be of equal or of more importance.

A related system to the EGFR is that of the c-*erbB*-2 proto-oncogene, which codes for a 185 kDa tyrosine kinase receptor that is structurally related to the EGFR. In invasive breast carcinomas, expression of c-*erbB*-2 is observed in 20–30% of tumours [37–39]. Normal and benign tissues show virtually no expression, and there is an inverse correlation between patient survival and expression of c-*erbB*-2, particularly in patients with no involved lymph nodes [38,39].

Fibroblast growth factors (FGFs) in normal development

The FGFs bind to two types of receptors: high-affinity tyrosine kinase receptors (FGFRs) that are ultimately responsible for the generation of primary intracellular signals, and low-affinity heparan sulphate proteoglycans (HSPGs), a type of glycosaminoglycan, which possess a storage function and an activation function. The latter enable binding of FGFs to the high-affinity receptor [40]. In cell lines from normal and benign rat and human mammary glands, basic FGF (bFGF) and the high-affinity (K_d 30–280 pM; ~5×10^4 per cell) and low-affinity (K_d 1–20 nM; ~3×10^6 per cell) receptors for bFGF are products of the myoepithelial-like cells and to a lesser extent the intermediate cells, but not of the epithelial cells [29,41–44]. The amounts of bFGF produced (6–7 ng/10^6 cells) are sufficient to stimulate the growth of the myoepithelial-like and intermediate cell lines [17], suggesting the possibility of autocrine/paracrine control of cell growth *in vivo*. The high-affinity receptors mainly correspond to FGFR-1 and the low-affinity receptors to HSPGs [42,44]. Approx. 50–66% of the low-affinity receptors are associated with the basement membrane/extracellular matrix *in vitro* and possess both storage and activation functions (Fig. 6) [42,45].

Confirmation of these results has been obtained by immunocytochemistry. In the resting glands, bFGF is associated with the myoepithelial cells/basement membrane [46], while in growing glands, particularly in intermediate

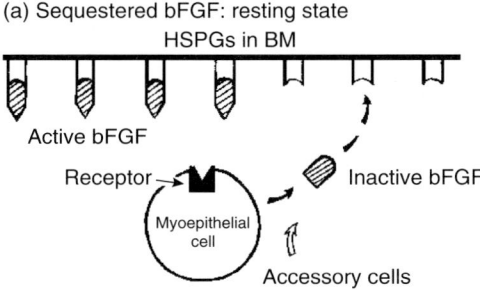

(a) Sequestered bFGF: resting state

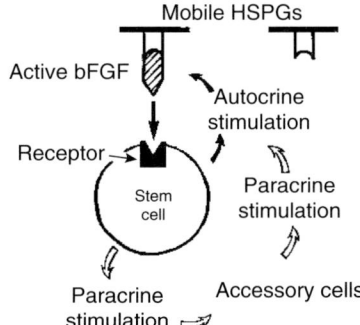

(b) Freely active bFGF: growing state

Fig. 6. Schematic representation of bFGF in breast tissues. (a) In non-growing tissues, bFGF is sequestered by the HSPGs, which occur mainly extracellularly in the basement membrane (BM) adjacent to the myoepithelial cells. Thus activated bFGF is in a separate compartment from its receptors on the plasma membrane. (b) In growing tissues in TEBs and in carcinomas, the HSPGs are considerably reduced in amount and are not immobilized in the basement membrane. Therefore the necessary activation of bFGF at the cell surface prior to its binding to its high-affinity tyrosine kinase receptor can take place. The active bFGF released can cause autocrine stimulation of its own cell's growth or paracrine stimulation of neighbouring cells, e.g. blood vessels in a carcinoma.

cells in TEBs, bFGF is more usually associated with individual cells. Moreover, blocking antibodies with bFGF dramatically increases the immunocytochemical staining of the basement membrane/myoepithelial cell region without any corresponding increase in the staining of the proliferating intermediate cells in growing regions of the glands [47]. These results suggest that in non-growing areas of the mammary gland there exists a considerable extracellular sink for bFGF which is not present in the growing areas (Fig. 6).

Ectopic expression of FGFs in malignant development

Receptors for bFGF have been found consistently on malignant epithelial mammary cell lines derived either from rodents or from humans with metastatic disease. These cell lines possess cell-surface, high-affinity receptors for bFGF with K_d values [43,48,49] that are comparable with the K_d values of these receptors found on the normal myoepithelial-like cells [29,42–44]. This expression of high-affinity FGFRs by malignant mammary cells is ectopic, since neither rat nor human mammary epithelial cells derived from the normal mammary gland or from benign tumours produce detectable levels of receptors for the FGFs, as described above.

In general, the malignant cells do not possess normal levels of low-affinity HSPG receptors ($<10^5$ per cell) for bFGF [43,48,49]. Nevertheless, bFGF is a potent stimulator of the growth of malignant mammary epithelial cells [48,50,51]. Moreover, at least in rat malignant mammary cells, the low levels of HSPGs that are produced by the malignant cells are able to activate bFGF [45]. This indicates that the dual receptor system for FGFs [40] is fully functional in the malignant cells, despite the apparent absence of most of the HSPG low-affinity receptors (Fig. 6), and these results have been confirmed on pilot studies of human breast specimens [48,52].

bFGF growth-promoting activity is found not only in extracts of rat mammary carcinoma cell lines but also in 25% of human mammary carcinoma cell lines [43,53,54]. mRNA encoding bFGF has been detected in human mammary carcinomas, but the level of expression relative to that in the benign/normal tissue is generally lower [53,54]. Since, in rat and human cell lines derived from the normal mammary gland and from benign tumours, bFGF is found in myoepithelial but not epithelial cells [41,43,44], this result is consistent with the loss of bFGF-producing myoepithelial cells in invasive carcinomas [8]. However, approx. 25% of the malignant tumours express bFGF mRNA at levels that are equivalent to, or higher than, those of the benign tissue [53]. bFGF has also been isolated from mammary carcinomas [55], so it is likely that the expression of bFGF mRNA by human carcinomas results in the synthesis of active bFGF polypeptides (Fig. 6).

Protein markers of differentiation into myoepithelial cells

Differentiation of our rat mammary epithelial cell lines into myoepithelial-like cells in culture is accompanied by changes in a small number of specific proteins which mark discrete cellular stages *in vitro* [56] prior to the major change of rearrangement of the cytoskeleton into that of a smooth muscle cell. For example, the calcium-binding regulatory protein p9Ka, now termed S100A4 [57], increases relatively early, keratin 14 increases in the middle stages, Thy-1 increases at later stages, and the basement membrane proteins laminin and type IV collagen increase relatively evenly along this *in vitro* pathway [58]. However, the level of their genetic regulation varies: p9Ka and Thy-1 are mainly regulated at the level of their mRNAs [59,60], while laminin and collagen type IV are regulated post-transcriptionally [58], probably at the level of intracellular breakdown [61]. Similar changes in immunocytochemically detected levels of these marker proteins are seen in the equivalent cells in the TEBs of growing rats [58] and in human intermediate cell types *in vitro* and *in vivo* [10,62]. Other, presumably early-marker, proteins of myoepithelial cells

Table 3. Summary of myoepithelial-associated proteins in TEBs and human carcinomas. The presence of myoepithelial-related proteins in other mammary cell types *in vivo* in either the cytoplasm (c) or in filaments (f) using immunocytochemical detection methods is shown. Key: + +, +, ± and −, present in 75–100%, 25–75%; 5–25% and <5% of cells or carcinomas respectively [10,72,73]. Immunocytochemical data for hyaluronectin [77] from P.S. Rudland and D. West (unpublished work).

Marker protein	Myoepithelial	TEB	Epithelial	Carcinoma
p9Ka	+ +f	+c	−	+c
Cathepsin D	+ +c	+c	−	+c
Hyaluronectin	+ +f	+c	−	+c
Keratin 14	+ +c	±c	−	±c
Laminin	+ +f	+c,f	−	+c,f
Type IV collagen	+ +f	+c,f	−	+c,f

in human breasts *in vivo* include the protease cathepsin D and the extracellular protein hyaluronectin, and these are also observed at lower levels in intermediate cells in TEBs, but not in epithelial cells *in vivo* (Table 3).

Since the increase in p9Ka was one of the earliest detectable changes in rat cell lines intermediate between epithelial and myoepithelial cells [56], it warranted further investigation. Transfection of p9Ka cDNA [63,64] into rat mammary epithelial cells produced intermediate cell/myoepithelial cell colonies at a higher frequency than in controls (Table 4). Antibodies to rat p9Ka predominantly stained the cellular cytoskeleton in cultured rat myoepithelial-like cells (Figs. 7A and 7B) [63], and scrape-loading of recombinant p9Ka into the epithelial cells caused similar changes in the cellular cytoskeleton within 48 h (Fig. 7C). These results suggest that, at least in culture, p9Ka may be capable of triggering differentiation along the myoepithelial cell pathway by

Table 4 Effect of DNA transfection of p9Ka on cultured rat epithelial cells. Rat mammary epithelial cells were scored for epithelial, intermediate or more-elongated, myoepithelial-like cell colonies [56] after DNA transfection with Ha-*ras*-1 cDNA or rat p9Ka cDNA coupled to the selectable vector pSV2*neo*, as described previously [63,64].

Transfecting DNA	Fraction of cell colonies (%)		
	Epithelial	Intermediate	Myoepithelial-like
None	244/250 (97%)	4/250 (2%)	2/250 (1%)
Vector alone	64/72 (89%)	5/72 (7%)	3/72 (4%)
Ha-*ras*-1 cDNA	99/120 (82%)	12/120 (10%)	9/120 (8%)
p9Ka cDNA	5/72 (7%)	20/72 (28%)	47/72 (65%)

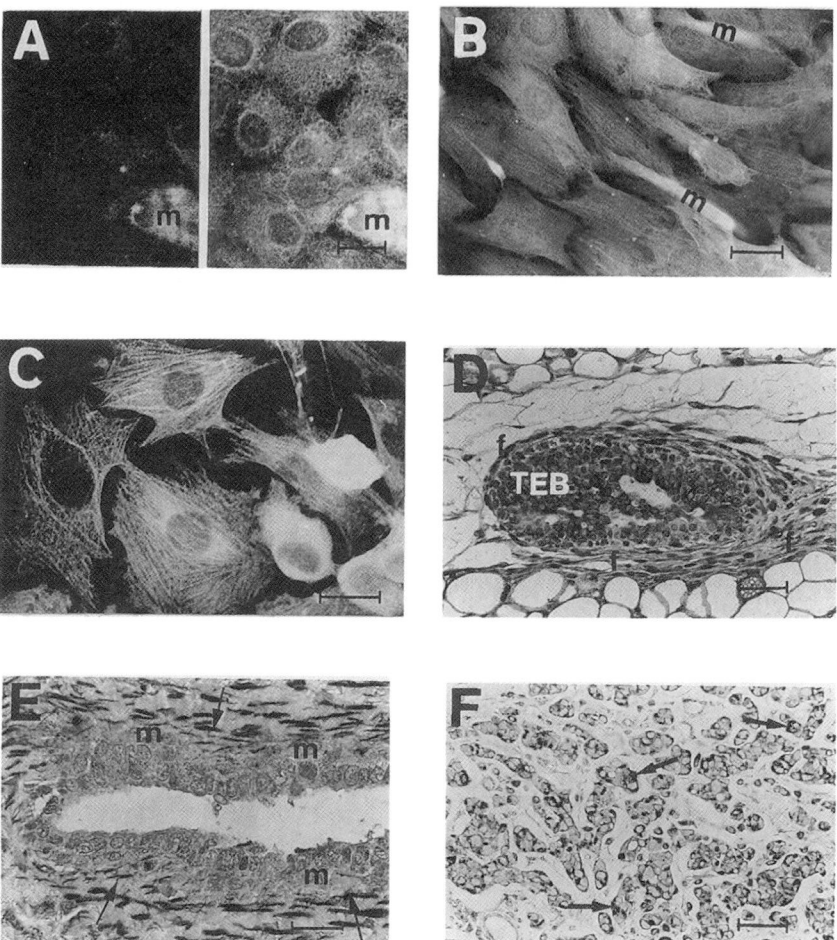

Fig. 7. Immunostaining of mammary tissues by anti-p9Ka. (A) Immunofluorescent staining of rat epithelial cells showing weak immunofluorescence, except where they are converting into intermediate/myoepithelial-like cells (m) in culture. The right panel shows an overexposure to enhance the weak intracellular staining of the epithelial cells, showing circumferentially arranged filaments. (B) Immunofluorescent staining of rat myoepithelial-like cells in culture showing longitudinal arrays of filaments corresponding to the cellular cytoskeleton; mitotic cells (m) are stained still more intensely. (C) Immunofluorescent staining of scrape-loaded rat epithelial cells showing rearrangment of the cellular cytoskeleton into that of intermediate/myoepithelial-like cells after 48 h [80]. (D) Immunocytochemical staining of the cytoplasm of cells in the TEB of a 21-day-old rat. Fibroblasts external to the TEB are also stained (f). (E) Immunocytochemical staining of extracellular filamentous arrays adjacent to the myoepithelial cells (m) in the rat mammary gland (arrows). (F) Immunocytochemical staining of the cellular cytoplasm of human invasive ductal carcinoma (arrows). Scale bars: 20 μm for (A)–(C) and (E); 50 μm for (D) and (F).

binding to the cellular cytoskeleton. That the intracellular cytoskeleton is the site of action for p9Ka inside the cell has been suggested from its stimulation of actin bundling [65] and its interaction with non-muscle tropomyosin [66] and smooth muscle myosin [67,68]. Although in growing rat mammary glands p9Ka also occurs cytoplasmically in intermediate cells in TEBs (Fig. 7D), in resting glands it predominantly occurs extracellularly, associated with filamentous material adjacent to the myoepithelial cells (Fig. 7E) [67]. The relationship between the intracellular and extracellular forms of p9Ka is unknown, although variant forms that can be detected in different subcellular fractions [68] could possibly explain its unusual topographical distribution in mammary cells [69].

Appearance of intermediate markers of the myoepithelial pathway in carcinomas

With the loss of the myoepithelial cell in frankly malignant carcinomas of rats and humans, it may be anticipated that protein markers along the myoepithelial cell pathway would also be entirely lost. This is true for the smooth-muscle-related proteins actin and myosin [70,71]. However, carcinoma cells in humans have shown a limited differentiating ability with respect to the above markers of the myoepithelial cell pathway; those produced evenly (e.g. the basement membrane proteins laminin/type IV collagen) were present in 39–42%, those intermediate (e.g. keratin 14) were present in 14% [10] and those produced early (e.g. p9Ka) were present in about 60% of breast carcinomas (Fig. 7F) [72]. Other, presumably early-marker, proteins of the myoepithelial cell, e.g. cathepsin D and hyaluronectin, were also observed in 50–60% of breast carcinomas [73] (Table 3). All such marker proteins were present in benign breast disease and benign tumours [10,72]. Production of these markers can also be observed in some human breast carcinoma cell lines (P.S. Rudland, unpublished work). These results suggest that vestiges of the differentiating ability to myoepithelial cells are variably retained by malignant carcinoma cells; those for basement membrane proteins and keratin 14 are associated with a lower (less malignant) grade [10], and those for p9Ka and cathepsin D with a more aggressive disease [72,73]. However, as for bFGF, the topographical location of p9Ka and hyaluronectin changes from predominantly extracellular in normal glands and benign tumours to predominantly intracellular in malignant carcinomas of rats and humans (Table 3). The clinical significance of intracellular p9Ka and cathepsin D is described by Barraclough et al. [72] and by Leinster [74] in this volume.

Conclusion

In the normal mammary gland, epithelial stem cells capable of giving rise to all of the parenchymal cell types probably correspond to the cells intermediate between epithelial and myoepithelial cells seen in growing areas of the mammary glands, particularly in TEBs, and to the corresponding intermediate cell lines in culture [8]. In normal development they, and/or associated cells, presumably require both systemic and local factors to enable them to replicate and cause mammary growth. However, the requirement for systemic ovarian, adrenal and pituitary hormones is largely lost in 70–75% of invasive carcinomas. If steroid hormones such as oestrogen stimulate cell growth indirectly through intermediary growth factors such as transferrin, TGFα and/or IGFs [75], then overexpression of these growth factors and/or their receptors would impart both a degree of growth autonomy on and hormonal independence of the malignant cells. This may be the case with certain breast cancers, and could be caused, among other things, by partial differentiation of the malignant cell along the myoepithelial pathway, at least for the TGFα/EGFR autocrine loop. Moreover, overexpression of closely related receptors, such as the EGFR-related *c-erbB-2*, would also impart both growth autonomy and hormonal independence. This is largely so for the 20% or so of breast carcinomas expressing this receptor [62]. In the case of pituitary-independent growth, differentiation of epithelial cells along the myoepithelial-like cell pathway yields an ever declining response to the growth-stimulatory ability of PMGF. Hence retention of vestiges of differentiation along this pathway by malignant cells could account for the refractory nature of most carcinoma cells to hormonal control of their growth (Fig. 8).

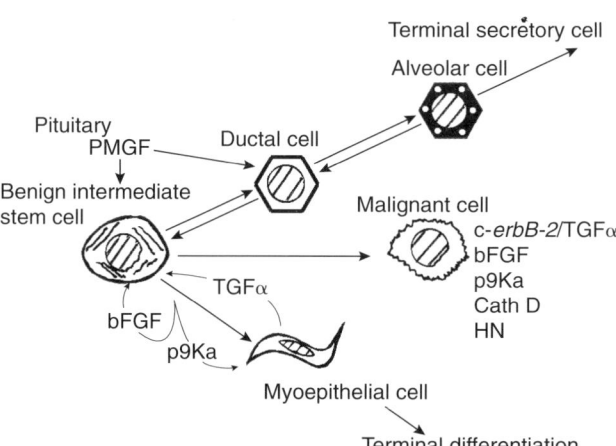

Fig. 8. Possible molecular model for mammary development and cancer. The normal and benign stem cells in terminal ductal structures and elsewhere in the mammary gland can differentiate into ductal epithelial and then into alveolar-like cells (⇄), or into myoepithelial-like cells (→). When fully differentiated, both secretory alveolar and myoepithelial cell types fail to divide and are terminally differentiated. This differentiating ability, particularly the terminal phases, is largely lost in the malignant state. Some of the growth factors, their receptors and other molecules [e.g. cathepsin D (Cath D) and hyaluronectin (HN)] produced by the myoepithelial cells are compensated for in the malignant state by their ectopic production and/or the production of related molecules in some rat and human mammary carcinomas.

Since intermediate stem cells may require bFGF and functional receptors for normal growth, the fact that some of the malignant cell lines and primary invasive carcinomas also produce both bFGF and its high-affinity receptors may suggest that the initially insulted cell bears some similarities to the normal intermediate stem cell. Moreover, both the carcinoma cells and the intermediate stem cells have a much lower level of production of HSPG low-affinity receptors than the myoepithelial cells, the bulk of which serve to sequester this family of growth factors and so prevent them from activating the high-affinity receptors that trigger cell proliferation. Thus the FGF sink provided by the HSPGs present in the basement membrane/extracellular matrix adjacent to the myoepithelial cells is reduced or lost in growing TEBs and in invasive carcinomas. Thus bFGF is then free to act in an autocrine manner by stimulating such cells to grow, and/or in a paracrine manner, e.g. by stimulating neovascularization and the influx of circulating systemic hormones and growth factors (Fig. 6).

In normal development, autocrine and paracrine loops involving growth factors and their receptors provide explanations for the enhancement of growth rates, but provide none for their cessation. The mechanism for limitation of normal glandular growth may be provided, in part, by the differentiation of the secretory alveolar and myoepithelial cells into a non-proliferating phenotype [76], as well as by the sequestration of certain growth factors through HSPGs [74]. Thus, in addition to enhancing existing autocrine and/or paracrine loops, this loss of the ability of the malignant cell to produce terminally differentiated secretory alveolar and myoepithelial cells may also contribute to its tendency towards self-perpetuating and continuous growth *in vivo* (Fig. 8). The significance of the retention and overproduction of early markers of myoepithelial cell differentiation, i.e. p9Ka and cathepsin D, will be described later in this volume [72,74].

This work was supported by grants from The Cancer and Polio Research Fund, The North West Cancer Research Fund, and The Cancer Research Campaign.

References

1. Russo, J., Tay, L.K. and Russo, I.H. (1982) Breast Cancer Res. Treat. **2**, 5–73
2. Topper, Y.J. and Freeman, C.S. (1980) Physiol. Rev. **60**, 1049–1105
3. DeOme, K.B., Faulkin, L.J., Bern, H.A. and Blair, P.B. (1959) Cancer Res. **19**, 515–520
4. Huggins, C., Grand, L.C. and Brillantes, F.P. (1961) Nature (London) **189**, 204–207
5. Hinton, C.P., Bishop, H.M., Holliday, H.W., Doyle, P.L. and Blamey, R.W. (1986) Br. J. Clin. Pract. **40**, 326–330
6. Williams, J.C., Gusterson, B.A., Monaghan, P., Coombes, R.C. and Rudland, P.S. (1985) J. Natl. Cancer Inst. **74**, 415–428
7. Vorherr, H. (1980) in Breast Cancer: Epidemiology, Endocrinology, Biochemistry and Pathobiology, pp. 374–408, Urban and Schwarzenberg, Baltimore
8. Rudland, P.S. (1993) Histol. Histopathol. **8**, 385–404
9. Folkman, J., Watson, K., Ingber, D. and Hanahan, D. (1989) Nature (London) **339**, 58–61
10. Aung, W., Zakhour, H.D., Platt-Higgins, A. and Rudland, P.S. (1993) The Breast **2**, 165–170
11. Ozzello, L. (1971) Pathol. Annu. **6**, 1–39
12. Rudland, P.S. (1987) Cancer Metastasis Rev. **6**, 55–83

13. Rudland, P.S. (1992) J. Cell. Physiol. **153**, 157–168

14. Kano-Sueoka, T., Cambell, G.R. and Gerber, M. (1977) J. Cell. Physiol. **93**, 417–424

15. Rudland, P.S., Hallowes, R.C., Durbin, H. and Lewis, D.J. (1977) J. Cell Biol. **73**, 561–577

16. Sirbasku, D.A., Officer, J.B., Leland, F.E. and Iio, M. (1982) in Growth of Cells in Hormonally Defined Media, vol. B (Sato, G.H., Pardee, A.B. and Sirbasku, D.A., eds.), pp. 765–788, Cold Spring Harbor Laboratory, Cold Spring Harbor

17. Smith, J.A., Winslow, D.P. and Rudland, P.S. (1984) J. Cell. Physiol. **119**, 120–126

18. Rudland, P.S., Durbin, H., Clingan, D. and Jiminez de Asua, L. (1977) Biochem. Biophys. Res. Commun. **75**, 556–562

19. Wilkinson, M.C., Nunez de Croker, C.A., Fernig, D.G., Rudland, P.S. and Smith, J.A. (1996) In Vitro, in the press

20. Walker, R.A. and Day, S.T. (1986) J. Pathol. **148**, 217–224

21. Keon, B.H. and Keenan, T.W. (1993) Protoplasma **172**, 43–48

22. Vandewalle, B., Hornez, L., Revillion, F. and Lefebvre, J. (1989) Biochem. Biophys. Res. Commun. **163**, 149–154

23. Warburton, M.J., Head, L.P., Ferns, S.A. and Rudland, P.S. (1983) Eur. J. Biochem. **133**, 707–715

24. Kim, U. (1979) in Breast Cancer, vol. 3 (McGuire, W.L., ed.), pp. 1–36, Plenum Press, New York

25. Segaloff, A. (1978) in Breast Cancer: Advances in Research and Treatment, vol. 2 (McGuire, W.L., ed.), pp. 1–22, Plenum Press, New York

26. Smith, J.A., Barraclough, R., Fernig, D.G. and Rudland, P.S. (1989) J. Cell. Physiol. **141**, 363–370

27. McAndrew, J., Rudland, P.S., Platt-Higgins, A.M. and Smith, J.A. (1994) Histochem. J. **26**, 355–366

28. McAndrew, J., Fernig, D.G., Rudland, P.S. and Smith, J.A. (1994) Growth Factors **10**, 281–287

29. Fernig, D.G., Smith, J.A. and Rudland, P.S. (1990) J. Cell. Physiol. **142**, 108–116

30. Salomon, D.S., Zwiebel, J.A., Bano, M., Losonczy, I., Fehnel, P. and Kidwell, W.R. (1984) Cancer Res. **44**, 4069–4077

31. Kidwell, W.R. (1986) in Hormones, Oncogenes, Growth Factors, Proc. Inst. Sci. Roussel Symp. p. 14, Paris

32. Ennis, B.W., Valverius, E.M., Bates, S.E., et al. (1989) Mol. Endocrinol. **3**, 1830–1838

33. Bjorge, J.D., Paterson, A.J. and Kudlow, J.E. (1989) J. Biol. Chem. **264**, 4021–4027

34. Lundy, J., Schuss, A., Stanick, D., McCormack, E.S., Kramer, S. and Sorvillo, J.M. (1991) Am. J. Pathol. **138**, 1527–1534

35. Umekita, Y., Enokizono, N., Sagara, Y., Kuriwaki, K., Takasaki, T., Yoshida, A. and Yoshida, H. (1992) Virchows Arch. A. Pathol. Anat. **420**, 345–351

36. Cowley, G., Gusterson, B.A., Smith, J.A., Headler, F. and Ozanne, B. (1984) in Cancer Cells, The Transformed Phenotype, pp. 5–10, Cold Spring Harbor Laboratory, Cold Spring Harbor

37. McCann, A., Johnston, P.A., Dervan, P.A., Gullick, W.J. and Carney, D.N. (1989) Ir. J. Med. Sci. **158**, 137–140

38. Winstanley, J.H.R., Cooke, T., Murray, D.G., et al. (1991) Br. J. Cancer **63**, 447–450

39. Slamon, D.J., Clark, G.M., Wong, S.G., Levin, W.J., Ullrich, A. and McGuire, W.L. (1987) Science **235**, 177–182

40. Fernig, D.G. and Gallagher, J.T. (1994) Prog. Growth Factor Res. **5**, 353–377

41. Barraclough, R., Fernig, D.G., Rudland, P.S. and Smith, J.A. (1990) J. Cell. Physiol. **144**, 333–344

42. Fernig, D.G., Rudland, P.S. and Smith, J.A. (1992) Growth Factors **7**, 27–39

43. Fernig, D.G., Barraclough, R., Ke, Y.Q., Wilkinson, M.C., Rudland, P.S. and Smith, J.A. (1993) Int. J. Cancer **54**, 629–635

44. Ke, Y., Fernig, D.G., Wilkinson, M.C., Winstanley, J.H.R., Smith, J.A., Rudland, P.S. and Barraclough R. (1993) J. Cell Sci. **106**, 135–143

45. Chen, H.-L., Rudland, P.S., Smith, J.A. and Fernig, D.G. (1995) in Intercellular Signalling in the Mammary Gland (Wilde, C.J., Peaker, M. and Knight, C.H., eds.), pp. 73–74, Plenum Press, New York

46. Gomm, J.J., Smith, J., Ryall, G.K., Baillie, R., Turnbull, L. and Coombes, R.C. (1991) Cancer Res. **51**, 4685–4692

47. Rudland, P.S., Platt-Higgins, A.M., Wilkinson, M.C. and Fernig, D.G. (1993) J. Histochem. Cytochem. **41**, 887–898

48. Peyrat, J.P., Bonneterre, J., Hondermarck, H., Hecquet, B., Adenis, A., Louchez, M.M., Lefebvre, J., Boilly, B. and Demaille, A. (1992) J. Steroid Biochem. Mol. Biol. **43**, 87–94

49. Peyrat, J.P., Hondermarck, H., Hecquet, B., Adenis, A. and Bonneterre, J. (1992) Bull. Cancer **79**, 251–260

50. Karey, K.P. and Sirbasku, D.A. (1988) Cancer Res. **48**, 4083–4092

51. Stewart, A.J., Johnson, M.D., May, F.E. and Westley, B.R. (1990) J. Biol. Chem. **265**, 21172–21178

52. Takahashi, K., Suzuki, K., Kawahara, S. and Ono, T. (1989) Int. J. Cancer **43**, 870–874

53. Anandappa, S.Y., Winstanley, J.H.R., Leinster, S., Green, B., Rudland, P.S. and Barraclough, R. (1993) Br. J. Cancer **69**, 772–776

54. Luqmani, Y.A., Graham, M. and Coombes, R.C. (1992) Br. J. Cancer **66**, 273–280

55. Rowe, J.M., Kasper, S., Shiu, R.C. and Friesen, H.G. (1986) Cancer Res. **46**, 1408–1412

56. Paterson, F.C. and Rudland, P.S. (1985) J. Cell. Physiol. **125**, 135–150

57. Schäfer, B., Wicki, R., Englekamp, D., Mattei, M. and Heizmann, C. (1995) Genomics **25**, 638–643

58. Rudland, P.S., Paterson, F.C., Monaghan, P., Twiston-Davies, A.C. and Warburton, M.J. (1986) Dev. Biol. **113**, 388–405

59. Barraclough, R., Kimbell, R. and Rudland, P.S. (1984) Nucleic Acids Res. **12**, 8097–8114

60. Barraclough, R., Kimbell, R. and Rudland, P.S. (1987) J. Cell. Physiol. **131**, 393–401

61. Warburton, M.J., Kimbell, R., Rudland, P.S., Ferns, S.A. and Barraclough, R. (1986) J. Cell. Physiol. **128**, 76–84

62. Rudland, P.S., Barraclough, R., Fernig, D.G. and Smith, J.A. (1996) in The Stem Cell Handbook (Potton, C., ed.), pp. 147–232, Academic Press, London

63. Davies, B.R., Davies, M.P.A., Gibbs, F.E.M., Barraclough, R. and Rudland, P.S. (1993) Oncogene **8**, 999–1008

64. Davies, B.R. (1993) Ph.D. Thesis, University of Liverpool

65. Watanabe, Y., Usuda, N., Minami, H., et al. (1993) FEBS Lett. **324**, 51–55

66. Takenaga, K., Nakamura, Y., Sakiyama, S., Hasegawa, Y., Sato, K. and Endo, H. (1994) J. Cell Biol. **124**, 757–768

67. Gibbs, F.E.M., Barraclough, R., Platt-Higgins, A., Rudland, P.S., Wilkinson, M.C. and Parry, E.W. (1995) J. Histochem. Cytochem. **43**, 169–180

68. Barraclough, R. and Rudland, P.S. (1994) Eur. J. Cancer **30A**, 1570–1576

69. Haigler, H.T. and Schlaepfer, D.D. (1992) in The Annexins (Moss, S.E., ed.), pp. 11–22, Portland Press, London

70. Gusterson, B.A., Warburton, M.J., Mitchell, D., Ellison, M., Neville, A.M. and Rudland, P.S. (1982) Cancer Res. **42**, 4763–4770

71. Dunnington, D.J., Kim, U., Hughes, C.M., Monaghan, P., Ormerod, E.J. and Rudland, P.S. (1984) J. Natl. Cancer Inst. **72**, 455–466

72. Barraclough, R., Chen, H.-J., Davies, B.R., Davies, M.P.A., Ke, Y., Lloyd, B.H., Oates, A. and Rudland, P.S. (1997) Biochem. Soc. Symp. **63**, 273–294

73. Winstanley, J.H.R., Leinster, S.J., Cooke, T.G., Westley, B.R., Platt-Higgins, A.M. and Rudland, P.S. (1993) Br. J. Cancer **67**, 767–772

74. Leinster, S. (1997) Biochem. Soc. Symp. **63**, 185–191

75.   Westley, B.R., Clayton, S.J., Daws, M.R., Molloy, C.A and May, F.E.B (1997) Biochem. Soc. Symp. **63**, 35–44

76.   Joshi, K., Smith, J.A., Perusinghe, N. and Monaghan, P. (1986) Am. J. Pathol. **124**, 199–206

77.   Bertrand, P., Girard, N., Delpech, B., Duval, C., D'Anjou, J. and Dauce, J.P. (1992) Int. J. Cancer **82**, 1–6

78.   Russo, J. and Russo, I.H. (1987) in The Mammary Gland: Development, Regulation and Function (Neville, M.C. and Daniels, C.W., eds.), pp. 67–93, Plenum Press, New York

79.   Lyons, R.W., Li, C.H. and Johnson, R.E. (1958) Recent Prog. Horm. Res. **14**, 219–254

80.   Gibbs, F.E.M. (1993) Ph.D. Thesis, University of Liverpool

Biochem. Soc. Symp. **63**, 21–34
Printed in Great Britain

2

Control of the three-dimensional growth pattern of mammary epithelium: role of genes of the *Wnt* and *erbB* families studied using reconstituted epithelium

Paul A. W. Edwards

Division of Cellular Pathology, Department of Pathology, University of Cambridge, Tennis Court Road, Cambridge CB2 1QP, U.K.

Abstract

The mammary gland is possibly the best system in which to study the three-dimensional organization of tissues and how that organization is disrupted in tumour development. The principal approach used has been to express genes such as oncogenes and growth factor genes in mammary epithelium *in vivo*, by using mammary-specific promoters in germ-line transgenic mice; by injecting virus vectors into the lumen of the mammary gland; or by transplanting genetically manipulated mammary epithelial cells into a mammary fat pad from which the natural epithelium has been removed. This chapter focuses on the last approach. The *Wnt* genes are short-range signalling molecules related to *Wnt-1*, which was discovered as an oncogene in mouse mammary tumours. Several Wnt proteins are expressed in the mammary gland; notably, Wnt-4 is normally expressed in early pregnancy. Introducing Wnt-4 into the mammary epithelium of virgin mice induces a growth pattern very similar to that of mid-pregnancy. Wnt-4 may therefore be a local signal driving epithelial branching in pregnancy. ErbB/epidermal growth factor receptor and ErbB-2 are receptors that may be important in breast tumour development and normal mammary growth control. Overactive mutants of them, i.e. the genes v-*erbB* and *neu*, disturb the growth pattern of the mammary epithelium in quite distinct ways. Overactive ErbB-2 causes local development of alveoli, suggesting that it may be involved in normal alveolus development. The varied effects of these gene products show the complexity of the control of the three-dimensional growth pattern, and encourage the idea that we may be able to relate oncogenic effects to normal growth controls.

Introduction

As well as being a tissue of great medical and commercial importance, the mammary gland is possibly the best model system in which to study the three-dimensional organization of tissues and how that organization is disrupted in tumour development.

One crucial advantage of the mammary gland for studying three-dimensional growth patterns is that it can be whole-mounted (see Figs. 2 and 3). The mammary gland consists of a tree-like array of epithelial tubes leading from the nipple into a fat pad. When the whole gland is fixed, stained with a nuclear stain such as haematoxylin or carmine, dehydrated and immersed in methyl salicylate, the tissue becomes completely transparent, and all the individual cell nuclei can be seen. As the epithelium has a higher density of nuclei than the fat, it dominates the whole mount (see Figs. 2 and 3) and its three-dimensional arrangement can be seen with a stereo microscope in great detail, permitting small, local disturbances (e.g. Fig. 3) to be seen. Using whole-mount preparations and conventional histology, the organization of growth and the variety of controls that are needed to give the epithelium its form can be appreciated. For example, the epithelium is made up of two layers of cells with distinct phenotypes; the ducts have a precise diameter; they branch fairly regularly and grow until the spacing between epithelial tubes is almost the same throughout the gland; and so on. In addition, the pattern of the epithelium changes in pregnancy and lactation, and returns to something like its original virgin pattern after lactation has finished. The challenge is to understand how such patterning is controlled, and how it is disrupted in neoplasia.

Much of the current work in this field centres on expressing genes, or abolishing the expression of genes, in mammary epithelium to see what this does to the pattern of growth. Some years ago we developed a technique for introducing genes into mammary epithelium by transplantation, known as the 'tissue reconstitution' or 'transgenic tissue' method [1–3]. This chapter describes this experimental approach and compares it with other methods available for expressing genes in mammary epithelium; then I describe our recent work on the control of normal development, and its relationship to neoplastic growth, using members of the *Wnt* and *erbB* gene families.

Expressing genes in the mammary gland

Three methods have been used to introduce genes into the mammary epithelium. The most widely known is the germ-line transgenic mouse approach, in which a gene is expressed from a mammary-specific promoter such as the mouse mammary tumour virus (MMTV) promoter or whey acidic protein (WAP) promoter (reviewed by Muller et al. and Jolicoeur et al. elsewhere in this volume; see also [4,5]). A second approach is to introduce genes directly into the lumen of the mammary gland, by injecting viruses that carry genes of interest via the nipple [6,7]. The third approach, which is the main subject of this chapter, is to place mammary epithelial cells in culture, introduce genes into them, and then transplant them back into the mammary fat pad of a host mouse, where they reconstitute a genetically manipulated epithelium [1,8].

The tissue reconstitution method

Fig. 1 shows the details of the method. Mammary epithelium develops postnatally by growing from the nipple into the mammary fat pad. If the nipple region is removed 3 weeks after birth, the gland has no endogenous epithelium and is known as a 'cleared mammary fat pad' [9]. A remarkable property of mammary epithelial cells is that if they are transplanted into such an empty fat

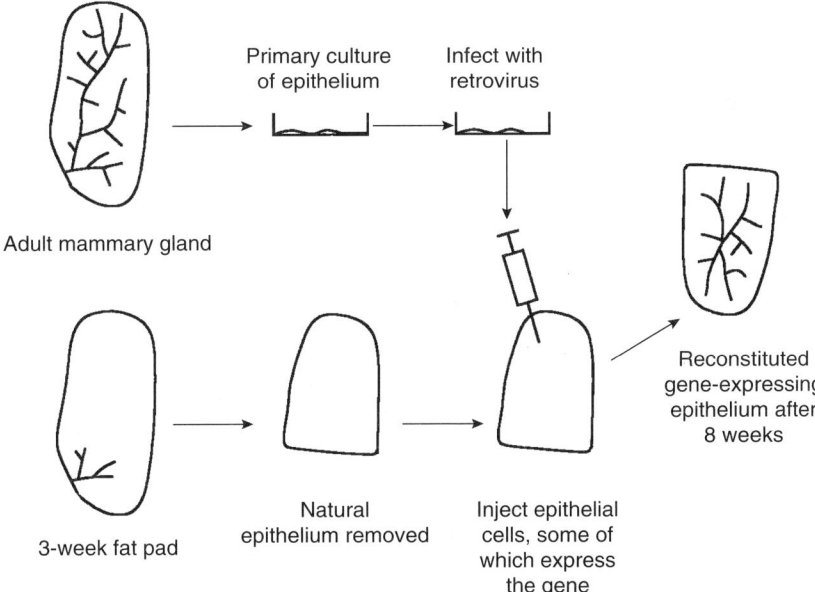

Fig. 1. Tissue reconstitution method for introducing genes into mouse mammary epithelium *in vivo*. Mammary epithelial cells are prepared from an adult female gland by collagenase digestion and placed in primary culture. They are infected with helper-free retrovirus and then transplanted into a 'cleared' mammary fat pad *in vivo*. The cleared fat pad is prepared from a 3-week-old female mouse. At this age the epithelium, represented in the diagram by lines, is a small cluster of ducts that has grown only a short way in from the nipple. It can be removed by cutting off the top of the fat pad. The genetically manipulated cells are injected into this 'cleared fat pad', where they re-form an epithelium which branches and fills the fat pad over about 10 weeks. The whole gland can then be whole-mounted (see Figs. 2 and 3). In our lab, cells are infected with retrovirus by subculturing the primary cells on to irradiated retrovirus-producing cells. The total time in culture is 4 days. For details, see [3].

pad, they grow to re-form a ductal epithelium which is indistinguishable from the normal ductal tree, in terms of duct diameter and branching pattern, extent of growth and histology (e.g. see Figs. 2 and 3). The reconstituted gland shows normal hormone responsiveness. However, the epithelium is not connected to a nipple and so secreted milk cannot be removed by suckling. Lactation normally terminates in a gland that is not drained, so, in a transplanted gland, lactation terminates at parturition rather than at weaning [10]. To produce genetically manipulated epithelium, primary cultures of mammary epithelial cells are prepared from a mature donor mouse. After infection with a non-replicating retrovirus carrying the gene of choice, the cells are injected into a cleared fat pad. The primary cells need only be kept in culture for a few days (typically 4 days), minimizing the risk of any other changes occurring in the cells [3].

Similar reconstitution methods have been described for skin, colon and the haemopoietic system [2].

The tissue reconstitution method compared with other methods of introducing genes into the epithelium

The three methods for introducing genes into mammary epithelium have various advantages and disadvantages. Perhaps the most important difference between the transgenic approach and the tissue reconstitution and direct introduction methods is that in the transgenic all cells in the mammary epithelium can express the introduced gene, while in the other two approaches only some cells take up the introduced gene, probably at most a few per cent. This is a major issue in the study of neoplasia, where, to model tumour development accurately, genes should be introduced into clones of cells surrounded by normal cells. In the germ-line transgenic model the entire mammary epithelium may be abnormal, so interactions between abnormal and adjacent normal cells are lost. There is evidence that the behaviour of abnormal cells is regulated by neighbouring normal cells. For example, by altering the ratio between normal and oncogene-expressing cells in reconstituted prostate, Thompson et al. [11] obtained different patterns of preneoplastic and neoplastic changes. Furthermore, the generalized hyperplasia that may be induced in the transgenic mammary epithelium may obscure early, subtle changes in the growth pattern induced by a cancer mutation, such as those shown induced by *erbB*-2 (see below). This makes the germ-line transgenic an unsatisfactory model of tumour development. Another problem with the transgenic model is that the tissue-specific promoters may be leaky and allow expression in other tissues. For example, the MMTV promoter can drive expression in kidney and lung, and this can lead to kidney and lung lesions that kill the mice before mammary gland changes can be studied [12]. In experiments on metastatic potential, primary tumours arising in the lung could be confused with metastases.

An additional advantage of the transplant system is flexibility in the promoter used to drive gene expression. Expression of a gene in the mammary gland of a germ-line transgenic mouse requires a mammary-specific promoter, and the available promoters have significant limitations. The promoters in use are the MMTV promoter [4] and milk-protein promoters such as those for β-lactoglobulin [13] and WAP [14]. Unfortunately, all of these promoters are hormone sensitive, and are only fully active during pregnancy and lactation, while the resting gland is of most relevance to human cancer development [5]. In contrast, in the other two techniques, expression is limited to the mammary epithelium by the method of introduction, so any promoter can be used to drive expression of the gene of interest. When retrovirus vectors are used, there is a choice between using the retrovirus' own promoter, the long terminal repeat promoter of the Moloney leukaemia virus or a close relative (these are quite distinct from MMTV), or any chosen internal promoter. For example, most of our recent work has used the β-actin promoter, a ubiquitously active promoter, in the retrovirus vector INA [15].

The tissue reconstitution approach is probably also cheaper and quicker than making transgenic mice, especially as any individual transgenic line may show effects specific to the integration site of the transgene, and at least two lines have to be compared. In transplants, many different sites of retrovirus integration are generated within one experiment, so integration-specific effects do not influence the overall picture.

A limitation of the reconstitution and direct introduction approaches is that there may be immune responses to the introduced gene product. For example, we have seen obvious lymphocyte infiltration around epithelium that expressed the MC29 gag–myc fusion protein [1] and the large-T antigen of simian virus 40 (P.A.W. Edwards, unpublished work), both highly immunogenic viral proteins. Other oncogenes have not elicited a detectable response, notably OK10 v-myc. One solution is to use mouse genes; another may be to induce tolerance to the introduced protein.

General limitations of all the methods

A subtler issue about which we know rather little is the cell types in the mammary epithelium in which the introduced gene is expressed. The two main types of cell in the epithelium are the inner luminal or secretory cell and the outer basal or myoepithelial cell. There are probably other types, e.g. precursor or stem cell types, such as the 'cap cells' of the terminal end bud in the growing duct [16] and the 'clear cell' [17]. Breast tumours mostly show cytokeratins characteristic of luminal cells, but other markers suggest that they are often intermediate in phenotype between luminal and basal cells, as argued elsewhere in this volume by Rudland et al. In the germ-line transgenic, expression driven by the MMTV and WAP promoters is presumably limited to the luminal cells, although this does not seem to have been explicitly determined. In the reconstitution model certain cells may be more prone to infection in culture or may transplant better. All we know at present, from sections stained with antibody, is that the luminal cells at least express introduced genes. The direct introduction approach presumably introduces genes selectively into luminal epithelial cells, which line the ducts. In future the precise pattern of expression achieved by the various approaches needs to be determined [5].

Another advance in the genetic manipulation of the mammary epithelium will be methods for tissue-specific inhibition of expression. So far only overexpression of genes has been achieved, or germ-line knockout. The most promising approach would seem to be use of the *lox–cre* system, in which genes are eliminated by recombination between flanking *lox* sequences mediated by the *cre* recombinase [18]. The *cre* recombinase would be expressed specifically in mammary epithelium, either in a transgenic animal from a promoter such as the MMTV promoter or in the transplant system using a retrovirus that expresses *cre*.

Genes that control normal development and are implicated in neoplasia: the *Wnt* genes

Wnt-1 was originally discovered as *int-1*, a gene whose expression is often activated in mammary tumours induced by MMTV [19]. It proved to be homologous to the *wingless* gene of *Drosophila*, which is involved in patterning of the *Drosophila* embryo, and so was renamed *Wnt-1*. The Wnt-1/Wingless proteins are secreted glycoproteins that carry short-range signals between cells. Subsequently a large family of closely related glycoproteins, the Wnt family, has been discovered, and they seem to be involved in controlling a wide range of developmental processes [20]. (The *Wnt* family of genes should not be confused with the *int* genes. Although *Wnt-1* is *int-1*, the *Wnt* genes are homologues of *Wnt-1*, while the other *int* genes are a list of unrelated genes that were discovered as consistent integration sites of MMTV in mouse mammary tumours).

Is Wnt-1 an oncogene because it mimics other Wnts?

For some time the oncogenic activity of Wnt-1/*int*-1 was a puzzle: it was not expressed in normal mammary gland, so why should there be a receptor for it? This was solved when other members of the Wnt family were discovered, and several of them proved to be expressed in the mammary gland in various stages of normal development [21,22]. Wnt-1 might therefore alter the mammary growth pattern by mimicking one or more of the other Wnt glycoproteins that are normally involved in regulating mammary development.

Wnt-4 may drive epithelial proliferation in (normal) pregnancy

We had noticed that the hyperplastic epithelium induced by expressing Wnt-1 looked rather like a mid-pregnant epithelium (Figs. 2c and 2d) [15]. In early pregnancy, new side-branches and alveoli develop on the duct framework laid down in the virgin animal. To show the resemblance, transplants of normal mammary epithelium were grown in a pregnant mouse, and their growth pattern was quite similar to the Wnt-1-expressing transplant in a virgin mouse (Figs. 2c and 2d) [15]. The effect of Wnt-1 was local, not systemic, as we will discuss later.

It followed that one or more of the Wnt gene products might be responsible for directing side-branch and alveolus growth in early pregnancy, so we expressed some of the likely Wnts in transplants. Wnt-4 seemed to fulfil the prediction [23]. In the normal mammary gland, it is expressed only weakly in the virgin and expression increases early in pregnancy [22]. Reconstituted epithelium expressing Wnt-4, in the virgin gland, showed an over-branched

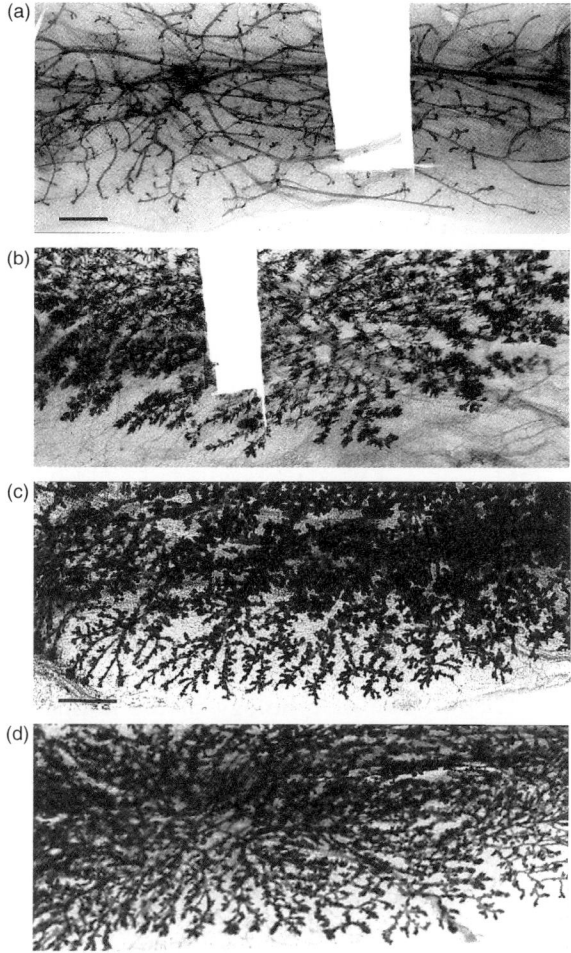

Fig. 2. Reconstituted mammary epithelium expressing *Wnt* genes in comparison with virgin and pregnant controls. Whole-mounts of reconstituted glands, prepared as described in Fig. 1, are shown. Whole glands were stained with the nuclear stain haematoxylin or carmine and then cleared by immersion in methyl salicylate. The epithelium appears as dark tree-like structures within clear adipose tissue. (a) Control transplanted epithelium, infected with control retrovirus that does not express an oncogene, grown in a virgin host (and contralateral to a Wnt-4-expressing gland such as that shown in b). The white area is where part of the transplant has been taken for histology. (b) Transplanted epithelium expressing Wnt-4, in a virgin host [23]. Again, part has been removed. Note the extensive branching of the epithelium, as in the pregnant epithelium below. (c) Pregnant epithelium, in the form of a transplant of normal epithelium into a host that was mated after transplantation. The transplant was whole-mounted between 14 and 17 days of pregnancy [15]. (d) Transplant expressing Wnt-1 in a virgin host, showing how the hyperplasia induced by expressing Wnt-1 is similar, although not identical, to that in both the pregnant and Wnt-4-expressing epithelia [15]. The magnification in (a) is the same as in (b); in (c) and (d) it is about 15% greater. Scale bars are 1 mm.

pattern of growth close to, but not identical to, that in early pregnancy (Figs. 2b and 2c). On comparing the patterns of growth induced by Wnt-4 and Wnt-1, the Wnt-4 pattern was closer to that of early pregnancy (Figs. 2b–2d). Although much more needs to be done, it seems likely that Wnt-4 plays a key role in pregnancy, changing the growth pattern of the epithelium, and that the oncogenic effect of Wnt-1 occurs at least in part through its ability to mimic Wnt-4. Wnt-1 may also mimic other Wnt proteins that are normally expressed in the mammary gland, such as Wnt-6 and Wnt-7b [21,22]. Wnt-1, Wnt-6 and Wnt-7b transform fibroblasts, while Wnt-4 has little or no effect [24], suggesting that Wnt-1 is a ligand for a receptor that binds Wnt-6 and Wnt-7b.

Hormone-independent growth of epithelium that expresses Wnt-1

Since the dependence of mammary growth on ovarian hormones is a major practical issue in breast cancer, any situations where the growth of mammary epithelium is independent of ovarian hormones are of interest. When Tsukamoto et al. [25] expressed Wnt-1 in mammary epithelium in transgenic mice, they found that the hyperplastic epithelium developed in male mice as well as in females, so its growth was independent of ovarian hormones. In the transgenic mice the effect could have been systemic. To show that it was local, Wnt-1-expressing epithelium and normal epithelium were transplanted into opposite ends of the same fat pad in normal mice [15,26]. The two epithelial outgrowths grew until they confronted each other in the fat pad, with a separation of about 100–200 μm. The morphology of the normal epithelium was completely unaffected, showing not only that the effect of Wnt-1 was not systemic, but also that it was of very limited range within the fat pad, as expected from the behaviour of Wnts in other systems [20].

In normal mice, the growth of epithelial tubes can be divided into two phases: growth of the major ducts in the virgin animal, and growth of side-branches in pregnancy. These two growth phases have different hormone/growth factor sensitivities; for example, they respond differently to transforming growth factor β [27]. The growth of major ducts occurs at characteristic terminal end bud structures, but these are not found in side-branch growth. Wnt-1-expressing epithelium has terminal end buds when growing in intact females, but these are absent during growth in males or ovariectomized females, showing that Wnt-1 does not simply substitute for ovarian hormones. We suggested an alternative, if speculative, interpretation, based on our hypothesis that Wnt-1 causes side-branch growth that would normally occur in pregnancy (see above): that growth of the side-branch type might be independent of ovarian hormones, and so Wnt-1-driven growth is also ovarian-independent [15]. If this is correct, then oestrogen-independent tumour growth might be driven by signals that would normally only be issued in pregnancy or lactation.

Genes that control normal development and are implicated in neoplasia: the erbB genes

To model the development of breast cancer, we [1,2,15,23,28–31] and others [32–35] have introduced tumour mutations into individual clones of cells in mouse mammary epithelium. Introducing oncogenes in this way allows us to address basic questions such as: what does an individual oncogene do to three-dimensional growth control? Do related oncogenes have similar or different effects? The tissue reconstitution method also allows sequential introduction of more than one oncogene to follow tumour development, by introducing one oncogene, harvesting the resulting preneoplastic epithelium, introducing a second oncogene into a few of the cells, and re-transplanting [29].

Among oncogenes suspected to play a role in the development of human breast cancer, erbB-2/HER-2 and other members of the erbB/HER family are perhaps the best established candidates. The four members of this family are the epidermal growth factor (EGF) receptor, known as ErbB or HER, and its homologues ErbB-2/HER-2 (the rat form of which is also known as Neu), ErbB-3/HER-3 and ErbB-4/HER-4. They are discussed in detail elsewhere in this volume by Muller et al., Gullick and Cohen et al.

ErbB-2: focal development of a spectrum of lesions

ErbB-2 has long been thought to be involved in the development of a subset of human breast cancers, with around 20% of breast carcinomas, and a high proportion of carcinomas in situ, expressing high levels of the protein [36]. Several groups have shown that the overactive mutant form of rat erbB-2, neu, is very effective at causing carcinoma in situ and frank carcinoma when expressed in mammary epithelium, as discussed elsewhere in this volume by Muller et al. and Jolicoeur et al. Wild-type erbB-2 was also reported to result in tumours when expressed in mammary epithelium in transgenic mice, but subsequently the introduced erbB-2 was found to have acquired activating mutations during tumour development [37], so exactly how much overexpression of the normal form can contribute to tumour development is uncertain.

When we introduced neu into reconstituted epithelium, focal lesions developed in the transplanted epithelium (Fig. 3a) [30]. The focal distribution of abnormal growth was as expected from parallel experiments in which β-galactosidase was expressed in a similar way: β-galactosidase-positive cells were distributed in clusters in the transplant [3]. In whole-mounts, the more obvious lesions were dense aggregates of cells, often of rather ill-defined shape, although some suggested the 'bunch-of-grapes' shape formed by clusters of alveoli in the lactating gland (Fig. 3a) [30,31]. The various lesions were classified by the standard criteria of human histopathology as hyperplasias with or without atypia, sclerosing adenosis, carcinoma in situ and frank carcinoma [30].

To try and understand the development of these lesions, we have examined whole-mounts and sections for mild disturbances of the growth pattern [3,31]. Many whole-mounts showed alveoli on ducts in the virgin gland, apparently representing inappropriate development of alveoli. They occurred either focally as distinct lesions, or peripherally to more advanced lesions. Alveoli

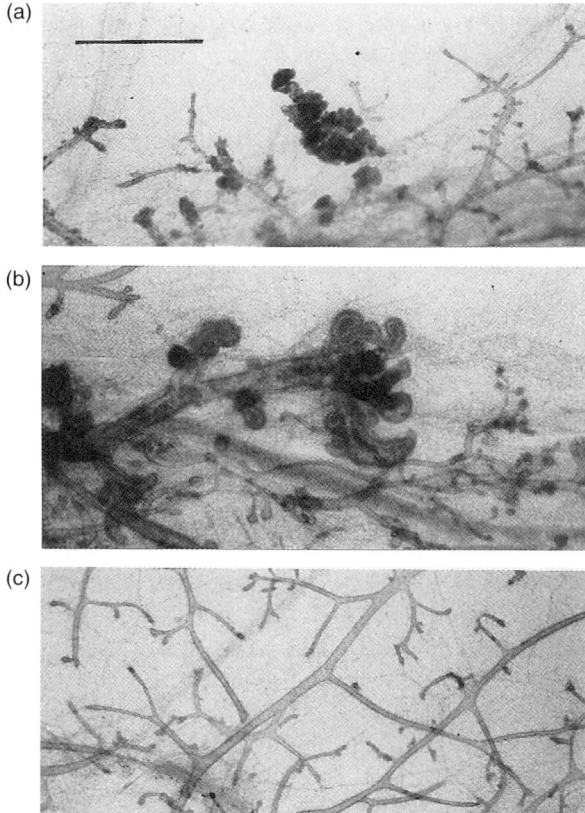

Fig. 3. Reconstituted mammary epithelium expressing genes of the erbB family. Whole-mounts of reconstituted glands, stained as in Fig. 2, expressing activated erbB-2 and erbB are shown. (a) Disturbance of growth pattern caused by expression of the activated c-erbB-2 oncogene *neu* [30]. The lesion resembles a tightly packed cluster of alveoli. The retrovirus that was used expresses *neu* from a β-actin promoter. (b) Different alteration of growth pattern resulting from expressing activated EGF receptor, in the form of the chicken retrovirus oncogene v-erbB [28]. Ducts are enlarged and have aberrant termini, and sectioning shows that the dark material in the lumen of the ducts represents epithelial cells that appear to have been shed from the ductal epithelium. (c) Control transplant infected with a retrovirus that carries no oncogene. The magnification is the same in all the photographs; scale bar = 1 mm.

were also often prominent in glands that had been taken through lactation and involution [3,30]. In this case they could have been present as inappropriate alveoli before lactation or they could have arisen normally in lactation but been retained as a result of *erbB-2/neu* expression. Antibody staining of sections through clusters of alveoli showed expression of ErbB-2 [30]. Histologically, a continuum of morphologies was seen, from essentially normal clusters of alveoli through to more advanced lesions [30,31].

One interpretation of these observations is that ErbB-2 is normally involved in initiating or maintaining alveoli in lactation, and that inappropriate activation of the receptor leads to inappropriate alveolus formation. This is consistent with evidence from Birchmeier's laboratory that expression of heregulin, a ligand that can activate ErbB-2 when heterodimerized to ErbB3 or ErbB4, can induce alveolus formation in mammary glands in organ culture [38]. In other words, the consequence of overactivity of ErbB-2 in breast tumour development may be to set up a lactation-like pattern of growth, or to protect epithelial cells against apoptosis in involution.

ErbB-2 compared with ErbB: do related oncogenes have similar or different effects?

ErbB and ErbB-2 are closely related growth factor receptors that can heterodimerize, so it was of interest to ask whether constitutively active mutants of them would have the same effect on mammary growth pattern. We expressed v-erbB, the original retrovirus oncogene version of the overactive chicken EGF receptor, in transplants, and found that it gave a quite distinct alteration of the growth pattern [28]. In contrast with the alveolar lesions produced by expressing neu, v-erbB produced enlarged ducts in which the luminal surface was fragmented, and there were frequently loose epithelial cells in the lumen (Fig. 3b). There was little alteration to the surrounding stroma [28]. Thus two closely related oncogenes have different effects, although we do not yet know whether this is because ErbB and ErbB-2 activate different signal transduction pathways, or because the mode of activation of the oncogenes was different – v-erbB is the chicken gene with both ends truncated, while neu is rat c-erbB-2 with a point mutation in the transmembrane domain. This is currently under investigation.

General conclusions about oncogene action in the mammary epithelium

Several oncogenes and growth factors have now been expressed in the mammary epithelium (reviewed in [5,8], and elsewhere in this volume). Their effects are strikingly diverse; for example altered branching of ducts, inappropriate alveolus formation and changes in hormone responsiveness, which draws our attention to the complexity of the growth controls operating in mammary epithelium and the variety of signals that can alter these controls in specific ways. The take-home message is that in vitro studies of the actions of cancer mutations are of little value in understanding cancer development – v-erbB, erbB-2/neu and (contrary to older literature; see [24]) Wnt-1 all transform fibroblasts in culture, but their effects in vivo are completely different. Another lesson is that it is generally of more interest to study the preneoplastic growth patterns induced by oncogene expression, without subsequent tumour progression, than to study tumours themselves, where undefined additional events have occurred. The altered growth patterns produced by oncogenes are in most cases quite well ordered and stable, rarely progressing to tumours on the time scale of the experiments (usually 3–4 months), and the changes in growth pattern can be interpreted in terms of alteration of normal growth controls, as we have seen in the examples above.

There is some controversy about the relationship between oncogene expression in the mammary gland and the appearance of an altered growth pattern. Cardiff [5], reviewing tumour development in transgenic mice, has concluded that expression of a single oncogene alone is not enough to disturb the growth pattern, and that some additional stochastic event is required. Our work, in which expression of the marker gene β-galactosidase matches the distribution of lesions induced by mutant *erbB-2*, suggests to us that he is mistaken. We believe that his 'additional event' is switch-on, by an epigenetic event, of the MMTV promoter that drives oncogene expression in the transgenic system. There is evidence that transgene expression in MMTV-driven transgenics is patchy. For example, *in situ* hybridization [39] suggests locally patchy expression. In some transgenics this patchiness seems quite clear; for example in those expressing heregulin from the MMTV promoter, only one eye may be affected by hyperplasia of the Harderian gland, and only this eye expresses the transgene, again suggesting that MMTV promoter switches on stochastically. This controversy should be resolved when oncogenes are co-expressed with a histochemical marker gene.

Conclusion

Why has expressing genes in the mouse mammary epithelium proved to be such a powerful tool for investigating the normal control of growth pattern and its subversion in cancer development? The answer in part is that we have been able to express genes in virgin epithelium and create some of the changes that occur in pregnancy and lactation. In other words, mammary epithelium has the unique property that we can mimic a natural change of growth pattern by turning on the expression of genes. In other tissues, 'normal' changes in growth pattern can only be obtained by knocking out function, which is difficult to do in a tissue-specific way. This is in addition to the advantage of being able to view the three-dimensional structure of the mammary epithelium by whole-mounting. The mammary gland is almost certainly the most amenable mammalian tissue for studies of the control of three-dimensional growth patterns.

I thank my co-workers, particularly those involved in our ErbB and Wnt family studies, Dr. Clare Abram, Dr. Jane Bradbury, Dr. Trevor Dale and Dr. Sue Hiby. Our work was supported by the Agriculture and Food Research Council, the Breast Cancer Research Trust, and the Cancer Research Campaign.

References
1.   Edwards, P.A.W., Ward, J.L. and Bradbury, J.M. (1988) Oncogene **2**, 407–412
2.   Edwards, P.A.W. (1993) Cancer Surv. **16**, 79–96

3.   Edwards, P.A.W., Abram, C.L. and Bradbury, J.M. (1996) J. Mammary Gland Biol. Neoplasia 1, 75–90

4.   Webster, M.A. and Muller, W.J. (1994) Semin. Cancer Biol. 5, 69–76

5.   Cardiff, R.D. (1996) J. Mammary Gland Biol. Neoplasia 1, 61–74

6.   Wang, B., Kennan, W.S., Yasukawa-Barnes, J., Lindstrom, M.J. and Gould, M.N. (1991) Cancer Res. 51, 2642–2648

7.   Yang, J., Tsukamoto, T., Popnikolov, N., Guzman, R.C., Chen, X.Y., Yang, J.H. and Nandi, S. (1995) Cancer Lett. 98, 9–17

8.   Edwards, P.A.W. (1996) Mammary Tumour Cell Cycle, Differentiation and Metastasis: Advances in Cellular and Molecular Biology of Breast Cancer (Dickson, R.B. and Lippman, M.E., eds.), pp. 23–36, Kluwer Academic, Boston

9.   DeOme, K.B., Faulkin, L.J.J., Bern, H.A. and Blair, P.B. (1959) Cancer Res. 19, 515–520

10.   Sekhri, K.K., Pitelka, D.R. and DeOme, K.B. (1967) J. Natl. Cancer Inst. 39, 491–527

11.   Thompson, T.C., Kadmon, D., Timme, T.L., et al. (1991) Cancer Surv. 11, 55–71

12.   Stocklin, E., Botteri, F. and Groner, B. (1993) J. Cell Biol. 122, 199–208

13.   Watson, C.J., Gordon, K.E., Robertson, M. and Clark, A.J. (1991) Nucleic Acids Res. 19, 6603–6610

14.   Andres, A.C., van der Walk, M.A., Schonenberger, C.A., Fluckiger, F., LeMeur, M., Gerlinger, P. and Groner, B. (1988) Genes Dev. 2, 1486–1495

15.   Edwards, P.A.W., Hiby, S.E., Papkoff, J. and Bradbury, J.M. (1992) Oncogene 7, 2041–2051

16.   Daniel, C.W. and Silberstein, G.B. (1987) in Mammary Gland: Development, Regulation and Function (Neville, M.C. and Daniel, C.W., eds.), pp. 3–36, Plenum Press, New York

17.   Smith, G.H. and Medina, D. (1988) J. Cell Sci. 89, 173–183

18.   Gu, H., Marth, J.D., Orban, P.C., Mossmann, H. and Rajewsky, K. (1994) Science 265, 103–106

19.   Nusse, R. and Varmus, H.E. (1992) Cell 69, 1073–1087

20.   McMahon, A.P. (1992) Trends Genet. 8, 236–242

21.   Gavin, B.J. and McMahon, A.P. (1992) Mol. Cell. Biol. 12, 2418–2423

22.   Weber-Hall, S.J., Phippard, D.J., Niemeyer, C.C. and Dale, T.C. (1994) Differentiation 57, 205–214

23.   Bradbury, J.M., Edwards, P.A.W., Niemeyer, C.C. and Dale, T.C. (1995) Dev. Biol. 170, 553–563

24.   Bradbury, J.M., Niemeyer, C.C., Dale, T.C. and Edwards, P.A.W. (1994) Oncogene 9, 2597–2603

25.   Tsukamoto, A.S., Grosschedl, R., Guzman, R.C., Parslow, T. and Varmus, H.E. (1988) Cell 55, 619–625

26.   Lin, T.-P., Guzman, R.C., Osborn, R.C., Thordarson, G. and Nandi, S. (1992) Cancer Res. 52, 4413–4419

27.   Daniel, C.W., Silberstein, G.B., Van Horn, K., Strickland, P. and Robinson, S. (1989) Dev. Biol. 135, 20–30

28.   Abram, C.L., Bradbury, J.M., Page, M.J. and Edwards, P.A.W. (1995) in Intercellular Signalling in the Mammary Gland (Wilde, C.J., Peaker, M. and Knight, C.H., eds.), pp. 67–68, Plenum Press, New York

29.   Bradbury, J.M., Sykes, H. and Edwards, P.A.W. (1991) Int. J. Cancer 48, 908–915

30.   Bradbury, J.M., Arno, J. and Edwards, P.A.W. (1993) Oncogene 8, 1551–1558

31.   Edwards, P.A.W., Abram, C.L., Hiby, S.E., Niemeyer, C.C., Dale, T.C. and Bradbury, J.M. (1995) in Intercellular Signalling in the Mammary Gland (Wilde, C.J., Peaker, M. and Knight, C.H., eds.), pp. 57–66, Plenum Press, New York

32.   Aguilar-Cordova, E., Strange, R., Young, L.J.T., Billy, H.T., Gumerlock, P.H. and Cardiff, R.D. (1991) Oncogene 6, 1601–1607

33.   Miyamoto, S., Guzman, R.C., Shiurba, R.A., Firestone, G.L. and Nandi, S. (1990) Cancer Res. 50, 6010–6014

34.   Smith, G.H., Gallaghan, D., Zweibel, J.A., Freeman, S.M., Bassin, R.H. and Callaghan, R.
       (1991) J. Virol. **65**, 6365–6370
35.   Strange, R., Aguilar-Cordova, E., Young, L.J.T., Billy, H.T., Dandekar, S. and Cardiff, R.D.
       (1989) Oncogene **4**, 309–315
36.   Varley, J.M. and Walker, R.A. (1993) Cancer Surv. **16**, 31–57
37.   Siegel, P.M., Dankort, D.L., Hardy, W.R. and Muller, W.J. (1994) Mol. Cell. Biol. **14**,
       7068–7077
38.   Yang, Y., Spitzer, E., Meyer, D., et al. (1995) J. Cell Biol. **131**, 215–226
39.   Stamp, G., Fantl, V., Poulsom, R., Jamieson, S., Smith, R., Peters, G. and Dickson, C. (1992)
       Cell Growth Differ. **3**, 929–938

Biochem. Soc. Symp. **63**, 35–44
Printed in Great Britain

3

Interactions between the oestrogen and insulin-like growth factor signalling pathways in the control of breast epithelial cell proliferation

B. R. Westley*, S. J. Clayton, M. R. Daws, C. A. Molloy and F. E. B. May

Department of Pathology, Royal Victoria Infirmary,
Newcastle upon Tyne NE1 4LP, U.K.

Abstract

There is increasing evidence for interactions between steroid and growth factor signalling pathways. Oestrogens modulate the responsiveness of breast epithelial cells to insulin-like growth factors (IGFs), and this may be the mechanism by which oestrogens modulate cell proliferation. Oestrogens appear to act at several points in the IGF signal transduction pathway. Despite earlier studies suggesting that breast epithelial cells do not synthesize IGF-I, we have shown by PCR that IGF-I is expressed and that its expression is regulated by oestrogen. IGF-II is expressed at markedly higher levels than IGF-I and is also regulated by oestrogen, consistent with it being an oestrogen-regulated autocrine growth factor. Oestrogens regulate the expression of IGF binding proteins and the type I IGF receptor. The biological significance of oestrogen regulation of IGF binding protein expression is not clear. Experiments in which the type I IGF receptor has been constitutively overexpressed have suggested that oestrogen regulation of the receptor is not involved in mediating the effects of oestrogen on cell proliferation. Recent studies have started to assess the effects of oestrogen on the expression of components of the IGF signal transduction pathway, and have shown that the expression of insulin receptor substrate-1, the principal substrate for the tyrosine kinase of the type I IGF receptor, is regulated by oestradiol.

* To whom correspondence should be addressed.

Introduction

Clinical studies on oestrogen deficiency syndromes in humans [1] and experiments in animals [2] have implicated oestrogens as important hormones in the normal development of the mammary gland. A large amount of clinical data has also shown that oestrogens are important hormones in the control of the growth of breast cancer cells, and therapeutic agents that inhibit the effects of anti-oestrogens and inhibit the synthesis of oestrogens are widely used in the treatment of breast cancer [3]. The mechanism by which oestrogens act on breast epithelial cells is not known, although they are thought to act in combination with other hormones and growth factors. The clearest example of this is in the development and differentiation of the mammary gland that occurs during pregnancy in preparation for lactation. Several groups of hormones, including oestrogens, are thought to be necessary to stimulate the massive proliferation of the ductular system and to prepare for the synthesis of large amounts of milk proteins during lactation.

One important group of growth factors that have been implicated in mammary gland development and lactation are the insulin-like growth factors (IGFs) [4–7]. Recent studies on transgenic mice expressing IGF-II in the mammary gland have shown an increased incidence of mammary tumours [8], suggesting that IGFs may also play a role in mammary carcinogenesis. Experiments on breast cancer cells have demonstrated that IGFs are important mitogens for tumour cells, suggesting that IGFs may play an important role in tumour growth and progression [9,10].

Evidence for interactions between oestrogens and the IGFs are emerging. This chapter reviews the effects of oestrogen on the various components of the IGF signal transduction pathway and the evidence suggesting that the effects of oestrogen on cell proliferation are mediated by controlling the responsiveness of cells to IGFs.

The IGFs

IGF-I and IGF-II are closely related and share homology with insulin. Whereas insulin is composed of two chains (A and B) of 21 and 30 amino acids, the IGFs are single-chain molecules that retain the equivalent of the C-peptide of pro-insulin (C domain) between the A and B domains. IGF-I has a C domain of 12 amino acids and a C-terminal extension (D domain) of 8 amino acids. NMR studies have shown that the structure of the IGF core is similar to that of insulin, with residues at the N-terminus and in the C and D domains being more mobile than those in the core of the molecule [11].

IGF receptors and IGF binding proteins (IGFBPs)

The IGFs interact with an array of cellular receptors: type I IGF, type II IGF, insulin and hybrid type I IGF/insulin receptors. The type I IGF receptor has the highest affinity for IGF-I and is generally considered to mediate the majority of the effects of the IGFs and insulin on growth. The type II IGF receptor is identical to the mannose 6-phosphate receptor and has a higher affinity for IGF-II than for IGF-I. The insulin receptor has the highest affinity for insulin, and primarily mediates the metabolic effects of these ligands. The type I IGF and insulin receptors are related and consist of two extracellular α subunits disulphide-linked to each other and to two transmembrane β subunits to form an $\alpha_2\beta_2$ heterotetramer [12]. The ligand binds to the α subunits and activates tyrosine kinase in the cytoplasmic portions of the β subunit.

IGFs, but not insulin, bind with high affinity to six related IGFBPs which are synthesized by a variety of cell types [13]. These proteins show limited sequence similarity overall, but the number and positions of their cysteine residues are conserved. IGFBP-3 is the most abundant IGFBP in adults, and most IGFs circulate as a complex of 150 kDa with IGFBP-3 (39–43 kDa) and an acid-labile protein (100–110 kDa). A principal function of the IGFBPs appears to be to stabilize IGFs. Free IGF-I has a half-life of less than 10 min in blood, but one of greater than 6 h when bound to IGFBP-3 as part of the 150 kDa complex. IGFBP-1 and IGFBP-2 are transported across intact endothelium and intact capillaries, whereas the IGFBP-3 complex, because of its large size, is not [14]. IGFBP-1 and -2 may therefore act to transport IGFs out of the vasculature. In experimental systems, addition of IGFBPs generally inhibits the activities of IGFs, presumably by sequestering a high proportion of free growth factor [15].

IGF signal transduction pathway

Intracellular components that interact with the type I IGF receptor and are phosphorylated by it have been partially elucidated during the past 5 years. Signal transduction from the insulin and type I IGF receptors have many components in common, and the differences between the two signalling pathways that result in the mitogenic effects of IGF-I and the metabolic effects of insulin have not been elucidated. The type I IGF receptor phosphorylates cytosolic proteins such as the insulin receptor substrate-1 (IRS-1) [16] and Src-homology/collagen (Shc) protein [17], which allows these proteins to bind to other signal transduction intermediates, thus forming multimeric signalling complexes. These proteins have no intrinsic enzymic activity, but are thought to act as linkers between the activated receptor and the downstream components of the signalling cascade.

IRS-1, with an apparent molecular mass of 185 kDa, has an immense capacity for phosphorylation. Human IRS-1 contains 14 potential tyrosine phosphorylation sites, including six Tyr-Met-Xaa-Met and three Tyr-Xaa-Xaa-Met motifs and more than 50 possible Ser/Thr phosphorylation sites. IRS-1 binds a number of proteins, including the p85 regulatory subunit of phosphatidylinositol 3'-kinase [18], a phosphotyrosine phosphatase (Syp) [19], Nck [20], CRk and Grb2 [21].

Shc exists in 46, 52 and 66 kDa isoforms produced from a single gene. It encodes a single SH2 domain, a glycine/proline-rich region and a tyrosine phosphorylation site.

The exact details of the interactions of these proteins remain to be elucidated, but the interaction of IRS-1, Shc and Grb2 appears to result in the recruitment and activation of guanine-nucleotide exchange factors which subsequently activate Ras. At least three such factors have been identified, and these interact with the SH3 domain of Grb2. p21^{ras}-GTP then activates Raf, which phosphorylates mitogen-activated protein kinase (MAP kinase)/extra-cellular-signal-related kinase (ERK). By this means, Raf initiates a cascade of intracellular phosphorylation events involving the MAP kinases, ultimately resulting in cell proliferation.

Interactions between oestrogens and IGFs in breast epithelial cells

Oestrogens, in common with other steroid hormones, control the expression of repertoires of cellular genes. They could, therefore, interact with IGFs by controlling the expression of components of the IGF signal transduction pathway, including the synthesis of the growth factors, IGFBPs, receptors and intracellular components of the pathway.

Effects of oestrogens on the synthesis of IGFs in breast cancer cells

Several groups have examined the possibility that IGFs are synthesized by malignant breast epithelial cells and that this synthesis is regulated by oestrogen. Huff et al. [22] identified IGF-I in conditioned medium from breast cancer cell lines by radioimmunoassay, and suggested that IGF-I secretion was under hormonal control, as it was inhibited by anti-oestrogens and stimulated by oestradiol [23]. These studies suggested a simple model of oestrogen-regulated proliferation in which IGF-I acts as an oestrogen-regulated autocrine growth factor; however, subsequent studies did not reinforce this view. van der Burg et al. [24] failed to detect IGF-I secretion using a bioassay, and Yee et al. [25] did not detect IGF-I mRNA using RNase protection. In contrast with the findings with cell lines, IGF-I expression was detected in most breast tumours, fibroadenoma and normal breast, and *in situ* hybridization demonstrated the presence of IGF-I RNA in stromal but not normal or malignant breast epithelial cells [25].

IGF-II, like IGF-I, is mitogenic for breast cancer cells. It is thought to act via the type I IGF receptor and it is somewhat less potent, reflecting its lower affinity [26]. In contrast to IGF-I, there is convincing evidence that IGF-II is expressed in a limited number of cell lines. Yee et al. [27] detected IGF-II mRNA in T47D and late-passage MCF-7 cells, whereas Osborne et al. [28] detected IGF-II secretion from all cell lines examined, but detected IGF-II mRNA in MCF-7 cells only. Both studies suggested that IGF-II expression is highest in the T47D cell line and that expression is increased by oestradiol.

We have now re-examined the expression of IGF-I and IGF-II in breast cancer cells using a quantitative competitive PCR assay based on the method of Becker-André and Hahlbrock [29]. The assay involves the reverse transcription of a series of aliquots of extracted cellular RNA to which known amounts of synthetic IGF-I and IGF-II RNAs have been added. The synthetic RNA is produced by *in vitro* transcription of plasmids containing IGF-I and IGF-II cDNAs which have been mutated at a single base to create a unique restriction site in the centre of the target PCR sequence. Following the PCR reaction, the products are digested at the unique restriction enzyme site in the centre of the target PCR sequence, separated by gel electrophoresis and then stained with ethidium bromide. The restriction enzyme digestion cuts the PCR product derived from the synthetic RNA so that it migrates as a single band that is half the size of the product derived from the cellular RNA. The amounts of product derived from the competitor and cellular RNAs are then determined by image analysis of the stained gel, and the amount of cellular mRNA in the original sample can be calculated after taking into account the formation of heteroduplex molecules between PCR products derived from the mutant competitor RNA and the cellular RNA, which are not digested by the restriction enzyme. The PCR assays detect less than 0.01 fg of IGF-I or IGF-II mRNA, and easily detect 2-fold differences in mRNA abundance [30].

IGF-I and IGF-II mRNAs were detected in all four of the oestrogen-responsive breast cancer cell lines tested (MCF-7, ZR-75, T47D and EFM-19). Quantification of the effects of oestradiol showed that oestrogen increased IGF-I mRNA levels 5-fold in T47D cells, but had no effect in MCF-7 cells. IGF-II was increased 2.5-fold in T47D cells, whereas it was increased 4.5-fold in MCF-7 cells. When the absolute amounts of IGF-I and IGF-II mRNAs were quantified, IGF-I mRNA levels were approx. 100-fold lower than those of IGF-II mRNA; if this difference in expression was reflected at the protein level, IGF-II expression would be of greater biological significance than IGF-I expression. Oestrogen-stimulated T47D cells express only 2-fold less IGF-II mRNA than liver, emphasizing the relatively high levels of expression in this cell line. The observation that IGF-II mRNA levels are increased by oestradiol suggests that IGF-II could act as an oestrogen-regulated autocrine growth factor.

Effects of oestrogens on IGFBPs

The possibility that the synthesis of one or more of the IGFBPs may be under the control of steroid hormones and therefore modulate the responsiveness of breast cancer cells to oestradiol has been examined. Clemmons et al. [31] concluded that oestrogen-receptor-negative cell lines secrete IGFBP-1, -3 and -4, whereas oestrogen-receptor-positive cell lines secrete IGFBP-2 and -4 but not -3 or -1. Shao et al. [32] and Pekonen et al. [33] have measured IGFBP expression in breast tumours. IGFBP-2 is expressed at higher levels in oestrogen-receptor-negative tumours. Oestrogen decreases IGFBP-3 but increases IGFBP-2 and -4, and has no effect on IGFBP-5. It would be expected that the oestrogen regulation of IGFBPs would influence the responsiveness of cells to IGFs, but direct evidence for this is still lacking.

Effects of oestrogens on the type I IGF receptor and components of the IGF signal transduction pathway

In oestrogen-free culture medium, insulin or IGFs have very little effect on cell proliferation and cannot replace oestradiol, implying that oestrogen regulation of IGF-I or IGF-II expression is not completely responsible for the increased proliferation of oestrogen-responsive breast cancer cells by oestradiol. The proliferative effects of both IGF-I and IGF-II are mediated by the type I IGF receptor. Blockade of this receptor by anti-receptor antibodies (α-IR3) inhibits the proliferation of breast cancer cells and inhibits IGF-I- and IGF-II-stimulated proliferation [34–37]. Several lines of evidence have suggested that oestrogen-stimulated proliferation of breast cancer cells might result from regulation of the responsiveness of breast cancer cells to IGFs. Four groups independently, although under rather different experimental conditions, have observed a synergistic effect between oestrogens and IGFs on cell proliferation, which suggests that oestrogen increases the responsiveness of cells to IGFs [26,38–40]. Dose–response experiments with insulin, IGF-I and IGF-II suggested that this effect was mediated through the type I IGF receptor [26].

Measurement of receptor expression by ligand binding, receptor cross-linking and mRNA hybridization suggested that the expression of the type I IGF receptor is increased by oestrogen [26]. This has also recently been observed for endometrial carcinoma cells [41].

To investigate the possibility that regulation of the type I IGF receptor could mediate the increased response of breast cancer cells to IGFs, a retroviral expression vector was used to constitutively overexpress the type I IGF receptor in oestrogen-responsive breast cancer cells [42]. Clones of infected cells were isolated that expressed up to 4.5-fold more receptors than the oestradiol-induced level in untransfected cells. These cells contained oestrogen receptors, and overexpression of the receptor had little effect on the induction of an oestrogen-regulated gene (pS2) by oestradiol. The three clones analysed did, however, show altered proliferative responses to IGFs in the presence of oestradiol (see Figs. 1 and 2).

Fig. 1(a) shows that IGF-I alone increased proliferation slightly, but the increase was no greater in cells overexpressing the type I IGF receptor than in control cells. This demonstrated that increased expression of the type I IGF receptor did not increase the magnitude of the proliferative response to IGF-I alone. Fig. 1(b) shows that oestradiol alone increased proliferation approx. 5-fold in the control cells and in the three clones overexpressing the type I IGF receptor. If oestrogen increases the response of breast cancer cells to the low concentrations of IGF-I in the culture medium, then increasing the constitutive expression of the type I IGF receptor would be expected to increase the proliferation of cells to the oestrogen-induced level in the absence of oestrogen. The results shown in Fig. 1(b) are not consistent with this model, and suggest that the stimulation of proliferation by oestradiol alone requires more than the induction of the type I IGF receptor. Fig. 1(c) shows that overexpression of the type I IGF receptor resulted in a marked attenuation of the synergistic effect between IGFs and oestradiol. In clone G10, the mitogenic effects of IGF-I and oestradiol were additive, whereas in the other two clones the effect was more dramatic, and proliferation in the presence of IGF-I and oestradiol was slower than in the presence of oestradiol alone.

As the oestrogen-responsiveness of the cloned cells was not adversely affected by overexpression of the type I IGF receptor, we also investigated whether these cells had an altered sensitivity to IGF-I. Cells infected with control retrovirus responded as previously reported for uninfected MCF-7 cells

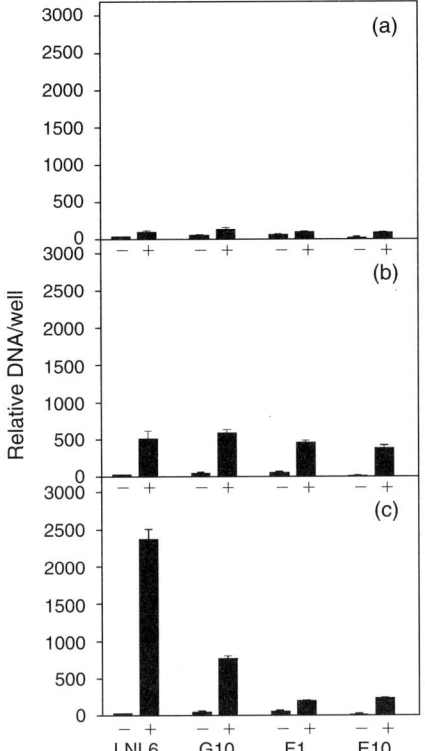

Fig. 1. Effects of IGF-I and oestradiol on the growth of MCF-7 cells and of three clones in which the type I IGF receptor is constitutively overexpressed. MCF-7 cells infected with control retrovirus (LNL6) and three clones infected with the LISN retrovirus (G10, F1 and E10) which over-express the type I IGF receptor were withdrawn from the effects of oestrogens in the culture medium and then treated with IGF-I (50 ng/ml) alone (a), oestra-diol (10 nM) alone (b) or oestradiol and IGF-I together (c). The bars show the relative amounts of DNA/well; — indicates the number of cells in wells receiv-ing control medium; + represents the number of cells in treated wells. Reproduced with permission from [42], ©1996, The Endocrine Society.

and showed a marked concentration-dependent increase in proliferation in response to IGF-I in the presence of oestradiol. The clones overexpressing the type I IGF receptor showed increased cell proliferation at low IGF-I concen-trations, but at high IGF-I concentrations the effect was reversed (Fig. 2). These results show that there are two effects of overexpression of the type I IGF receptor: a decrease in the concentration of IGF-I required to stimulate cell proliferation in the presence of oestradiol, and an unexpected paradoxical attenuation of the combined effect of oestradiol and IGF-I at concentrations above 10 ng/ml IGF-I.

Collectively, these experiments show that the level of expression of the type I IGF receptor is an important determinant in the responsiveness of breast

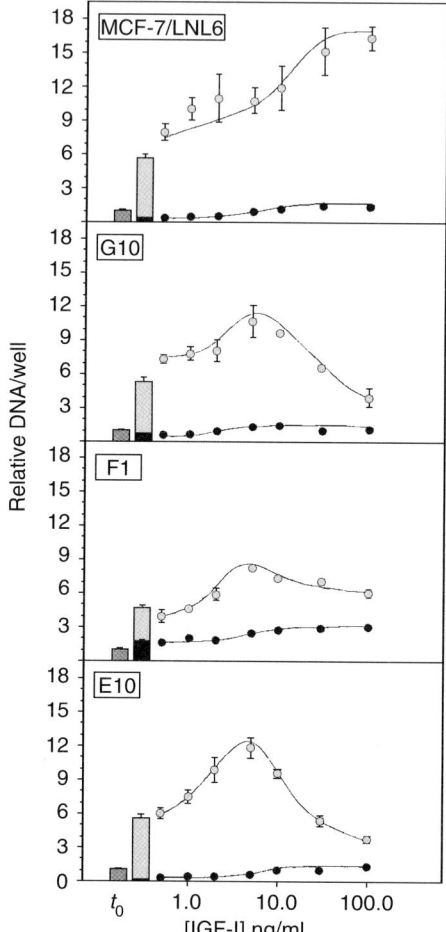

Fig. 2. Dose–response curves for MCF-7 cells and three clones in which the type I IGF receptor is constitutively overexpressed. MCF-7 cells infected with control retrovirus (MCF-7/LNL6) and three clones infected with the LISN retrovirus (G10, F1 and E10) which overexpress the type I IGF receptor were withdrawn from the effects of oestrogens in the culture medium and then treated with various concentrations of IGF-I alone (●) or in the presence of 10 nM oestradiol (○). The bars indicate the standard errors. Reproduced from [42], ©1996, The Endocrine Society.

cancer cells to oestrogen. However, the observation that the response of cells to oestradiol alone is not affected by constitutive overexpression of the type I IGF receptor suggests that oestrogens stimulate the proliferation of breast cancer cells by regulating the expression of genes in addition to that encoding the type I IGF receptor.

A small number of studies have examined the effects of oestrogens and IGF-1 on components of signal transduction pathways leading to cell proliferation. Two studies have examined the regulation of Fos and Jun, which are components of the AP-1 activity. van der Burg et al. [43] have argued that oestrogen and IGF-I induce the expression of Fos and Jun respectively and that together these increase AP-1 activity. Philips et al. [44] have shown that oestrogens and anti-oestrogens regulate AP-1 activity in breast cancer cells.

We have investigated the possibility that components downstream of the type I IGF receptor could mediate the effects of oestradiol on the responsiveness of breast cancer cells to oestradiol. cDNA probes for a number of components of the IGF signal transduction pathway were hybridized to RNA extracted from control and oestrogen-treated oestrogen-responsive breast cancer cells. Of the mRNAs examined, only IRS-1 expression was affected by oestradiol. IRS-1 mRNA was not detected in cells that had been cultured in oestrogen-free medium, but was detected in cells that had been treated with oestradiol. The concentration of oestradiol required to induce IRS-1 mRNA was consistent with the effect being mediated by the oestrogen receptor, and the induction by oestradiol was inhibited by anti-oestrogens. These experiments suggest that oestrogens may regulate the responsiveness of breast cancer cells to IGFs by regulating the expression of IRS-1, a key molecule in the signal transduction pathway of IGFs. The extent to which IRS-1 is regulated by oestrogens in normal breast epithelial cells and other oestrogen-responsive cells and controls their responsiveness to IGFs should now be examined.

References

1. Laron, Z., Kauli, R. and Pertzelan, A. (1989) in Oestrogen and the Human Breast (Beck, J.S., ed.), pp. 13–22, The Royal Society of Edinburgh, Edinburgh

2. Silberstein, G.B., Van Horn, K., Shyamala, G. and Daniel, C.W. (1994) Endocrinology **134**, 84–90

3. Early Breast Cancer Trialists' Collaborative Group (1992) Lancet **339**, 71–85

4. Ruan, W., Newman, C.B. and Kleinberg, D.L. (1992) Proc. Natl. Acad. Sci. U.S.A. **89**, 10872–10876

5. Prosser, C.G., Fleet, I.R., Corps, A.N., Froesch, E.R. and Heap, R.B. (1990) J. Endocrinol. **126**, 437–443

6. Kleinberg, D.L. (1996) Endocrinology **137**, 1–2

7. Hadsell, D.L., Greenberg, N.M., Fligger, J.M., Baumrucker, C.R. and Rosen, J.M. (1996) Endocrinology **137**, 321–330

8. Bates, P., Fisher, R., Ward, A., Richardson, L., Hill, D.J. and Graham, C.F. (1995) Br. J. Cancer **72**, 1189–1193

9. Westley, B.R. and May, F.E.B. (1994) J. Steroid Biochem. Mol. Biol. **51**, 1–9

10. Rosen, N., Tee, D., Lippman, M.E., Paik, S. and Cullen, K.J. (1991) Breast Cancer Res. Treat. **1**, 55–62

11. Cooke, R.M., Harvey, T.S. and Campbell, I.D. (1991) Biochemistry **30**, 5484–5491

12. Ullrich, A., Gray, A., Tam, A.W., et al. (1986) EMBO J. **5**, 2503–2512

13. Cohick, W.S. and Clemmons, D.R. (1993) Annu. Rev. Physiol. **55**, 131–153

14. Bar, R.S., Clemmons, D.R., Boes, M., Busby, W.H., Booth, B.A., Dake, B.L. and Sandra, A. (1990) Endocrinology **127**, 1078–1086

15. McCusker, R.H. and Clemmons, D.R. (1992) in The Insulin-Like Growth Factors (Schofield, P., ed.), pp. 110–150, Oxford University Press, Oxford

16. White, M.F., Maron, R. and Kahn, C.R. (1985) Nature (London) **318**, 183–186

17. Pelicci, G., Lanfrancone, L., Grignani, F., et al. (1992) Cell **70**, 93–104

18. Myers, M., Wang, L.M., Xiao, J.S., Zhang, Y., Yenush, L., Schlessinger, J., Pierce, J.H. and White, M.F. (1994) Mol. Cell. Biol. **14**, 3577–3587

19. Kuhne, M.R., Pawson, T., Lienhard, G.E. and Feng, G.S. (1993) J. Biol. Chem. **268**, 11479–11481
20. Lee, C.H., Li, W., Nishimura, R., et al. (1993) Proc. Natl. Acad. Sci. U.S.A. **90**, 11713–11717
21. Skolnik, E.Y., Lee, C.H., Batzer, A., et al. (1993) EMBO J. **12**, 1929–1936
22. Huff, K.K., Kaufman, D., Gabbay, K.H., Spencer, E.M., Lippman, M.E. and Dickson, R.B. (1986) Cancer Res. **46**, 4613–4619
23. Huff, K.K., Knabbe, C., Lindsey, R., Kaufman, D., Bronzert, D., Lippman, M.E. and Dickson, R.B. (1988) Mol. Endocrinol. **2**, 200–208
24. van der Burg, B., Isbrucker, L., van Selm-Miltenburg, A.J.P., de Laat, S.W. and van Zoelen, E.J.J. (1990) Cancer Res. **50**, 7770–7774
25. Yee, D., Paik, S., Lebovic, G.S., et al. (1989) Mol. Endocrinol. **3**, 509–517
26. Stewart, A.J., Johnson, M.D., May, F.E.B. and Westley, B.R. (1990) J. Biol. Chem. **265**, 21172–21178
27. Yee, D., Cullen, K.J., Paik, S., Perdue, J.F., Hampton, B., Schartz, A. and Lippman, M.E. (1988) Cancer Res. **48**, 6691–6696
28. Osborne, C.K., Coronado, E.B., Kitten, L.J., Arteaga, C.I., Fuqua, S.A.W., Ramasharma, M.M. and Li, C.H. (1989) Mol. Endocrinol. **3**, 1701–1709
29. Becker-André, M. and Hahlbrock, K. (1989) Nucleic Acids Res. **17**, 9437–9446
30. Carr, M., May, F.E.B., Lennard, T.W.J. and Westley, B.R. (1995) Br. J. Cancer **72**, 1427–1434
31. Clemmons, D.R., Camacho-Hubner, C., Coronado, E. and Osborne, C.K. (1990) Endocrinology **127**, 2679–2686
32. Shao, Z.-M., Sheikh, M.S., Ordonez, J.V., et al. (1992) Cancer Res. **52**, 5100–5103
33. Pekonen, F., Nyman, T., Ilvesmaki, V. and Partanen, S. (1992) Cancer Res. **52**, 5204–5207
34. Rohlik, Q.T., Adams, D., Kull, F.C. and Jacobs, S. (1987) Biochem. Biophys. Res. Commun. **149**, 276–281
35. Arteaga, C.L. and Osborne, C.K. (1989) Cancer Res. **49**, 6237–6241
36. Cullen, K.J., Yee, D., Sly, W.S., Perdue, J., Hampton, B., Lippman, M.E. and Rosen, N. (1990) Cancer Res. **50**, 48–53
37. Arteaga, C.L., Kitten, L.J., Coronado, E.B., Jacobs, S., Kull, F.C., Allred, D.C. and Osborne, C.K. (1989) J. Clin. Invest. **84**, 1418–1423
38. Thorsen, T., Lahooti, H., Rasmussen, M. and Arkvaag, A. (1992) J. Steroid Biochem. Mol. Biol. **41**, 537–540
39. van der Burg, B., Rutteman, G.R., Blakenstein, M.A., de Laat, S.W. and van Zoelen, E.J.J. (1988) J. Cell. Physiol. **134**, 101–108
40. Surmacz, E. and Burgaud, J.-L. (1995) Clin. Cancer Res. **1**, 1429–1436
41. Kleinman, D., Karas, M., Roberts, C.T., LeRoith, D., Phillip, M., Segev, Y., Levy, J. and Sharoni, Y. (1995) Endocrinology **136**, 2531–2537
42. Daws, M.R., Westley, B.R. and May, F.E.B. (1996) Endocrinology **137**, 1177–1186
43. van der Burg, B., de Groot, R.P., Isbrucker, L., Kruijer, J. and De Laat, S.W. (1991) J. Steroid Biochem. Mol. Biol. **40**, 215–221
44. Philips, A., Chalbos, D. and Rochefort, H. (1993) J. Biol. Chem. **268**, 14103–14108

Biochem. Soc. Symp. **63**, 45–50
Printed in Great Britain

4

Transcriptional activation by oestrogen receptors

M.G. Parker

Molecular Endocrinology Laboratory, Imperial Cancer Research Fund,
London WC2A 3PX, U.K.

Abstract

The oestrogen receptor belongs to a superfamily of nuclear receptors that function as hormone-dependent transcription factors. Transcriptional activation is mediated by two activation regions: AF-1 in the N-terminal domain and AF-2 in the ligand binding domain. AF-1, whose activity is also regulated by epidermal growth factor and insulin-like growth factor-I, varies considerably between receptors, whereas AF-2 seems to be conserved in nuclear receptors. From recent structural analysis of the ligand binding domains of two retinoid receptors and the thyroid hormone receptor, it appears that this domain contains a common fold that generates a conserved ligand binding pocket. As a consequence of ligand binding, a C-terminal helix is realigned over the ligand binding pocket to form a novel interacting surface to which co-activators are likely to bind. Several candidate proteins have been identified, including receptor-interacting protein (RIP)-140, RIP-160, transcription intermediary factor (TIF)-1, suppressor of gal4D lesions (SUG)-1 and steroid receptor co-activator (SRC)-1. These proteins interact with receptors only in the presence of their respective hormonal ligands; moreover, their interaction with a series of mutant receptors correlates with their transcriptional activity, suggesting that they may play a role in transcriptional activation. However, only SRC-1 stimulates the transcriptional activity of receptors in transfected mammalian cells, implying that the proteins have different functions. The properties of RIP-140 and SRC-1 will be described and their potential role and mechanism of action discussed.

Introduction

Many, if not all, of the actions of oestrogens in the mammary gland are mediated by oestrogen receptors acting as ligand-dependent transcription factors to regulate specific gene expression. Until recently it was assumed that there was only one form of the oestrogen receptor, but it is now realized that there is a second receptor, referred to as the β form [1], encoded by a distinct gene from that of the original, now called the α form. The ligand binding and target gene specificity of the two receptors are similar, but their relative cellular distribution differs. This chapter outlines the molecular mechanism of transcriptional activation by oestrogen receptors, based entirely on work carried out on the α form; in view of the sequence similarities, the molecular mechanisms of action are likely to be conserved between the two forms.

Alternative mechanisms of receptor activation

Oestrogen receptors are classically activated by the binding of their normal hormonal ligand, 17β-oestradiol, but a number of alternative signalling pathways have also been implicated. Additional stimuli include the neurotransmitter dopamine [2] and epidermal growth factor (EGF) [3,4], but with the possible exception of EGF it is not clear whether their effects are direct or whether they modulate the activity of other proteins involved in receptor activity. Clearly, the ability of growth factors to activate the oestrogen receptor in target tissues has far-reaching implications and may well play a role in the aetiology of breast and endometrial cancer.

The process of receptor activation upon ligand binding is relatively well understood and, since dopamine and EGF appear to activate the receptor in the absence of hormone, they may be able to mimic certain aspects of oestrogen-dependent activation. Initially, the receptor was found to exist as an oligomeric complex that contains the heat-shock protein hsp90 [5–7], one of whose roles seems to be the maintenance of the receptor in an inactive state. Upon oestrogen binding, the complex dissociates and allows the formation of receptor homodimers which are capable of binding to DNA with high affinity. During this process a conformational change in the receptor is likely to take place which allows it to trigger, by an extremely ill-defined process, an alteration in the transcriptional initiation of specific genes.

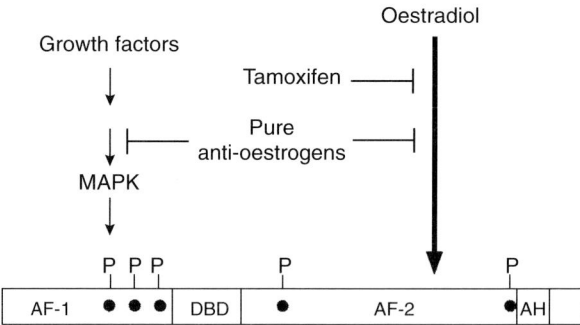

Fig. 1. Scheme to show that the oestrogen receptor is a target for growth factors as well as for its normal cognate ligand, 17β-oestradiol. The receptor contains two activation functions, AF-1 and AF-2. AF-1 is a target for phosphorylation and is activated via the MAP kinase (MAPK) pathway by growth factors, while the activity of AF2, upon hormone binding, is dependent on the integrity of an amphipathic α-helix (AH). DBD, DNA binding domain.

Two transcriptional activation functions (AFs) have been defined in the oestrogen receptor (Fig. 1): AF-1 in the N-terminal domain and AF-2 in the hormone binding domain [8–11]. AF-1 is the target for EGF [12,13], which, by means of the mitogen-activated protein kinase (MAP kinase) pathway, stimulates the phosphorylation of serine-118 [14,15] in the human receptor and thereby increases its activity. AF-2 is dependent on the binding of oestrogen for full activity and can be blocked by oestrogen antagonists such as tamoxifen and the so-called pure anti-oestrogens (Fig. 1). In contrast, AF-1 is unaffected by tamoxifen and seems to be responsible for the agonist activity of this drug. The activities of AF-1 and AF-2 vary depending upon the responsive promoter and cell type and, in some cases, both are required for full transcriptional stimulation [11].

The activity of AF-2 depends on a number of dispersed elements throughout the hormone binding domain that are brought together upon oestrogen binding [16]. The best defined element is an amphipathic α-helix near the C-terminus of nuclear receptors [17], which is essential for ligand-dependent transcriptional activity. This region is absolutely conserved in

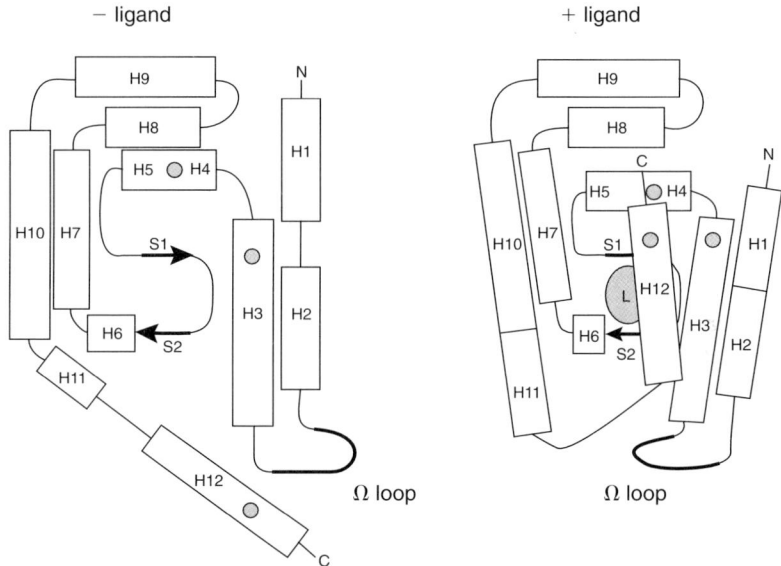

Fig. 2. Schematic representation of the ligand binding domains of the oestrogen receptor in the absence and presence of ligand. The diagram, based on crystal structure of the ligand binding domains of the retinoic X and retinoic acid receptors [21,22] and the thyroid hormone receptor [23], shows 12 α-helical regions, H1–H12 (open boxes), anti-parallel β-strands (S1 and S2; shaded arrows) and an Ω loop between helices 2 and 3. Following the binding of ligand (L), the structure compacts, and it is proposed that helices 10 and 11 become continuous, releasing helix 12 from the Ω loop and allowing its realignment with helices 3 and 4 [22,23]. The shaded circles mark helices shown by mutagenesis to contain residues required for transcriptional activity [17–20,22,39].

oestrogen receptors (both the α and β forms from all species analysed) and highly conserved in all transcriptionally active nuclear receptors [18–20]. Structural analysis of the ligand binding domains of the retinoid X and retinoic acid receptors and the thyroid hormone receptor [21–23] have led to a general model to account for ligand-dependent AF-2 activity [24]. The ligand binding domain of nuclear receptors appears to contain a common fold that generates a conserved ligand binding pocket. Their transcriptional activity seems to be induced by ligand following the rearrangement of helices 10 and 11 to form a continuous helix, which then allows the realignment of the C-terminal helix. This helix, together with helix 3 and/or helix 4, is likely to form a novel interacting surface (Fig. 2) that interacts directly either with proteins in the general transcription apparatus or with intermediary factors which act as bridging proteins between the receptor and the basic transcription machinery.

Transcriptional activation by the oestrogen receptor

The ability of the oestrogen receptor to stimulate transcription is likely to involve the recruitment of the basal transcription machinery into a preinitiation complex. Although receptors bind directly with a number of basal transcription factors *in vitro*, including the TATA box binding protein (TBP) [25], transcription factor IIB [26,27] and TBP-associated factor (hTAF$_{II}$30) [28], these interactions are unaffected by ligand binding or by mutations in the AF-2 amphipathic α-helix that abolish transcriptional activity, suggesting that receptors are likely to interact with alternative proteins. Furthermore, the observation that AF-2 activity can be inhibited by overexpressing the hormone binding domain in 'squelching' experiments [29] suggests that AF-2 is likely to interact with target proteins that are distinct from basal transcription factors.

In order to search for additional target proteins, two approaches have been used. The first was a 'far-western blotting' technique [30] in which the hormone binding domain was radiolabelled with ^{32}P and used as a probe to screen nuclear extracts and subsequently cDNA expression libraries for receptor-interacting proteins (RIPs). The second, more popular, approach has been to use two hybrid screening in yeast. The initial far-western blotting indicated the presence of two RIPs with molecular masses of 140 and 160 kDa [31], but we now know that the 160 kDa band comprised several proteins and that there are also some higher-molecular-mass proteins. cDNA clones have now been isolated for many of these proteins (Table 1), including RIP-140 [32], TIF-1 [33], a number of isoforms of SRC-1 [34,35], thyroid hormone receptor interacting protein (TRIP)-1/SUG-1 [36,37] and TIF-2 [38]. These proteins are likely to play a role in oestrogen receptor activity for two reasons. First, their interaction with the receptor is ligand-dependent and is abolished by hormone antagonists. Secondly, their interaction is also reduced when mutations are introduced into the receptor that disrupt its transcriptional activity, suggesting that they play a role in transcriptional activation. The surprising finding is that so many such interacting proteins have already been identified.

There are several possibilities to account for the number of RIPs. One group, which includes SRC-1 and TIF-2, appears to comprise *bona fide* co-

Table 1. RIPs for steroid hormone receptors. Proteins for which cDNA clones are available are listed. The receptor that was used to isolate the interacting protein is marked with an asterisk, and other receptors subsequently found to interact with the protein are also listed. OR, oestrogen receptor; RAR, retinoic acid receptor; TR, thyroid hormone receptor; RXR, retinoid X receptor; PPAR, peroxisome-proliferator-activated receptor; PR, progesterone receptor; GR, glucocorticoid receptor; VDR, vitamin D receptor.

RIP	Size (kDa)	Receptor specificity	References
RIP-140	140	OR*, RAR, TR, RXR, PPAR	[32]
SRC-1	125/159	PR*, OR, TR, RXR, GR	[34,35]
RIP-160	160	OR*, RAR, TR, RXR, PPAR	[31]
ERAP-160	160	OR*	[30]
TIF-1	112	RXR*, RAR, OR, TR, VDR	[33]
TRIP-1	46	TR*, RXR	[36]
SUG-1	45	RAR*, RXR, OR, VDR, TR	[37]
TRIP-1–14	Various	TR*, RXR	[36]
GRIP-170	170	GR*	[40]
TIF-2	160	OR*, RAR, RXR, TR, AR, PR	[38]

activators that play a role in ligand-dependent activation when the receptor binds to simple response elements. Since the conformation of the receptor can be modified by the binding site (composite versus simple response elements) and by associated transcription factors such as AP-1, it is possible that the recruitment of co-activators depends on the precise binding site. Secondly, SRC-1 and TIF-2 may be recruited to the receptor when it is activated by ligand binding and a different set of co-activators may be recruited when it is activated by alternative signalling pathways. Finally, some of the interacting proteins, such as TIF-1, might have completely different roles, for example in chromatin remodelling. Further work is clearly required to elucidate the role of these proteins in oestrogen receptor function.

References

1. Kuiper, G.G.J.M., Enmark, E., Pelto-Huikko, M., Nilsson, S. and Gustafsson, J.-A. (1996) Proc. Natl. Acad. Sci. U.S.A. **93**, 5925–5930
2. Power, R.F., Mani, S.K., Codina, J., Conneely, O.M. and O'Malley, B.W. (1991) Science **254**, 1636–1639
3. Ignar-Trowbridge, D.M., Nelson, K.G., Bidwell, M.C., Curtis, S.W., Washburn, T.F., McLachlan, J.A. and Korach, K.S. (1992) Proc. Natl. Acad. Sci. U.S.A. **89**, 4658–4662
4. Ignar-Trowbridge, D.M., Teng, C.T., Ross, K.A., Parker, M.G., Korach, K.S. and McLachlan, J.A. (1993) Mol. Endocrinol. **7**, 992–998
5. Catelli, M.G., Binart, N., Jung, T.I., Renoir, J.M., Baulieu, E.E., Feramisco, J.R. and Welch, W.J. (1985) EMBO J. **4**, 3131–3135
6. Sanchez, E.R., Toft, D.O., Schlessinger, M.J. and Pratt, W.B. (1985) J. Biol. Chem. **260**, 12398–12401
7. Redeuilh, G., Moncharmont, B., Secco, S. and Baulieu, E.E. (1987) J. Biol. Chem. **262**, 6969–6975

8. Kumar, V., Green, S., Stack, G., Berry, M., Jin, J.R. and Chambon, P. (1987) Cell **51**, 941–951
9. Webster, N.J.G., Green, S., Jin, J.R. and Chambon, P. (1988) Cell **54**, 199–207
10. Lees, J.A., Fawell, S.E. and Parker, M.G. (1989) J. Steroid Biochem. **34**, 33–39
11. Tora, L., White, J., Brou, C., Tasset, D., Webster, N., Scheer, E. and Chambon, P. (1989) Cell **59**, 477–487
12. Kato, S., Endoh, H., Masuhiro, Y., et al. (1995) Science **270**, 1491–1494
13. Bunone, G., Briand, P.-A., Miksicek, R.J. and Picard, D. (1996) EMBO J. **15**, 2174–2183
14. Ali, S., Metzger, D., Bornert, J.-M. and Chambon, P. (1993) EMBO J. **12**, 1153–1160
15. Aronica, S.M. and Katzenellenbogen, B. (1993) Mol. Endocrinol. **7**, 743–752
16. Webster, N.J., Green, S., Tasset, D., Ponglikitmongkol, M. and Chambon, P. (1989) EMBO J. **8**, 1441–1446
17. Danielian, P.S., White, R., Lees, J.A. and Parker, M.G. (1992) EMBO J. **11**, 1025–1033
18. Saatcioglu, F., Bartunek, P., Deng, T., Zenke, M. and Karin, M. (1993) Mol. Cell. Biol. **13**, 3675–3685
19. Barettino, D., Ruiz, M.D.M.V. and Stunnenberg, H.G. (1994) EMBO J. **13**, 3039–3049
20. Durand, B., Saunder, M., Gaudon, C., Roy, B., Losson, R. and Chambon, P. (1994) EMBO J. **13**, 5370–5382
21. Bourguet, W., Ruff, M., Chambon, P., Gronemeyer, H. and Moras, D. (1995) Nature (London) **375**, 377–382
22. Renaud, J.-P., Rochel, N., Ruff, M., Vivat, V., Chambon, P., Gronemeyer, H. and Moras, D. (1995) Nature (London) **378**, 681–689
23. Wagner, R.L., Apriletti, J.W., McGrath, M.E., West, B.L., Baxter, J.D. and Fletterick, R.J. (1995) Nature (London) **378**, 690–697
24. Wurtz, J.-M., Bourguet, W., Renaud, J.-P., Vivat, V., Chambon, P., Moras, D. and Gronemeyer, H. (1996) Nature Struct. Biol. **3**, 87–94
25. Sadovsky, Y., Webb, P., Lopez, G., Baxter, J.D., Cavailles, V., Parker, M.G. and Kushner, P.J. (1995) Mol. Cell. Biol. **15**, 1554–1563
26. Ing, N.H., Beekman, J.M., Tsai, S.Y., Tsai, M.-J. and O'Malley, B.W. (1992) J. Biol. Chem. **267**, 17617–17623
27. Baniahmad, A., Ha, I., Reinberg, D., Tsai, S., Tsai, M.J. and O'Malley, B.W. (1993) Proc. Natl. Acad. Sci. U.S.A. **90**, 8832–8836
28. Jacq, X., Brou, C., Lutz, Y., Davidson, I., Chambon, P. and Tora, L. (1994) Cell **79**, 107–117
29. Tasset, D., Tora, L., Fromental, C., Scheer, E. and Chambon, P. (1990) Cell **62**, 1177–1187
30. Halachmi, S., Marden, E., Martin, G., MacKay, H., Abbondanza, C. and Brown, M. (1994) Science **264**, 1455–1458
31. Cavaillès, V., Dauvois, S., Danielian, P.S. and Parker, M.G. (1994) Proc. Natl. Acad. Sci. U.S.A. **91**, 10009–10013
32. Cavaillès, V., Dauvois, S., L'Horset, F., Lopez, G., Hoare, S., Kushner, P.J. and Parker, M.G. (1995) EMBO J. **14**, 3741–3751
33. Le Douarin, B., Zechel, C., Garnier, J.M., et al. (1995) EMBO J **14**, 2020–2033
34. Onate, S.A., Tsai, S.Y., Tsai, M.-J. and O'Malley, B.W. (1995) Science **270**, 1354–1357
35. Kamei, Y., Xu, L., Heinzel, T., et al. (1996) Cell **85**, 403–414
36. Lee, J.W., Ryan, F., Swaffield, J.C., Johnston, S.A. and Moore, D.D. (1995) Nature (London) **374**, 91–94
37. vom Baur, E., Zechel, C., Heery, D., et al. (1996) EMBO J. **15**, 110–124
38. Voegel, J.J., Heine, M.J.S., Zechel, C., Chambon, P. and Gronemeyer, H. (1996) EMBO J. **15**, 101–108
39. O'Donnell, A.L. and Koenig, R.J. (1990) Mol. Endocrinol. **4**, 715–720
40. Eggert, M., Mows, C.C., Tripier, D., Arnold, F., Michel, J., Nickel, J., Schmidt, S., Beato, M. and Renkawitz, R. (1995) J. Biol. Chem. **270**, 30755–30759

Biochem. Soc. Symp. **63**, 51–69
Printed in Great Britain

5

Local control of mammary gland differentiation: mammary-derived growth inhibitor and pleiotrophin

A. Kurtz*, E. Spitzer†, W. Zschiesche†, A. Wellstein*
and R. Grosse†

Georgetown University, Lombardi Cancer Center, The Research Building W208,
3970 Reservoir Rd. N.W., Washington, DC 20007, U.S.A., and †Institute for
Medical Molecular Diagnostics, Gotlindestrasse 2-22, 10365 Berlin, Germany

Abstract

Mammary gland development is controlled by systemic hormones and by growth factors that might complement or mediate hormonal action and provide the signalling basis for mesenchyme–epithelial cross-talk. Two locally expressed factors, pleiotrophin and mammary-derived growth inhibitor (MDGI), their hormonal regulation and proposed functions will be discussed. Pleiotrophin expression in non-tumorigenic, attachment-dependent epithelial cells leads to an attachment-independent, highly tumorigenic phenotype. The fatty acid binding protein MDGI specifically inhibits growth of normal mouse mammary epithelial cells, whereas growth of stromal cells is not suppressed. In mammary gland organ culture, inhibition of ductal growth by MDGI is associated with the appearance of bulbous alveolar end buds and formation of fully developed lobulo-alveolar structures. In parallel, MDGI stimulates its own epithelial-restricted expression and promotes milk protein synthesis. Selective inhibition of endogenous MDGI expression suppresses the appearance of alveolar end buds and lowers the β-casein level in organ cultures. MDGI activity can be antagonized by epidermal growth factor (EGF); reciprocally, MDGI can suppress the mitogenic effects of EGF. An MDGI-derived C-terminal 11-amino-acid peptide is able to mimic MDGI activity *in vitro*. In conclusion, members of the family of fatty acid binding proteins are able to regulate mammary gland differentiation locally, and fatty acid binding is not required for this activity.

* To whom correspondence should be addressed.

Introduction

The developmental balance between growth and differentiation of the mammary epithelium is locally tuned by a multitude of autocrine and paracrine acting growth factors, receptors, and extracellular matrix components and modulators. Fluctuation of this local net balance between stimulatory and inhibitory factors determines developmental decisions that ultimately lead to mammary morphogenesis, terminal differentiation or involution.

A number of growth-stimulatory factors and their receptors are expressed in the normal mammary gland [1]. Some of these growth factors have been implicated in mammary tumorigenesis, indicating the sensitivity of the system to balance changes in favour of growth stimulation, which can be due to up-regulation of only one or two stimulating principles. Examples of growth factors that induce hyperproliferation and that are overexpressed in breast cancer are members of the epidermal growth factor (EGF) family and their receptors, heparin binding growth factors such as fibroblast growth factors, or pleiotrophin and midkine [2–5]. In contrast, only a few factors have been described to show growth-inhibitory activity on mammary epithelial cells. Examples are mammastatin [6], transforming growth factor β (TGF-β) [7], neuregulin [8,9] and mammary-derived growth inhibitor (MDGI) [10]. TGF-β was shown to inhibit ductal growth in prepubertal mice, and overexpression of TGF-β in transgenic mice inhibits the formation of lobulo-alveolar structures [7].

Few data are available that describe the role of growth inhibitors during the later stages of mammary gland development. In particular, it is poorly understood which locally acting factors are involved in the developmental switch from massively proliferating mammary epithelium to terminal differentiation during pregnancy. To elucidate whether MDGI and pleiotrophin are involved in this process, we studied their hormonal regulation, their expression patterns in normal mammary gland and breast cancer and their physiological activities. Furthermore, the interactions of EGF and MDGI during pregnancy are discussed, and a model for MDGI activity in the mammary gland will be proposed.

Pleiotrophin

Pleiotrophin is a secreted, heparin binding protein of molecular mass 18 kDa that has been isolated from the conditioned medium of MDA MB 231 breast cancer cells [11]. Pleiotrophin is highly conserved between organisms from *Xenopus* to human, and shares about 50% sequence identity with the heparin binding protein midkine. All ten cysteine residues are conserved between pleiotrophin and midkine, and they are thought to form five disulphide bridges, dividing the proteins into two cysteine-rich domains. The C-terminal domain contains the heparin binding site, whereas the function of the N-terminal domain is not clear, but its presence is necessary for the neuronal survival activity of midkine. Pleiotrophin and midkine form a novel protein family of developmentally regulated proteins with high expression during embryogenesis and only rudimentary expression in adult tissues. Both proteins have been implicated in the promotion of angiogenesis and cell migration. Their expression pattern suggests a function in mesenchyme–epithelial induction (for a review, see [12]).

Pleiotrophin expression and hormonal regulation

Pleiotrophin is expressed in epithelial cells of the mammary glands of virgin mice. Expression of pleiotrophin continues at high levels during pregnancy until day 15. After day 15, pleiotrophin expression is undetectable by Northern analysis and continues to be absent during lactation. However, pleiotrophin expression reappears in the mammary gland of ex-breeder mice and the mRNA levels are comparable with those found in virgin animals (Table 1). This temporally regulated expression pattern of pleiotrophin suggests a function during ductal proliferation and tissue remodelling, and its down-regulation coincides with terminal differentiation of the mammary gland (see Fig. 2). Furthermore, pleiotrophin expression seems to be hormonally regulated.

The hormone-dependence of pleiotrophin expression was studied. Mice were treated with different lactogenic hormones and hormone combinations and the expression of pleiotrophin mRNA was determined by Northern analysis. Our preliminary data indicate rapid and reversible down-regulation of pleiotrophin transcript levels after treatment with dexamethasone. In addition, a combination of oestrogen and progesterone was able to down-regulate pleiotrophin with a half-maximal effect after 7 days of treatment. Oestrogen or progesterone alone had no effect on pleiotrophin expression (Table 1). These preliminary data indicate that pleiotrophin expression in the mammary gland is indeed regulated by hormones. The hormonal effect is specific, since pleiotrophin expression in the brain is not influenced by systemic hormone application.

Pleiotrophin, like its homologue, midkine, is overexpressed in several mammary tumour cell lines and in the majority of breast cancer samples tested (Table 1). Since one of the essential requirements for the development of breast cancer is circulating steroid hormones, the correlation between hormone receptor levels and pleiotrophin expression in breast cancer cell lines and breast cancer samples was tested.

Constitutive expression of pleiotrophin in breast cancer cell lines (Table 1) indicates that the presence of the oestrogen receptor does not correlate with expression of pleiotrophin. Furthermore, when more aggressive and drug-resistant pleiotrophin-positive clonal cell lines were derived from the wild-type oestrogen- or progesterone-responsive and pleiotrophin-negative MCF-7 and T47D human breast cancer cells, the pleiotrophin-positive clones were tumorigenic in nude mice without hormone supplementation. In contrast, the tumorigenic potential of the parental cell lines is hormone-dependent.

When breast cancer samples were studied it was found that, in pleiotrophin-positive tumours, the median oestrogen receptor level (25 fmol/mg) was higher than in pleiotrophin-negative tumours. Further *in vivo* data from rats also indicate that pleiotrophin expression may be affected by oestrogenic regulation. Pleiotrophin was expressed in all carcinogen-induced, oestrogen-

Table 1. Expression and hormonal regulation of pleiotrophin mRNA.
Expression was analysed in normal mouse mammary gland, rat and human
breast cancers and human breast cancer cell lines. Oestrogen receptor status is
indicated when determined.

Cell line/tissue	Pleiotrophin expression	Oestrogen receptor
Mouse mammary gland		
Virgin	+++	
Pregnancy day 13	+++	
Pregnancy day 16	−	
Lactation	−	
Ex-breeder	+++	
Virgin + dexamethasone	−	
Virgin + oestrogen	+++	
Virgin + progesterone	+++	
Virgin + oestrogen + progesterone	+	
Breast cancer		
Rat mammary tumour ($n = 8$)	+ ($n = 8$)	(+)
Human breast cancer ($n = 44$)	+ ($n = 25$)	(+)
Mammary tumour cell lines		
MCF-7	−	+
MCF-7/ADr	++	+
MDA MB 231	++	−
MDA MB 361	−	−
MDA MB 134	−	−
MDA MB 435	−	−
MDA MB 453	−	−
MDA MB 468	−	−
SK-BR-3	−	−
HS-578T	++	−
T47Dco	++	+
T47Dwz	−	+
ZR-75-1	−	+
BT 474	−	−
BT 549	−	−

responsive rat breast tumours studied (a total of eight). No correlation was
found between pleiotrophin expression and progesterone receptor expression.

Pleiotrophin is a tumour growth factor

Pleiotrophin expression in breast cancer samples is not correlated with
the proliferation rate of the tumours, as determined by correlation with the
number of cells in S phase. This is not surprising, given the data on pleiotrophin
expression in different breast cancer cell lines (Table 1). Pleiotrophin mRNA
was expressed in five of 15 breast cancer cell lines, and all of these lines were in

a proliferative state in culture when analysed. Obviously, pleiotrophin is a growth factor that is not expressed as a indicator gene of cell proliferation.

To elucidate the possible function of pleiotrophin for tumour growth, non-tumorigenic epithelial SW-13 cell were transfected with pleiotrophin and their tumorigenic potential was tested. The results obtained from this experiment show that pleiotrophin expression alone is able to phenotypically transform SW-13 cells to grow anchorage independent and to form highly vascularized, metastatic tumours in nude mice [13,14]. When transfected, pleiotrophin-positive SW-13 cells were mixed with pleiotrophin-negative non-tumorigenic parental SW-13 cells and then grafted onto nude mice, a ratio of less than 25% pleiotrophin positive cells in the mixture promoted tumour formation (unpublished data). Furthermore, targeting of pleiotrophin by specific ribozymes in SW-13 pleiotrophin cells or in tumorigenic, pleiotrophin-positive choriocarcinoma cell line JEG-3, completely abolished the tumorigenic potential of these cells [14a].

In conclusion, these data show that pleiotrophin can act as a tumour growth factor *in vivo* and that its expression is sufficient to induce a tumorigenic phenotype. This effect is not due to a stimulation of mitosis. Our current working model suggests that pleiotrophin might promote tumour growth by stimulation of angiogenesis. Another possible mechanism might involve pleiotrophin-stimulated cell interactions with the extracellular matrix leading to enhanced cell attachment and spreading.

MDGI

Protein structure

The 14 kDa protein MDGI was originally isolated from bovine mammary gland in an attempt to identify growth-inhibitory factors of the normal mammary gland. Subsequently, MDGI-homologous proteins were identified in all other mammals studied, and it was shown that MDGI is identical to the heart-type fatty acid binding protein (h-FABP) (for reviews, see [15,16]). FABPs form an evolutionarily highly conserved family of intracellular proteins

Heart FABP-subtype	C-terminal sequence (exon 4)
mouse heart (MDGI)	T L T H G S V V S T R T Y E K E A
mouse brain	T L T F G D I V A V R C Y E K - A
mouse adipocyte	E C V M K G V T S T R V Y E R - A
mouse MyP2	E C I M K G V V C T R I Y E K - V
mouse keratinocyte	E C V M N N A T C T R V Y E K V Q
bovine heart (MDGI)	T L T H G T A V C T R T Y E K Q A
rat heart (MDGI)	T L T H G N V V S T R T Y E K E A
human heart (MDGI)	T L T H G T A V C T R T Y E K E A
human keratinocyte	E C V M N N V T C T R I Y E K V E
rat keratinocyte	E C V M N N A I C T R V Y E K V Q
chick retina	T L T F G D V V A V R H Y E K - A

Fig. 1. Sequence comparison of h-FABP subtype C-terminal amino acid sequences. Highly conserved amino acids are in bold. FABPs of the same subtype are more conserved between species than FABPs of different subtypes within the same species, indicating highly conserved tissue-specific functions.

which are commonly characterized by their binding affinity for hydrophobic ligands such as fatty acids, eicosanoids and retinoids. Structural analysis revealed a hydrophobic pocket for ligand binding which is formed by an anti-parallel array of β-sheets (β-clam-shell-like structure) [17,18]. The FABP family can be divided into four subfamilies based on degree of identity and evolutionary relationship: the h-FABPs, the liver-type FABPs, the intestinal-type FABPs and the cellular retinoid binding proteins [17]. Within the h-FABP subfamily, the amino acid identity is highest in the N-terminal half and decreases significantly at the C-terminus (Fig. 1).

MDGI expression and hormonal regulation

For the adipocyte, brain, intestinal and liver FABPs, a relationship between their expression and the differentiated stage of the tissue has been documented [19–23]. Association with the induction of differentiation seems to be a common characteristic of members of the FABP family. Despite their high degree of identity and frequent association with differentiation, FABPs seem to be functionally distinguished. This is emphasized by their reciprocal expression patterns in different cell types or at different stages in the same tissue. For example, MDGI is expressed in the trigeminal ganglion in neurons, whereas the highly related brain FABP is expressed in the surrounding glial satellite cells (A. Kurtz, unpublished work). In the mammary gland, expression of adipocyte FABP and keratinocyte FABP was detected in the mammary fat pad and in epithelial cells respectively. MDGI is expressed in epithelial cells of the mammary gland in a temporally and spatially restricted pattern, as shown by *in situ* hybridization and immunohistochemistry [24].

In the adult, MDGI is expressed at very low levels in virgin mammary gland tissue. During pregnancy, expression increases dramatically as lobulo-alveolar structures start to emerge. At this stage, the ductal proliferation rate reaches its maximum and morphological and functional differentiation, as indicated by initial β-casein expression, is becoming obvious. Furthermore, the destruction of stromal tissue and its replacement by lobulo-alveolar structures is advanced at this stage. MDGI expression is localized to epithelial cells of emerging alveoli, which are preferentially found at the epithelial–stroma junction. These cells are the primary elements to undergo terminal differentiation, in contrast with adjacent ductal epithelial cells, which are characterized by continuing proliferation and which do not directly contact the stromal compartment [24]. Thus MDGI expression appears to be correlated with a reduced proliferative potential of epithelial cells and the initiation of differentiation (Fig. 2).

During terminal differentiation in late pregnancy, MDGI expression reaches peak levels, and levels remain high during lactation. At this stage, MDGI is found in epithelial cells of alveoli and ductules. The highest levels of expression are found in epithelial cells lining the terminal regions of ducts. During late pregnancy and lactation, MDGI transcript and protein levels are increased about 5-fold compared with mid-pregnancy and comprise about 0.5–0.8% of total mRNA. MDGI protein is found in the basal extracellular

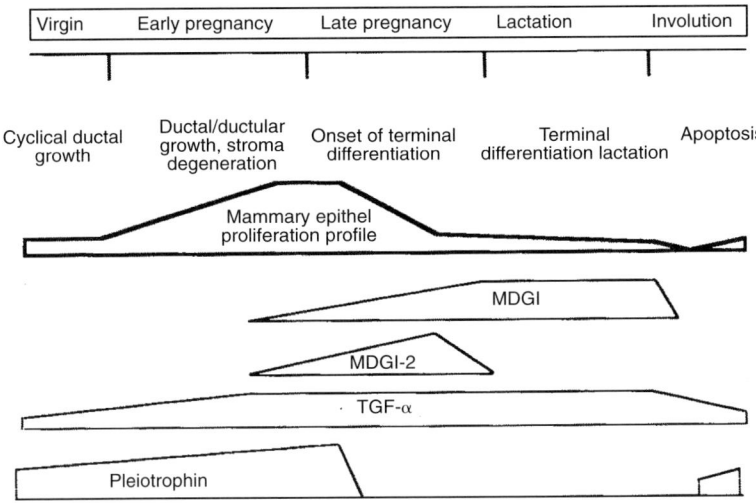

Fig. 2. Schematic diagram of the time courses of the phases of mammary gland differentiation and of the expression of MDGI, MDGI-2, pleiotrophin and TGF-α. The proliferation rate for mammary epithelial cells at different stages is indicated.

matrix and in the lumen of alveoli and ductules, where it appears associated with milk fat globule membranes [24,25].

The onset of MDGI expression around mid-pregnancy implies its regulation by mammogenic hormones. Hormonal stimulation of MDGI expression is also indicated by its embryonic expression. When we studied MDGI expression in the embryonic mammary gland at late stages of fetal development, MDGI was detected in epithelial cells of mammary gland anlagen. This expression is most probably induced by maternal hormones such as prolactin, which crosses the placental blood barrier and effects embryonic gene expression.

To address the relationship between MDGI expression and the hormonal milieu, an *in vitro* mammary organ culture system was used. Virgin-mouse-derived mammary gland organ cultures that are cultivated in a serum-free medium containing aldosterone (A), prolactin (P), insulin (I) and cortisol (hydrocortisone; H) (APIH medium) undergo morphological and functional differentiation *in vitro* and mimic the *in vivo* MDGI expression pattern. Cultivation of the explants in medium containing EGF and insulin maintained the lobulo-alveolar structure of the mammary explant, but MDGI expression was suppressed. Subsequent supplementation of the culture medium with prolactin and cortisol re-induced MDGI in the same mammary explant culture [16].

Finally, when mouse mammary gland organ cultures cultivated in APIH medium were treated with anti-progestins (i.e. ZK 114043), MDGI expression was dramatically up-regulated, and this up-regulation was accompanied by a marked inhibition of DNA synthesis (Fig. 3a). Up-regulation of MDGI by anti-progestins precedes functional differentiation, as determined by β-casein

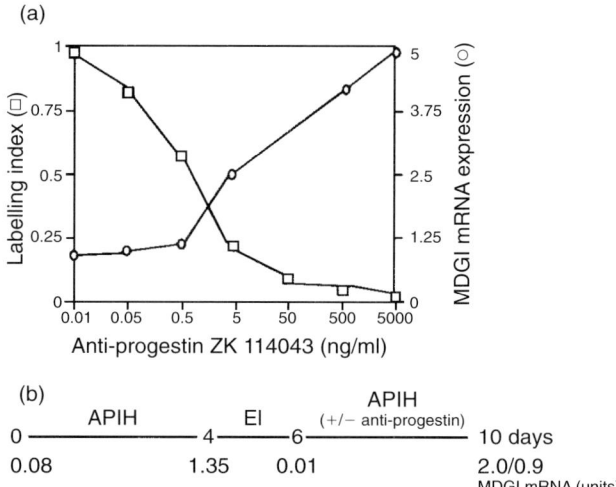

Fig. 3. Effects of anti-progestins on cell proliferation and MDGI expression in mammary gland organ culture. (a) Mammary gland organ cultures were maintained in serum-free APIH medium and treated with the anti-progestin ZK 114043 (Schering AG) for 2 days. The labelling index and mRNA expression levels were analysed. (b) Mammary gland organ cultures were maintained in serum-free APIH medium for 4 days. Under these conditions, mammary glands differentiate. At day 4, the hormones were replaced by EGF and insulin (EI), which led to marked de-differentiation and induced proliferation of epithelial cells. After 2 days in EI, the medium was replaced by APIH medium as before, either supplemented with 5 ng/ml ZK 114043 or not supplemented with ZK 114043. MDGI mRNA expression was analysed after 0, 4, 6, and 10 days.

induction. The effect of ZK 114043 on MDGI up-regulation is not due to an anti-glucocorticoid effect, since cortisol is present at 1000-fold higher concentrations than the IC_{50} of the ZK compound. Likewise, competition of anti-progestins with progesterone for the progesterone receptor could be excluded. Fig. 3(b) shows the strong hormonal dependence of the induction of MDGI expression [26].

Effects of MDGI on mammary gland proliferation

MDGI was detected by screening mammary proteins for their growth-inhibitory activities on tumour cells *in vitro* [16]. It was shown that inhibition is reversible, can be blocked by neutralizing anti-MDGI antibodies and is antagonized by insulin, EGF or platelet-derived growth factor. Furthermore, screening of different mammary cell lines and primary cell cultures indicates that non-transformed, primary mammary epithelial cells respond to a greater extent to the inhibitory effect of MDGI than do tumour cells (Table 2). The IC_{50} is approx. 1 nM in all cell lines tested.

MDGI is expressed exclusively in epithelial cells of the mammary gland, and expression is pronounced in epithelial cells that border stromal compart-

Table 2. Effects of MDGI, MDGI-derived peptides and intestinal- and liver-type FABPs on proliferation of normal mammary epithelial cells, breast cancer cell lines and normal mammary stromal cells. n.d., not determined.

Cell type	Growth inhibition (%)				
	MDGI	P108	P14	Liver FABP	Intestinal FABP
MA-Ca; mouse adenocarcinoma	5–10	n.d.	n.d.	n.d.	n.d.
MCF-7; human ductal carcinoma	0–10	0–10	n.d.	n.d.	n.d.
T47D; human ductal carcinoma	0–30	n.d.	n.d.	n.d.	n.d.
MaTu; human ductal carcinoma	0–30	10–30	0	n.d.	n.d.
Ehrlich ascites tumour cells	20–40	20–40	0	n.d.	n.d.
A184; normal human epidermoid	40–50	n.d.	n.d.	n.d.	n.d.
BME; normal pregnant bovine mammary	30–50	30–50	0	n.d.	n.d.
MAC-T; normal lactating bovine mammary	40–60	40	0	n.d.	n.d.
Mouse; normal virgin mammary epithelial cells	45–60	50	0–5	0	0
Mouse; normal virgin stromal cells	0	0	0	0	0

ments during pregnancy [24]. This pattern of expression suggests a paracrine mode of action of MDGI on stromal cells of the developing mammary gland. However, when primary mammary cultures were treated with MDGI, a strong inhibitory effect on DNA synthesis could only be observed for the epithelial cells, but not for the stromal cells, which are also present in the primary cultures used (Table 2). This strongly supports an autocrine mechanism of MDGI action in the mammary gland.

An autocrine growth-inhibitory activity could also be shown in transfection experiments. Bovine MDGI cDNA under the control of the inducible mouse mammary tumour virus promoter was transfected in the MDGI-negative mammary epithelial cell lines MaTu (human) and HC11 (mouse). Induction of MDGI expression by dexamethasone resulted in a maximal decrease of cell number of 50% compared with control-transfected dexamethasone-treated cells (Fig. 4). This experiment suggests that the mechanism of action of MDGI is conserved between mouse and human. This is also indicated by the high degree of identity of MDGI from different species (Fig. 1). In contrast, identity with other members of the FABP family is less conserved. Indeed, when the growth-modulating effects of intestinal and liver FABPs

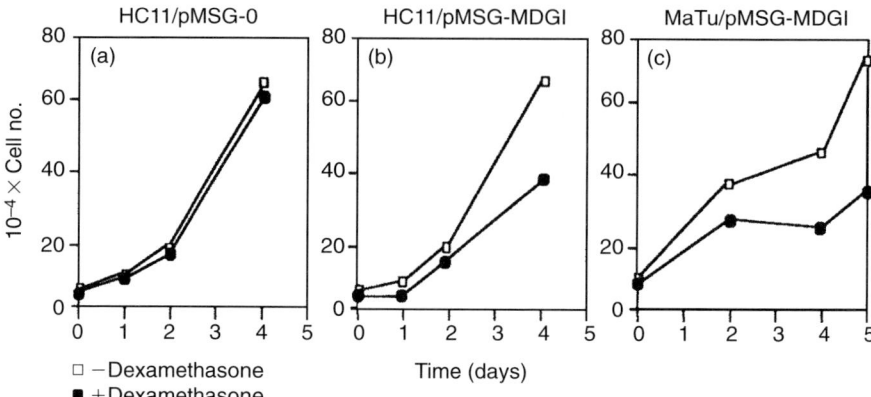

Fig. 4. **Transfection of MDGI into mammary epithelial cell lines inhibits cell proliferation.** Cell lines HCII (mouse mammary epithelial cell line) and MaTu (human ductal carcinoma cell line) were transfected with an expression plasmid (pMSG) containing bovine MDGI cDNA under the control of the dexamethasone-inducible mouse mammary tumour virus promoter. Controls were transfected with the empty vector. Stable mass-transfected cells were treated with dexamethasone for up to 5 days and the cell number was determined at the time points indicated. (a) Mock-transfected control HCII cells; (b) MDGI-transfected HCII cells; (c) MDGI-transfected MaTu cells.

were analysed on mammary epithelial and stromal cells respectively, no growth-inhibitory activity was found (Table 2).

To ascertain if MDGI is able to inhibit proliferation of mammary epithelial cells in the context of the intact mammary tissue, whole-organ mammary glands derived from virgin mice were used. As mentioned above, these organ cultures undergo complete lobulo-alveolar development of the gland and functional differentiation as characterized by milk protein production after 5 days when cultivated in serum-free APIH medium [9]. Addition of MDGI at 1 nM to these organ cultures for 5 days results in the appearance of smaller ducts and ductules when compared with the control. Numerous short side branches are formed that terminate in alveolar structures. When labelling indices were determined in alveoli, ducts and ductules of MDGI-treated and control glands, the strongest inhibition of proliferation was found in ductular epithelial cells. Inhibition was less pronounced in ductal epithelial cells (Table 3) [9]. Interestingly, MDGI can first be detected in mammary gland organ culture under APIH conditions after 3 days. *In vivo*, MDGI expression starts around day 10 of pregnancy in the mouse mammary gland and is localized to emerging alveolar structures, but is not found in ductular epithelium [9,27]. Expression of MDGI in ducts and ductular epithelial cells starts around day 15 of pregnancy in the mouse mammary gland. In late pregnancy and lactation, MDGI expression is most pronounced in ductules and terminal parts of ducts. Thus *in vivo* expression of MDGI in ductules coincides with decreased proliferation and the beginning of terminal differentiation. Furthermore, the presence of MDGI at

Table 3. Effects of MDGI and EGF on cell proliferation and functional differentiation in mammary organ culture. n.d., not determined.

	MDGI/P108 (5 ng/ml)	EGF (1 ng/ml)	MDGI (3 ng/ml) + EGF (1 ng/ml)
Growth inhibition (%)			
Overall mammary gland	45	−160% (stimulation)	30
Alveoli	10	n.d.	n.d.
Ducts	33	n.d.	n.d.
Ductuli	60	n.d.	n.d.
Relative mRNA levels (% of control)			
MDGI	290	60	250
β-Casein	275	<10	245
WAP	295	80	250

earlier time points during organ culture results in diminished ductular elongation and a reduced proliferation rate of ductular mammary epithelial cells. Finally, MDGI is expressed in differentiating alveolar epithelial cells as soon as they emerge, and consequently the growth-inhibitory effect of additional MDGI on these cells is minimal.

In agreement with the proposed growth-inhibitory function of MDGI, blocking of MDGI expression by antisense oligonucleotides in organ culture leads to a 4-fold increase in the labelling index of ductal and ductular epithelial cells, and prevents alveolar differentiation [9].

Effects of MDGI on mammary gland differentiation

A decreasing rate of proliferation of ducts and ductules in late pregnancy is accompanied by terminal differentiation of lobulo-alveolar mammary epithelial cells. This functional shift is characterized by the appearance of monolayered alveoli with enlarged luminal spaces, the synthesis and secretion of milk proteins such as α- and β-casein, lactoglobulin and whey acidic protein (WAP), and the apical secretion of milk fat globules. Since MDGI expression coincides with the onset of functional and morphological differentiation, its potential as a differentiation factor was studied. When mammary gland organ cultures were treated with MDGI under the same conditions as described above (1 nM for 5 days), ducts and ductules were smaller than in the control gland. Under the influence of MDGI, numerous bulbous alveolar end buds formed which represent a developmental stage that ultimately undergoes functional and morphological differentiation. These alveolar structures consist of monolayered secretory epithelial cells which enclose enlarged luminal spaces that are filled with secretion [9] and resemble those found in fully differentiated mammary glands. To quantify differences in the degree of functional differentiation between MDGI-treated and control glands, the levels of expression of β-casein and WAP were analysed (Table 3). The results indicate that MDGI treatment leads to increased levels of differentiation markers and produces autostimulation of its own expression.

MDGI is expressed in mammary gland organ culture under APIH medium conditions starting at around day 3. To elucidate the role of endogenous MDGI during mammogenesis, antisense oligonucleotides against MDGI were developed to 'knock out' MDGI expression in mammary organ culture. Addition of these specific antisense oligonucleotides to the organ culture medium completely inhibits MDGI expression. This blockade results in developmentally degenerated glandular structures and the prevention of alveolar end-bud formation [9]. Furthermore, intraluminal β-casein levels were significantly decreased. Interestingly, intracellular β-casein levels were less severely affected, suggesting an effect of MDGI on maturation of the alveolar secretory pathway rather than on β-casein gene transcription. The independent control of milk protein expression and secretion has also been suggested by other groups. For example, WAP transcription was detected in the mammary glands of virgin mice in oestrus in a limited number of cells, but secretion was only found after terminal differentiation in late pregnancy and during lactation. Furthermore, an autocrine negative-feedback mechanism for milk proteins has been shown to exist for WAP and for the feedback inhibitor of lactation [28]. Similar to MDGI, the early production of WAP disrupts the timing of milk gene activation. However, in contrast with MDGI, which promotes the terminal differentiation of alveoli, precocious WAP expression leads to a premature termination of the differentiation programme, and alveolar development is impaired [29].

A C-terminal MDGI-derived peptide mimics MDGI activities

The high degree of identity between FABP family members suggests similar and redundant functions. However, their exclusive tissue distributions indicate additional specialization. Identity between FABP family members decreases from the N- to the C-terminus, which hints that the C-terminal region is the carrier of these specialized functions (Fig. 1). The less conserved C-terminal region is encoded by a separate exon on the FABP genes (exon 4), also indicating that this region represents a functional domain within the MDGI protein. Furthermore, the common denominator of FABP function, i.e. the binding of long-chain fatty acids, is structurally preserved in the more N-terminal regions of the proteins, but also involves critical amino acids within the C-terminus [30]. Thus the C-terminal peptide domain of MDGI might carry functions other than fatty acid binding.

Interestingly, MDGI has been isolated in two different isoforms [31,32]. The full-length 14.5 kDa MDGI protein was found throughout pregnancy and lactation within the mammary gland. In contrast, a low-molecular-mass C-terminally truncated MDGI isoform (MDGI-2) was only found during pregnancy. In addition to its lack of the C-terminal sequence, MDGI-2 is associated with a glycosylated complex. Thus it was tempting to speculate that, during pregnancy,

MDGI is proteolytically processed to release a bioactive C-terminal peptide. In addition, C-terminal truncation will also result in the loss of the ligand binding properties of MDGI. MDGI might thus play a dual role, one exerted by the full-length protein and the second one by the C-terminal sequence. Intriguingly, the C-terminal MDGI sequence contains a potential tyrosine-phosphorylation site (Tyr[128]), and it was shown that the insulin receptor is able to phosphorylate a small proportion of MDGI in the mammary gland [33].

To test the hypothesis that the C-terminal region of MDGI contains a separate functional domain, peptides of different lengths were synthesized, derived from the MDGI C-terminus (amino acids 121–131, designated P108; amino acids 126–130, designated P126) and from a more N-terminal region (amino acids 69–78; designated P14). P126 is a pentapeptide that contains a functional growth hormone domain and lies within P108. These peptides were tested for growth-inhibitory and differentiation-inducing activities on mammary gland organ cultures under the same conditions as used for full-length MDGI [9]. P108, but not P126 or P14, was able to strongly suppress the wave of DNA synthesis accompanying ductal growth when present for 3 days in organ culture at 1 nM. This is identical to the results obtained with MDGI at the same concentration. Thus P108 is as effective as MDGI in inhibiting ductal DNA synthesis. Prolonged treatment of organ cultures with P108 for 5 days resulted in the appearance of differentiated, secretory, active alveolar epithelium. In parallel, β-casein expression was markedly stimulated by P108. In addition, when Tyr[128] was replaced by Ala, the activity of P108 was abolished. However, it is not currently known if phosphorylation of Tyr[128] is necessary for peptide or MDGI activity. Taken together, these results strongly suggest that the C-terminal domain of MDGI alone is able to mimic its growth-inhibitory and differentiation-inducing functions, and that this peptide region determines the specialized role of MDGI in the mammary gland compared with other FABPs.

MDGI inhibitory and differentiation-inducing activities are ligand-independent

It is tempting to speculate that a diffusible hydrophobic ligand for MDGI is released by the stromal compartment during tissue remodelling. Binding of this putative hydrophobic ligand to MDGI might be a regulatory mechanism for the modulation of ligand levels in a manner that limits its association with alternative binding sites, in particular with members of the nuclear hormone receptor family. A similar mechanism of action was proposed for other members of the FABP family [17,34]. In the case of cellular retinoid binding protein, it was suggested that ligand–binding-protein complexes are direct substrates of retinoid conversion [35], and may serve to create retinoid gradients. Furthermore, fatty acids, prostaglandins and eicosanoids, which are FABP ligands, may activate the nuclear hormone receptors peroxisome-proliferator-activated receptor and retinoid X receptor [36,37].

To elucidate whether ligand binding is directly responsible for the growth-inhibitory and differentiation-inducing functions of MDGI, recombinant MDGI was produced that cannot bind fatty acid due to the substitution of

Arg[106] by Thr [9]. Although [Thr[106]]MDGI does not bind oleic acid, its biolog-ical activities are maintained. This result strongly suggests that the physiologi-cal function of MDGI in mediating mammary gland differentiation is independent from its fatty acid binding property. The same conclusion is sup-ported by the observation that P108 is able to completely mimic MDGI activi-ties. It has been shown that P108 is unable to bind hydrophobic ligands [9].

These findings, as well as the detection of two MDGI isoforms, support a model that proposes a dual function for MDGI (Fig. 5). One function might be dependent on the binding of hydrophobic ligands, thereby modulating their metabolism and accessibility to alternative binding sites within the cell. The second function might be the regulation of growth and differentiation during pregnancy in a tissue-specific manner by a proteolytically derived short C-ter-minal MDGI fragment; P108 is able to mimic this activity. The mechanism of

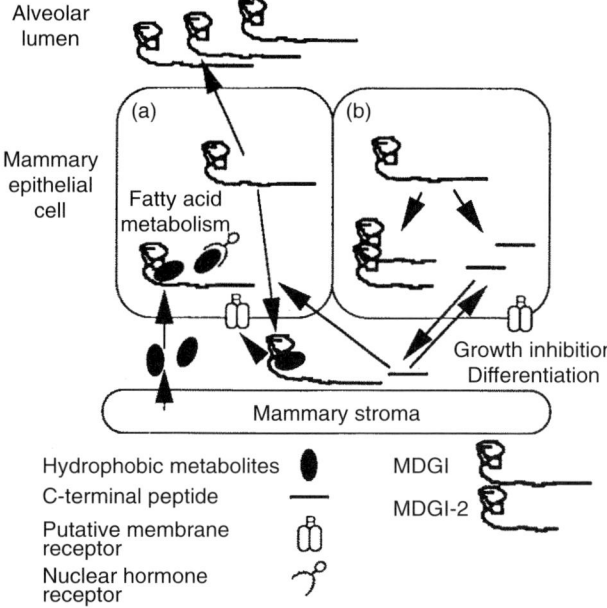

Fig. 5. Proposed model of MDGI function in the mammary gland during differentiation and lactation. This schematic diagram considers a dual function for MDGI. (a) MDGI is able to bind hydrophobic ligands and might act as a modulator of metabolite accessibility to alternative binding sites, such as members of the nuclear hormone receptor family. Those ligands might be released by stromal cells during glandular differentiation or, alternatively, pro-duced by epithelial cells, or both. Extracellularly, MDGI is found in the lumen of alveoli as well as in the basal extracellular matrix. (b) During pregnancy, MDGI is proteolytically cleaved into MDGI-2 and a bioactive C-terminal peptide which is not able to bind hydrophobic ligands. The C-terminal peptide might be secreted and act as an paracrine or autocrine signalling molecule. Although MDGI and P108 are able to enter the cell, it is not known if transport mecha-nisms are necessary for MDGI/P108 to cross the cell membrane. Alternatively, MDGI/P108 might bind to a putative membrane receptor.

action of P108 has not yet been identified; however, interactions with membrane receptors and second messenger pathways have been suggested [38].

MDGI and EGF are functional antagonists

Earlier studies showed that the effects of MDGI on the proliferation of mammary tumour cells *in vitro* can be blocked by growth factors such as EGF, TGF-α and platelet-derived growth factor [39]. TGF-α and EGF might serve as key mitogens for ductal and ductular growth during mammary gland differentiation. The EGF receptor and TGF-α are expressed during mammary gland development within ductal and alveolar epithelial cells. TGF-α expression is detectable in the virgin stage and increases during pregnancy and lactation about 3-fold (Fig. 2) [40–42]; it is a strong mitogen for the mammary epithelium, and overexpression in the mammary glands of transgenic mice results in a hyperproliferative phenotype [43]. The mitogenic effect of EGF and TGF-α on ductal, ductular and alveolar epithelial cells is associated with structural and functional de-differentiation [42]. In addition, MDGI mRNA expression is strongly inhibited by EGF and TGF-α in mammary epithelial cells *in vitro* and in organ culture. Finally, MDGI is able to inhibit EGF receptor expression by about 60% in 184 A1N4 cells [31] (A. Kurtz, R. Grosse, E. Spitzer and B. Binas, unpublished work). The effects of EGF on MDGI expression, the down-regulation of EGF receptors by MDGI, their partially overlapping expression patterns and their opposite activities on mammary development led to the assumption that EGF and MDGI interact functionally during growth and differentiation.

To study the physiological significance of the interaction between EGF and MDGI, mammary gland organ cultures were treated for 5 days with both factors at different concentrations ranging from 1 to 3 nM. As shown in Table 3, EGF exerts mitogenic activity and suppresses WAP gene expression. With increasing concentrations of MDGI the effects of EGF on growth and de-differentiation were gradually suppressed. MDGI at 3 nM completely prevented the activities of 1 nM EGF. On the other hand, stimulation of functional differentiation by MDGI could be completely blocked with 3 nM EGF. In conclusion, MDGI and EGF act as functional antagonists during mammary gland differentiation.

The point of the signalling pathway at which MDGI and EGF interact is only partially understood. However, several lines of evidence suggest that physiological metabolites generated downstream of the phospholipase pathways are involved in the regulation of MDGI expression. First, the growth factor-dependent MDGI down-regulation can be reversed by inhibitors of the lipoxygenase and cyclo-oxygenase pathways (A. Kurtz, R. Grosse, B. Binas and M.-L. Li, unpublished work). Secondly, in an assay using primary myocytes, MDGI is able to reverse arachidonic acid- and 15S-hydroxyeicosatetraenoic acid-induced hypersensitivity to β-adrenergic agents. Signalling through the lipoxygenase pathway was also suggested for the mammary growth inhibitor TGF-α [42]. Our current working model for MDGI signalling is shown in Fig. 6.

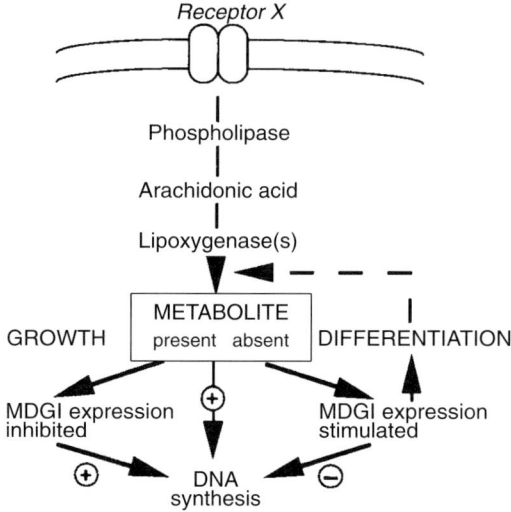

Fig. 6. Proposed model of MDGI signalling in mammary epithelial cells and heart myocytes. The model is based on the finding that MDGI affects signalling downstream of the lipoxygenase pathway.

MDGI expression in breast cancer

The mode of MDGI expression during normal mammogenesis and its biological activities prompted studies on MDGI expression in human breast cancer samples. These studies confirmed that MDGI expression was suppressed in more than 75% of all breast cancers analysed by immunohistochemistry. The remaining approx. 25% MDGI-positive breast cancer tissues were analysed for correlation of MDGI expression and hormone receptor levels as well as staging parameters. A significant negative correlation could only be found with progesterone receptor levels (W. Zschiesche, E. Spitzer and R. Grosse, unpublished work).

Expression of MDGI in carcinoma *in situ* shows restriction of the protein to the intraductal part of the carcinoma. The invasive part of the carcinoma is negative for MDGI (Fig. 7). The biological significance of this localized expression pattern is not clear. However, our data suggest that loss of MDGI expression is correlated with gain of an invasive phenotype.

Furthermore, it was shown in the laboratory of Pollak that expression of MDGI in tumorigenic breast cancer cell lines abolished their ability to form tumours in nude mice [44]. The same group reported that MDGI might be inactivated in breast cancers by an aberrant MDGI gene methylation mechanism [45]. In conclusion, our data support the thesis that MDGI might act as a growth inhibitor for mammary tumours *in vivo*.

(a)   (b)

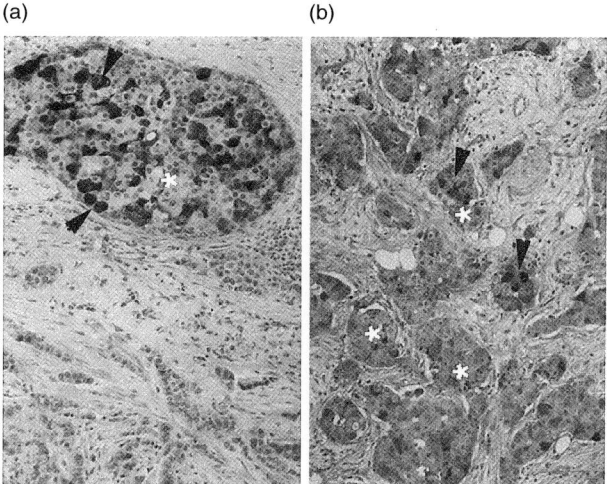

Fig. 7. MDGI expression in human breast carcinoma *in situ*. MDGI expression was detected by immunohistochemistry. (a) MDGI expression (arrowheads) is restricted to the ductal compartment (asterisk). (b) MDGI expression (arrowheads) occurs in ductal epithelial cells (asterisk).

Conclusions

The developmental decision that triggers terminal differentiation and inhibits proliferation in mid and late pregnancy is mediated by locally acting factors. Pleiotrophin is one hormonally regulated factor that might stimulate proliferation and tissue remodelling. The hormonally induced MDGI, on the other hand, induces terminal differentiation and inhibits proliferation. In addition, MDGI is a potent antagonist for the mitogenic and de-differentiating functions of EGF. Thus the balance between MDGI and EGF is exemplatory for a mechanistic model of dynamic regulation of mammogenesis that is at least partially due to the concentration gradients of growth stimulators and inhibitors. Furthermore, factors that potentially stimulate or inhibit proliferation of normal mammary epithelial cells are important players during breast cancer development. Indeed, pleiotrophin acts as a tumour growth factor, whereas MDGI is down-regulated in breast cancers and acts as a growth inhibitor.

We are grateful to Dr. Anke Schulte and Bryan Boyle for providing unpublished data regarding pleiotrophin expression and regulation. We thank the Biochemical Society, and in particular Professor P.S. Rudland, for making the Annual Symposium and this publication possible. This work was supported in part by grants from the National Cancer Institute (NIH) and the USAMRMC Breast Cancer Program (to A.W.).

References

1. Aaronson, S.A. (1991) Science **254**, 1146–1153
2. Clarke, R., Dickson, R.B. and Lippman, M.E. (1992) Crit. Rev. Oncol. Hematol. **12**, 1–23
3. Cross, M. and Dexter, T.M (1991) Cell **64**, 271–280
4. Liotta, L.A., Steeg, P.S. and Stetler-Stevenson, W.G. (1991) Cell **64**, 327–336
5. Wellstein, A. and Lippman, M.E. (1991) in Molecular Foundations of Oncology (Broder, S., ed.), pp. 403–418, Williams and Wilkins, Baltimore
6. Ervin, P.R., Kaminski, M.S., Cody, R.L. and Wicha, M.S. (1989) Science **244**, 1585–1587
7. Silberstein, G. and Daniel, C. (1987) Science **237**, 291–293
8. Peles, E., Bacus, S.S., Koski, R.A., et al. (1992) Cell **69**, 205–216
9. Yang, Y., Spitzer, E., Meyer, D., Sachs, M., Birchmeier, C. and Birchmeier, W. (1995) J. Cell Biol. **127**, 1120–1129
10. Zavizion, B., Politis, I., Gorewit, R.C., Turner, J.D., Spitzer, E. and Grosse, R. (1993) J. Dairy Sci. **76**, 3721–3726
11. Wellstein, A., Fang, W.J., Khatri, A., et al. (1992) J. Biol. Chem. **267**, 2582–2587
12. Kurtz, A., Schulte, A.M. and Wellstein, A. (1995) Crit. Rev. Oncog. **6(2)**, 151–177
13. Czubayko, F., Riegel, A.T. and Wellstein, A. (1994) J. Biol. Chem. **269**, 21358–21363
14. Fang, W.J., Hartmann, N., Chow, D., Riegel, A.T. and Wellstein, A. (1992) J. Biol. Chem. **267**, 25889–25897
14a. Schulte, A.M., Lai, S., Kurtz, A., Czubayko, F., Riegel, A.T., Wellstein, A. (1996) Proc. Natl. Acad. Sci. U.S.A. **93**, 14759–14764
15. Borchers, T. and Spener, F. (1994) Curr. Top. Membr. Transp. **40**, 261–294
16. Grosse, R., Bohmer, F.D., Binas, B., Kurtz, A., Spitzer, E., Muller, T. and Zschiesche, W. (1992) Cancer Treat. Res. **61**, 69–96
17. Bass, N.M. (1993) Mol. Cell. Biochem. **123**, 191–202
18. Grigsby, P.W., Pilepich, M.V. and Parsons, C.L. (1990) Am. J. Clin. Oncol. **13**, 28–31
19. Bernlohr, D.A., Angus, C.W., Lane, M.D., Bolanowski, M.A. and Kelly, Jr., T.J. (1984) Proc. Natl. Acad. Sci. U.S.A. **81**, 5468–5472
20. Gordon, J.I. (1989) J. Cell Biol. **108**, 1187–1194
21. Kaikaus, R., Bass, N.M. and Ockner, R.K. (1990) Experientia **46**, 617–630
22. Kurtz, A., Zimmer, A., Schnütgen, F., Brüning, G., Spener, F. and Müller, T. (1994) Development **120**, 2637–2649
23. Veerkamp, J., Peeters, R. and Maatman, R. (1991) Biochim. Biophys. Acta **1081**, 1–24
24. Kurtz, A., Vogel, F., Funa, K., Heldin, C.-H. and Grosse, R. (1990) J. Cell Biol. **110**, 1779–1789
25. Erdmann, B. and Breter, H. (1993) Cell Tissue Res. **272**, 383–389
26. Li, M., Spitzer, E., Zschiesche, W., Binas, B., Parczyk, K. and Grosse, R. (1995) J. Cell. Physiol. **164**, 1–8
27. Zschiesche, W., Kleine, A.H., Spitzer, E., Veerkamp, J.H. and Glatz, J.F. (1995) Histochem. Cell Biol. **103**, 147–156
28. Rennison, M.E., Kerr, M., Addey, C.V., Handel, S.E., Turner, M.D., Wilde, C.J. and Burgoyne, R.D. (1993) J. Cell Sci. **106**, 641–648
29. Robinson, G.W., McKnight, R.A., Smith, G.H. and Hennighausen, L. (1996) Development **121**, 2079–2090
30. Muller-Fahrnow, A., Egner, U., Johnes, T.A., Rudel, H., Spener, F. and Saenger, W. (1991) Eur. J. Biochem. **199**, 271–276
31. Binas, B., Spitzer, E., Zschiesche, W., et al. (1992) In Vitro Cell. Dev. Biol. **28A**, 625–634
32. Brandt, R. and Grosse, R. (1992) Biochem. Biophys. Res. Commun. **189**, 406–413
33. Nielsen, S.U., Rump, R., Hojrup, P., Roepstorff, P. and Spener, F. (1994) Biochim. Biophys. Acta **1211**, 189–197
34. Glatz, J.F.C., Vork, M., Cistola, D. and van der Vusse, G. (1993) Prostaglandins Leukotrienes Essential Fatty Acids **48**, 33–41

35. Napoli, J.L. (1993) J. Nutr. **123**, 362–366
36. Eager, N.S., Bricknell, P.M., Snell, C. and Wood, J.N. (1992) Proc. R. Soc. London B **250**, 63–69
37. Keller, H., Dreyer, C., Medin, J., Mahfoudi, A., Ozato, K. and Wahli, W. (1993) Proc. Natl. Acad. Sci. U.S.A. **90**, 2160–2164
38. Wallukat, G., Boehmer, F.D., et al. (1991) Mol. Cell. Biochem. **102**, 49–60
39. Grosse, R., Boehmer, F.D., Langen, P., Kurtz, A., Lehmann, W., Mieth, M. and Wallukat, G. (1991) Methods Enzymol. **198**, 425–440
40. Liscia, D.S., Merlo, G., Ciardiello, F., Kim, N., Smith, G.H., Callahan, R. and Salomon, D.S. (1990) Dev. Biol. **140**, 123–131
41. Plaut, K. (1993) J. Dairy Sci. **76**, 1526–1538
42. Spitzer, E., Zschiesche, W., Binas, B., Grosse, R. and Erdmann, B. (1995) J. Cell. Biochem. **57**, 495–508
43. Dickson, R.B. and Lippman, M.E. (1995) Endocr. Rev. **16**, 559–589
44. Huynh, H.T., Larsson, C., Narod, S. and Pollak, M. (1995) Cancer Res. **55(11)**, 2225–2231
45. Huynh, T.H., Alpert, L. and Pollak, M. (1996) Proc. Am. Assoc. Cancer Res. **87**, 536 (Abstract)

Biochem. Soc. Symp. **63**, 71–79
Printed in Great Britain

6

Local control of the mammary gland

Malcolm Peaker*, Colin J. Wilde and Christopher H. Knight

Hannah Research Institute, Ayr, Scotland KA6 5HL, U.K.

Abstract

Studies on increasing the frequency of milking in dairy animals have led to the uncovering of the mechanism by which tactical control of the rate of milk secretion is achieved locally within each mammary gland, against a strategic, systemic control by the hormones that maintain all glands in the secretory condition. Experiments *in vivo* established that the response is local, and were compatible with the hypothesis that milk contains an inhibitor of its own secretion which accumulates during storage within the lumen of the mammary gland and which acts in an autocrine manner on the secretory cells. Isolation of a protein, initially from goats' milk, called FIL (feedback inhibitor of lactation) has enabled, and is enabling, further studies to be done from the whole-animal down to the molecular level. Examples at the whole-animal level are: the effects of immunization against FIL on the rate of secretion; the concentration of FIL and the kinetics of its formation and breakdown; the importance of the internal structure of the mammary gland and the capacities of the alveolar and ductular storage regions in determining feedback inhibition; differences between individuals and species influencing the degree of control exerted by FIL in matching supply of milk to demand by the young. Other local control mechanisms at the onset and cessation of lactation, including mammary distension, are also discussed.

Introduction

The integration of processes within the body is usually considered to be that between the different tissues and organs of a single organism. However, in mammalian reproduction, another type of integration occurs: that between a mother and her offspring, both *in utero* and during lactation. This type of integrative control is different from that within a single organism because the mother and her offspring are not genetically identical. Therefore, in evolutionary terms, the interests of the mother are not identical with the interests of the

---

* To whom correspondence should be addressed.

young or, as Trivers [1] put it, "there is an overlap of self-interest between parent and offspring but not an identity of self-interest". A mother's evolutionary fitness is her lifetime reproductive success, and it may pay to invest resources in several offspring rather than in one, and the mother will be adapted to ration her expenditure on a single offspring beyond a certain level. The young, bearing its father's genes as well as its mother's, is adapted to ensuring its own success at the expense of possible future siblings by persuading its mother to invest more. Communications from mother to offspring and from offspring to mother are a vital part of the integration of the mutual self-interest in raising a successful offspring and in being raised successfully. Such signalling can, however, involve some degree of false signalling as, for example, when a young primate or dog tries to inveigle its mother into suckling during weaning.

In the present context, the communications between mother and offspring are confined to the mutual self-interest of producing milk and consuming milk. It is obvious that the rate of milk secretion must be controlled in some way, but what are the costs of the mother not producing enough or of her producing too much?

Costs of milk secretion and matching supply to demand

The metabolic demands of lactation depend on body size. In general, peak milk energy output and neonatal body weight are related in a similar manner as metabolic rate to body weight [2–5]. However, as more data became available, it was established that this relationship is not rigid and that differential selection pressures may increase or decrease the proportion of the mother's energy budget devoted to producing milk at any given maternal body size [4,5]. For example, altricial mammals have relatively small offspring at birth, while their daily milk energy output is greater than that in precocial mammals of the same size. By contrast, primates have a relatively low milk energy output but a longer period of lactation.

The substrates required for milk secretion and energy metabolism can be obtained from an increased rate of food intake and from body stores. Since the daily output of energy in milk is a significant proportion of the total energy content of a small mammal, but a much smaller proportion in a large mammal, increased food intake has to be the main source in small mammals, whereas large mammals can draw on body reserves, provided they have them, to a much greater extent. If this is so, then at one extreme it can be calculated that a pygmy shrew (*Sorex minutus*) weighing 5 g must more than double its food consumption during lactation and eat more than four times its own body weight per day [3]. At the other extreme, the interested reader can make similar calculations for the blue whale (*Balaenoptera musculus*) using the equations given in [5] (see also [6] for the importance of energy reserves for lactation in whales).

The major metabolic demands of lactation have been used to study the limits to metabolic rate and the performance and safety factors of different physiological systems [7,8]. In experiments with mice, food intake at peak lactation was increased more than 3-fold compared with that of virgins.

Given that lactation imposes great metabolic demands, it would be expected that there would be selective advantage in having a mechanism to prevent the overproduction of milk, even though some of that excess might be recovered by re-absorption and re-synthesis. Since the consequences of under-production are obvious for the viability and success of the young, it might be expected that some mechanism, or an array of mechanisms, might have evolved to prevent the wastage of maternal resources while providing the needs of the young; in other words, some means of matching supply of milk to demand.

In studying the supply of milk in relation to demand, it often has to be pointed out that the mammary gland is an unusual exocrine organ in two respects: (i) secretion is continuous during lactation, whereas most exocrine glands secrete intermittently in response to an acute stimulus; and (ii) secretion is stored in the lumen of the secretory alveoli and duct system until removed at intervals by the sucking young or, in dairy animals, by milking. Moreover, secretion does not simply flow from the glands but is assisted by the contraction of myoepithelial cells around each secretory alveolus under the influence of oxytocin in the systemic circulation, released as the efferent arm of the neuroendocrine milk-ejection reflex.

Supply and demand: early work by dairy scientists

That the rate of milk secretion changes with the frequency and completeness of milk removal has long been known by dairy farmers, with an increase in frequency eliciting an increase in the rate of secretion. As the pioneering research on the endocrine control of milk secretion unfolded, it was assumed that changes in the rate of secretion would be explained by surges of galactopoietic hormones produced as an offshoot of the milk-ejection reflex by the anterior pituitary. However, dairy scientists pointed out that the response to changing the frequency of milk removal could be elicited locally within the mammary gland, since, when one or more glands of cows were milked more frequently, then the increase in milk yield was confined to those glands rather than to all glands equally. In other words, the response was not elicited systemically, and a simple explanation based on the frequency of hormonal stimulation could not obtain. However, another explanation was offered by dairy scientists in the U.S.A. They suggested that an increase in intra-mammary pressure, brought about by the accumulating volume of milk, occurs between milkings and that the secretory rate is inhibited by higher pressures. According to this simple notion, frequent milking relieves the pressure and the secretory rate rises. There was, however, evidence that milk secretion between milkings was linear during a normal period between milkings and could not, therefore, have been gradually inhibited by increasing intra-mammary pressure. This does not mean to say that the raised intra-mammary pressure which occurs with even longer periods of milk accumulation does not inhibit secretion eventually: it does, and the mechanism is interesting (see below), but the early results did indicate that the effects of changing the milking frequency were unlikely to be due to relief of intra-mammary pressure. These early studies have recently been described in more detail [9].

Physiological studies on frequent milking

The search for the mechanism controlling the rate of milk secretion in response to changes in milking frequency stems from work in the 1960s by J.L. Linzell [10]. In order to study the acute effects of physiological factors on milk secretion, he developed the technique of milking goats every 1 h instead of twice daily. Because the milk-ejection reflex becomes refractory at such high rates in this species, he injected oxytocin in physiological amounts in order to obtain the milk that had been secreted during the previous 1 h. In such circumstances, an amount of milk was obtained each hour that equalled the average hourly yield before hourly milking began. However, in some of these animals and in subsequent experiments, it was found that the rate of secretion increased during hourly milking. Moreover, when only one of the two glands was milked hourly, the rate of secretion increased only in that gland [11]. Evidence was also obtained that the response was connected with the removal of milk rather than with an effect of the exogenous oxytocin.

In these short-term experiments and from the behaviour of milk flow between the secretory alveoli and mammary ducts, it was considered unlikely that the relief of mammary distension was involved. The most likely explanation was some form of local chemical feedback operating within each mammary gland and we proposed that "...it is possible that some local humoral factor may be involved in the local regulation of the rate of secretion" [11]. Testing of this hypothesis *in vivo* was performed in goats using either hourly milking, as in the original experiments, or thrice-daily instead of twice-daily milking.

Key evidence compatible with the hypothesis of a chemical inhibitor of milk secretion present in milk was obtained. For example, Henderson and Peaker [12] showed that the local response to increasing the frequency of milk removal from twice to thrice daily could not be explained by the relief of mammary distension. At one of the three milkings, an amount of inert, isotonic solution, equal in volume to the milk removed at that milking, was infused into the lumen of one gland. The rate of milk secretion still increased, showing that the composition of the stored secretion, rather than its physical presence, was the key determinant. Similarly, when milk stored in the mammary gland was diluted with isotonic sucrose or lactose solutions, the rate of milk secretion increased [13,14]. Therefore, even though the degree of distension increased, the rate of secretion increased in a manner compatible with the dilution of a chemical inhibitor.

Evidence was also obtained that it is the presence of milk in the secretory alveoli that is responsible for inhibition. When milk was drained from the duct system by catheter every 1 h, a procedure that does not elicit the milk-ejection reflex and evacuate the alveoli, the rate of milk secretion did not increase [14].

FIL, the feedback inhibitor of lactation

The isolation and characterization of the putative inhibitor of milk secretion present in milk is described in the following chapter ([15]; see also [16]).

Briefly, a hitherto-unknown milk protein has been found in milk which inhibits milk secretion *in vitro* and *in vivo*. This protein has been called FIL, i.e. feedback inhibitor of lactation [17].

Studies on the concentration of FIL in relation to the frequency and completeness of milk removal are under way in several species. This is an important aspect, because the mechanism cannot simply be one of secretion of inhibitor and its subsequent removal by milking or suckling. After milk ejection, some milk remains in the alveoli (the 'residual milk'), and the putative site of inhibition is never free from milk. Therefore an activation step leading to the formation in milk of FIL from a precursor, or a catabolic step in which a clearance mechanism is overwhelmed by secretion of FIL in milk, must be postulated.

The importance of FIL has been demonstrated by actively immunizing goats against caprine FIL [18]. The immunization was by three treatments during the declining phase of lactation. Only after the third immunization was antibody to FIL detected in milk (as opposed to plasma), and only then was a response to a change in milking frequency noted. Firstly, the decline in milk secretion with advancing lactation slowed. Secondly, when one gland of immunized goats was switched from twice- to once-daily milking, the ipsilateral decrease in the rate of milk secretion was reduced significantly compared with the response in sham-immunized animals. In other words, immuno-neutralization of FIL allowed milk secretion to continue over a period when FIL would normally have been acting to slow the rate of secretion.

Interactions with the internal structure of the mammary gland

Within the lumen of the mammary gland, milk is stored in two, connected, compartments, i.e. within the duct system (which has no secretory function) and within the secretory alveoli themselves. The capacity of the ducts as a percentage of the total capacity varies between species and between breeds and individuals within a species. One of the characteristics of dairy animals is the relatively large duct system. Since FIL operates in the alveoli, and assuming either that the concentration of FIL increases with storage or that FIL is somehow cleared from residual milk in the alveoli, it was predicted that dairy goats and cows, which store relatively more of their secretion in the enlarged ducts (the 'cistern' of the gland), would show less of a response of milk yield to increasing or decreasing the milking frequency. Such a relationship has been confirmed in both the goat and the cow [19].

Local control in late pregnancy

A characteristic of changing the milking frequency during lactation, treating with exogenous FIL or immunizing against FIL is that the milk composition is not affected. In other words, the synthetic and secretory pathways of all major milk components are affected equally. However, other cases of intra-mammary control are known in which changes in milk composition are manifest.

One of the physiological conditions in which the rate and composition of milk secretion are subject to local control is at the onset of copious secretion in the periparturient period (lactogenesis stage II). If, in goats, milk removal is started in late pregnancy, the composition of the secretion changes from that of colostrum to that of normal milk, and the rate of secretion increases. If early milk removal is confined to one gland, then only in that gland do the changes occur; the changes in the other gland still occur, but only at the normal time. Thus it possible by a local mechanism to accelerate the changes that occur during the onset of copious secretion.

The changes in milk composition are marked by increases in the concentrations of lactose and potassium and decreases in those of sodium and chloride. Evidence was obtained from studies on the permeability of the mammary epithelium *in vivo* that, during pregnancy, there is a paracellular pathway across the mammary epithelium, and that this pathway closes in the periparturient period [20].

In order to explain the local acceleration of an eventual systemically controlled event, it was suggested that a substance is produced by the mammary gland during pregnancy and that this substance acts to maintain the paracellular pathway. Near parturition, as hormonal changes occur, the substance is no longer produced and that remaining in the gland is catabolized, so that the paracellular pathway closes and the composition changes to that of normal milk. With regular and frequent milk removal *pre partum*, the substance is removed at a rate greater than its production, so that milk composition would alter only in the milked gland.

A possible candidate for the substance produced by the mammary gland in late pregnancy emerged later. During late pregnancy in the goat, prostaglandin $F_{2\alpha}$ is produced by the mammary gland. This output into milk and into venous blood ceases near term. However, catabolism of prostaglandin $F_{2\alpha}$ to an inactive form begins about 6 days *pre partum*. Since these changes coincide with the change in milk composition, the hypothesis that prostaglandin $F_{2\alpha}$ is responsible for maintaining the paracellular pathway was tested by injecting a long-lived analogue, cloprostenol, into the lumen of one mammary gland. Such treatment prevented the normal change in milk composition, indicating the possibility that prostaglandin synthesis and catabolism, under systemic hormonal control but subject to local influences, is responsible for controlling mammary epithelial permeability [21].

Whether the increase in the rate of secretion obtained on milk removal *pre partum* is also partly or wholly controlled by prostaglandin $F_{2\alpha}$, and whether FIL is also involved, is not known. However, preliminary studies were carried out on the inhibitory properties of mammary secretions from non-lactating goats in early pregnancy [22]. Small quantities of secretion were injected into the lumen of one mammary gland in lactating goats. In all animals, a shift in the permeability of the mammary epithelium, towards that obtaining in late pregnancy, was observed. In two of the five animals, the rate of secretion decreased. In mammary culture, lactose synthesis was inhibited. Whether these changes can be accounted for solely by the presence of prostaglandin $F_{2\alpha}$ and FIL, or whether different and/or additional factors are involved at different stages of the lactation cycle, needs to be investigated.

Local control in marsupials

Macropod marsupials, i.e. kangaroos and wallabies, provide the classic case of local mammary control of milk yield and composition [23,24]. The reproductive strategy of these animals operates like a conveyor belt, with young of different ages having overlapping periods of lactation. One of the four mammary glands within the pouch is feeding a young at heel, while another is feeding a newly born young only a few grams in weight. Then, when the older one is weaned, that gland regresses and another young attaches itself to another of the undeveloped glands. Obviously, the amounts of milk for the young of different ages are completely different, but so too is milk composition [25].

Mammary distension

There are important differences between species in the mechanism responsible for arresting milk secretion when milk removal is ceased during established or declining lactation. In the goat, clear evidence has been obtained that a local, physical mechanism, mammary distension, is responsible, rather than the withdrawal of galactopoietic hormones released in response to the suckling stimulus or the accumulation of chemical feedback inhibitors in milk [13]. For example, when milking of autotransplanted, and therefore denervated, glands was stopped while normal milking of the other normal gland *in situ* was continued, secretion was quickly arrested after the first 24 h. Since milking the denervated gland does not excite the milk-ejection reflex, the normal hormonal environment was maintained. In another experiment, not in autotransplanted glands, normal twice-daily milking was continued but, in one gland, isotonic lactose solution equal in volume to the volume obtained from the gland at that milking was injected into the lumen of the gland. This procedure was repeated at each milking (with the volume increasing each time as further milk was secreted) until the volume obtained was less than that at the previous milking (i.e. the fluid was being resorbed). The rate of secretion fell to zero within 1–2 days, while that of the untreated gland remained unchanged. Therefore it was the physical presence of milk, and not its chemical content, that was responsible for arresting secretion. Further, short-term direct studies on distension showed effects on mammary secretory and metabolic activity, followed by loss of integrity of the mammary epithelium [26].

While these experiments indicated the importance of mammary distension and the unimportance of the withdrawal of galactopoietic hormones in arresting secretion after the cessation of milk removal in the goat, they cannot be extrapolated necessarily to other species. In the rat, withdrawal of the suckling stimulus is clearly more important. Following separation from the young, the rate of milk accumulation in the glands decreases. However, when the young are not removed but removal of milk is prevented by sealing the teats with adhesive, the rate of milk secretion remains high [27]. Eventually, the rate of secretion falls in the rats with sealed teats but, clearly, mammary distension is of secondary importance to the withdrawal of hormones released at suckling. Therefore there is a hierarchy of control that differs between species, with FIL operating within the physiological range of normal suckling intervals. The order on an increasing time-scale in the goat is: FIL, mammary distension, hormonal withdrawal; in the rat the order is probably: FIL, hormonal withdrawal, mammary distension. Arguing teleologically, small animals have greater problems meeting the energy needs of lactation, and a 'belt and braces' approach cannot be unexpected.

The comparisons between species also stress the dangers of extrapolating from one species to another the quantitative aspects of intracellular signalling events that link hormone action and the synthesis and secretion of milk constituents. For example, in the rat, it would be expected that the overall intracellular message would be relatively short-lived (up to 4 h; [27]). It must be presumed that there will be some relationship between the length of the stimulatory message from a single episode of galactopoietic hormone release and the normal suckling interval, which varies from minutes in rats to hours in humans and goats, to 1 day in rabbits, to 2 days in tree shrews and to more than 4 days in fur-seals. Local control by FIL and by mammary distension must also take these differences into account.

The mechanism by which stretching the mammary epithelium arrests secretion is not known, although results from undifferentiated mammary cells subjected to mechanical formation on ion fluxes [28,29] indicate that such a study would be worthwhile.

Concluding comments

The above is an account of the major known mechanisms controlling milk secretion at the local, intra-mammary level. There may be others, since milk itself contains a vast array of known hormones and biologically active substances [30,31]. Only one of the mechanisms described, i.e. the search for the autocrine inhibitor FIL, has been subject to an explanatory reductionist approach as yet. If this chapter stimulates that approach to other established phenomena, such as the complex interaction between systemic and local factors at lactogenesis and the mechanism by which deformation of the secretory cells leads to the arrest of secretion, apoptosis and involution of the gland, then it will, in part, have served a purpose.

References
1.   Trivers, R.L. (1985) Social Evolution, Benjamin/Cummings, Menlo Park, CA
2.   Linzell, J.L. (1972) Dairy Sci. Abstr. 34, 351–360
3.   Hanwell, A. and Peaker, M. (1977) Symp. Zool. Soc. London 41, 297–312
4.   Martin, R.D. (1984) Symp. Zool. Soc. London 51, 87–117
5.   Oftedal, O.T. (1984) Symp. Zool. Soc. London 51, 33–85

6.   Lockyer, C. (1987) Symp. Zool. Soc. London 57, 343–361
7.   Hammond, K.A. and Diamond, J. (1992) Physiol. Zool. 65, 952–977
8.   Hammond, K.A., Konarzewski, M., Torres, R.M. and Diamond, J. (1994) Physiol. Zool. 67, 1479–1506
9.   Peaker, M. (1995) in Intercellular Signalling in the Mammary Gland (Wilde, C.J., Peaker, M. and Knight, C.H., eds.), pp. 193–202, Plenum, New York
10. Linzell, J.L. (1967) J. Physiol. (London) 190, 333–346
11. Linzell, J.L. and Peaker, M. (1971) J. Physiol. (London) 216, 717–734
12. Henderson, A.J. and Peaker, M. (1984) J. Physiol. (London) 351, 39–45
13. Fleet, I.R. and Peaker, M. (1978) J. Physiol. (London) 279, 491–507
14. Henderson, A.J. and Peaker, M. (1987) Q. J. Exp. Physiol. 72, 13–19
15. Wilde, C.J., Addey, C.V.P., Bryson, J.M., Finch, L.M.B., Knight, C.H. and Peaker, M. (1997) Biochem. Soc. Symp. 63, 81–90
16. Wilde, C.J., Addey, C.V.P., Boddy-Finch, L.M. and Peaker, M. (1995) in Intercellular Signalling in the Mammary Gland (Wilde, C.J., Peaker, M. and Knight, C.H., eds.), pp. 227–237, Plenum, New York
17. Wilde, C.J., Addey, C.V.P., Boddy, L.M. and Peaker, M. (1995) Biochem. J. 305, 51–58
18. Wilde, C.J., Addey, C.V.P. and Peaker, M. (1996) J. Physiol. (London) 491, 465–469
19. Knight, C.H. (1995) in Intercellular Signalling in the Mammary Gland (Wilde, C.J., Peaker, M. and Knight, C.H., eds.), pp. 1–11, Plenum, New York
20. Linzell, J.L. and Peaker, M. (1974) J. Physiol. (London) 243, 129–151
21. Maule Walker, F.M. and Peaker, M. (1980) J. Physiol. (London) 309, 65–79
22. Blatchford, D.R., Neville, M.C., Peaker, M. and Wilde, C.J. (1985) J. Physiol. (London) 361, 75P
23. Sharman, G.B. (1970). Science 167, 1221–1228
24. Findlay, L. and Renfree, M. (1984) Symp. Zool. Soc. London 51, 403–432
25. Green, B. (1984) Symp. Zool. Soc. London 51, 369–387
26. Peaker, M. (1980) J. Physiol. (London) 301, 415–428
27. Hanwell, A. and Linzell, J.L. (1973) J. Physiol. (London) 233, 111–125
28. Enomoto, K.-I., Furuya, K., Yamagishi, S. and Maeno, T. (1992) Cell Calcium 13, 501–511
29. Furuya, K., Enomoto, K.-I. and Yamagishi, S. (1993) Pflügers Arch. 422, 295–304
30. Peaker, M. and Neville, M.C. (1991) J. Endocrinol. 131, 1–3
31. Grosvenor, C.E., Picciano, M.F. and Baumrucker, C.R. (1992) Endocrinol. Rev. 14, 710–728

Biochem. Soc. Symp. **63**, 81–90
Printed in Great Britain

7

Autocrine regulation of milk secretion

Colin J. Wilde*, Caroline V.P Addey, Jane M. Bryson,

Lynn M.B. Finch, Christopher H. Knight and

Malcolm Peaker

Hannah Research Institute, Ayr, Scotland KA6 5HL, U.K.

Abstract

Mammary development and the rate of milk secretion are regulated by frequency and completeness of milk removal. This regulation occurs through chemical feedback inhibition by a milk constituent. Novel, immunologically related milk proteins able to perform this function have been isolated from caprine, bovine and human milk, based on their ability to inhibit milk constituent synthesis in mammary tissue and cell cultures, and to decrease temporarily milk secretion when added to milk stored in the mammary gland. Inhibition is concentration-dependent, suggesting that milk accumulation and removal is accompanied by cyclical changes in inhibitor accretion and depletion in milk. Feedback inhibition is an autocrine mechanism: the caprine inhibitor, termed FIL (feedback inhibitor of lactation) is synthesized by mammary epithelial cells in primary culture. Inhibition is by reversible blockade of the secretory pathway, an effect which, by down-regulating cell-surface hormone receptors, has longer-term consequences on epithelial cell differentiation. Treatment of goat mammary epithelial cell cultures with caprine FIL initially decreased milk protein secretion and subsequently reduced milk protein messenger RNA abundance. Thus the actions of a single milk constituent can bring about both the effect of milking frequency on milk secretion rate and a sequential modulation of cellular differentiation which acts to sustain the secretory response. Long-term regulation, through changes in galactopoietic hormone receptors, also provides an efficient mechanism for integrating acute intramammary regulation of lactation with strategic endocrine control of mammary tissue development.

* To whom correspondence should be addressed.

Introduction

Mammary development and milk secretion are regulated by a complex interaction of steroid and polypeptide hormones. Endocrine control is primarily strategic, signalling the limit to milk secretion set by the genetic background, nutrition and environment of the lactating animal. This strategic control of lactation is modulated by local mechanisms operating within each mammary gland. The classic example of mammary glands functioning independently is the macropod marsupial, which can produce milk of different compositions and at vastly different rates from adjacent mammary glands to feed young at different stages of development [1]. This functional asynchrony is apparent at the cellular and molecular levels: in the tammar wallaby, asynchronously lactating glands differ both in the number of secretory epithelial cells and in their pattern of milk protein gene expression [2]. The local mechanism underpinning this remarkable lactational strategy is not known, but may not be unique to the marsupial. The transition from low to high milk production in marsupials is associated with a change to less frequent but more vigorous (and presumably more efficient) suckling by the offspring. Similarly, in goat mammary glands, a unilateral change in milking frequency or efficiency regulates the rate of milk secretion, milk protein mRNA abundance and mammary cell number ([3–5]; J.M. Bryson and C.J. Wilde, unpublished work). Thus, across evolutionarily divergent mammals, each mammary gland operates with a degree of autonomy conferred by removal of product, which may be evident as different rates of milk secretion, differing degrees of mammary development, or both. The possibilities for the local control of mammary function by milk removal are myriad, since the gland accommodates the extracellular storage of a secretion rich in biologically active substances [6,7]. In this chaper we focus on one local mechanism which provides both a means of regulating milk supply according to milk removal and a mechanism for co-ordinating the local developmental adaptations which act to maintain the secretory response to a sustained change in suckling or milking.

Identification of FIL, the feedback inhibitor of lactation

The physiological basis for the local regulation of milk secretion by a chemical in milk has been discussed in the previous chapter [8]. Essentially, the frequent milking of one gland of lactating goats stimulated milk secretion ipsilaterally by a mechanism that was neither endocrine nor related to gland distension. Instead, the results were compatible with the presence in milk of a chemical inhibitor whose removal by frequent milking stimulated milk secretion. Experiments with lactating goats also identified several of the criteria expected of a chemical feedback inhibitor: its action should be rapid (able to regulate milk secretion within hours or less), readily reversible, and co-ordinate, such that secretion rate but not composition of secretion is altered.

Mammary tissue explants in organ culture provided a convenient means of screening milk constituents for a putative inhibitor of milk secretion. Tissue explants were prepared from mid-pregnant rabbits and stimulated by lactogenic hormones to synthesize milk constituents; milk fractions and then individual milk constituents were tested for their ability to inhibit casein and lactose synthesis [9]. To complement physiological observations *in vivo*, the first experiments were carried out with goat's milk [10,11]. Inhibitory activity identified in crude milk fractions was associated with the whey proteins [10], and subsequent resolution by anion-exchange chromatography and chromatofocusing identified a single fraction that was able to inhibit lactose and casein synthesis with equal potency. This fraction represented a 40000-fold purification of both inhibitory activities compared with unfractionated whey, and contained a single protein. Structural analysis showed the inhibitor to be a small, acidic glycoprotein of M_r 7600. N-terminal amino acid analysis indicated no sequence identity with known milk proteins or with any recorded sequence. Therefore, based on its novelty and biological activity, the protein was named FIL – feedback inhibitor of lactation [11]. Subsequent studies of cow's milk [12,13] and human milk (C.J. Henderson and C.J. Wilde, unpublished work) have identified proteins with similar biological activity that share a number of molecular characteristics and immunological epitopes.

This inhibitory protein fulfils many of the criteria predicted by experiments *in vivo*. Inhibition in explant culture was apparent within 1 h of exposure to the whey protein, reversible within 1 h of transferring explants to normal culture medium, and concentration-dependent when the whey protein was added at levels approximating those in milk. On the other hand, whereas the inhibitor was competent to inhibit aqueous milk constituents, it had no effect on milk lipid synthesis *in vitro* ([10,14]; but see below). Importantly, FIL is synthesized by the secretory epithelial cells of the mammary gland. Synthesis was demonstrated in goat mammary cells cultured on a reconstituted basement derived from the Engelbreth–Holm–Swarm tumour (EHS matrix). On this substratum, primary mammary cells form mammospheres, multicellular structures in which cells are arranged peripherally around a central luminal space. Cell polarization results in vectorial protein secretion, with milk proteins being secreted preferentially into the luminal space [15,16]. In goat mammosphere cultures, FIL was secreted along with other milk proteins via the apical cell membrane, and was recovered in the luminal secretion [11]. Therefore the protein fulfilled the principal criterion of feedback inhibition, that of being locally produced and, potentially, independently regulated in each mammary gland.

Confirmation of FIL's biological activity

Inhibition of tissue explant function could be a phenomenon of the culture system, and of no more significance than the effects obtained *in vitro* with numerous other milk components. Physiological relevance depended on establishing that FIL was active in lactating animals, and that its concentration changed with milk accumulation and removal in a manner consistent with the acute regulation of milk secretion. The first of these criteria was demonstrated by injecting purified FIL through the teat canal into the mammary cistern of lactating goats. FIL produced a dose-dependent inhibition of milk secretion which persisted for up to 3 days after a single injection [11,17]. The effect occurred ipsilaterally in the treated glands, and was specific to FIL; larger amounts of other milk proteins had no effect on the milk secretion rate when injected by the same route [17].

In contrast to its effect on tissue explants, FIL treatment of lactating goats appeared to regulate milk constituents co-ordinately: the milk secretion rate decreased but milk composition was unaffected. This inconsistency was not restricted to explant culture: lipid synthesis in lactating mammary acini was also insensitive to FIL at concentrations which inhibited protein synthesis and secretion by more than 50% within 2 h [14]. The reason for this inconsistency between observations *in vivo* and *in vitro* may lie in the culture conditions adopted. Explant and acini culture both took place in the absence of triacyl-glycerol synthesis from exogenous fatty acids, which normally accounts for a high proportion of total mammary triacylglycerol secretion [18], and which regulates *de novo* lipid synthesis through an inhibitory mechanism similar to that described for medium-chain fatty acids [19,20]. Without this modulating influence, *de novo* fatty acid synthesis *in vitro* may have been rendered insensitive to factors that would normally regulate its activity *in vivo*.

The persistence of inhibition induced by a single injection of FIL, despite regular milking and the presumed clearance of exogenous protein, implies that the inhibitor is not an acute regulator of milk secretion. However, the response to intraductal injection must be considered in its physiological context. The presence of 'residual milk' in the gland after milk ejection and the kinetics of milk flow between the alveoli and cistern during milk accumulation [21,22] both conspire to slow inhibitor clearance. Indeed, the site of inhibitor storage has an important influence on the susceptibility of secretion to feedback inhibition [23]. Therefore a slow response [17] or the persistence of an effect with FIL treatment *in vivo* [11] reflects as much the processes of milk movement and storage as cell responsiveness to FIL. Milk movement and storage also dictate that feedback inhibition cannot be simply a matter of secretion of the inhibitor and its removal during milking. Incomplete milking necessitates some form of inhibitor processing, either inactivation of secreted inhibitor or activation of a precursor form; otherwise FIL in residual milk would prevent cyclical variation in feedback with milk accumulation and removal [24]. How these factors together regulate the endogenous FIL concentration during milk accumulation and removal, or influence the clearance of exogenous FIL, is currently under investigation. However, measurement of bovine FIL has suggested that milk storage in the gland is accompanied by FIL accumulation. Conversely, continuous milk removal by catheter milking prevented any increase in feedback inhibition (P. Irving, K. Stelwagen, S.R. Davis and C.J. Wilde, unpublished work).

Mechanism of feedback inhibition

Feedback regulation by exogenous FIL in stored milk, and indeed the absolute requirement for milk removal in the local control of milk secretion [3], suggests that FIL acts after, rather than during, secretion. It also implies that the mammary epithelial cell possesses an apical receptor for the secreted inhibitor. The effectiveness of active immunization against FIL in lactating goats supports such a mechanism. Systemic antibody was ineffective, but when antibody against FIL was present in milk, the decline in milk yield expected in late lactation was slower, and immunized goats showed a greater tolerance of once-daily milking [25]. Therefore antibody against FIL acted to neutralize feedback inhibition and increase milk yield, but only when the antibody was present in milk.

Experiments with primary cultures of mammary epithelial cells suggest that the putative receptor is located predominantly on the apical surface of the luminal epithelial cell. Protein synthesis and secretion in mammary epithelial cells from lactating mice were inhibited by caprine FIL when the cells were cultured in suspension as acini [14]. In contrast, FIL preparations which potently inhibited acini function had a negligible effect on mouse mammary epithelial cells cultured as mammospheres on an EHS matrix (D.R. Blatchford and C.J. Wilde, unpublished work). Adjacent cells in mammospheres form tight intercellular junctions, such that proteins in the culture medium are excluded from the luminal space of the structure [15,16]. We have interpreted the apparent FIL-insensitivity of mammosphere cultures to indicate a lack of access to an apical receptor. Accordingly, when FIL was allowed access to the luminal space by transient opening of intercellular tight junctions, protein secretion was inhibited, as in acini cultures. Direct evidence for a cell-surface FIL receptor from radioligand binding studies is supportive but thus far not definitive. Only low specific radioactivities have been obtained with a variety of labelling methods, and alternative approaches are currently being tested.

The intracellular signal transduction of autocrine feedback is as yet uncharacterized and, in view of FIL's virtually unparalleled mode of action, is not easily predicted. The inhibitor acts primarily by inhibiting the constitutive secretion of milk constituents. This was demonstrated by pulse–chase radiolabelling experiments in mammary acini cultures. FIL inhibited the secretion of pre-formed radiolabelled secretory protein by blocking the early stages of the secretory pathway at the level of endoplasmic reticulum-to-Golgi transport [14]. Calcium-dependent regulated secretion, which involves the later stages of the secretory pathway [26], was independent of the actions of FIL [14]. Blockade of secretion was rapid (within 1 h) and accompanied by dramatic alterations in the cells' ultrastructure: the Golgi apparatus was dispersed through the cytoplasm, and the endoplasmic reticulum became vesiculated and in places distended. Nevertheless, within 1 h of FIL removal, the structural organization of lactating mammary epithelial cells was re-established. Concurrently, protein secretion, inhibited by up to 50% in the presence of FIL, recovered to its pretreatment level. This appears to be the first recorded example of the physiological regulation of a constitutive secretory pathway.

FIL's other effects on the mammary epithelial cell appear to be consequent upon the protein's primary action on the secretory pathway. By analogy with the effects of the fungal drug brefeldin A, an agent that disrupts membrane trafficking between the endoplasmic reticulum and the Golgi, FIL may also be competent to inhibit protein synthesis. Brefeldin A causes retrograde transport of *cis*-, medial and *trans*-Golgi elements (but not *trans*-Golgi network enzymes) back to the endoplasmic reticulum, and inhibits protein secretion in other cell types [27,28]. Brefeldin A mimicked the effect of FIL on mammary protein secretion and also inhibited mammary protein synthesis [14]. An effect of FIL on vesicular transport would then explain its co-ordinated effects on the synthesis and secretion of non-milk constituents. Early disruption of the secretory pathway may also explain FIL's ability to induce intracellular casein degradation *in vivo* and *in vitro* [29,30]. Intracellular degradation of secretory protein was observed in CHO and COS cell lines and in mouse L-cell cultures when protein transport between the endoplasmic reticulum and Golgi apparatus was inhibited [31].

Autocrine feedback in the regulation of mammary development

Autocrine disruption of membrane trafficking also affects the subcellular location of other constituents of the mammary cell, including its complement of hormone receptors. In mammary acini cultures, FIL not only inhibited protein secretion but also rapidly down-regulated mammary prolactin receptors [32]. Down-regulation of prolactin receptors was not itself the cause of inhibited secretion. Neither protein synthesis nor secretion in short-term acini cultures is prolactin-dependent. In the longer term, however, decreased sensitivity to circulating prolactin may have a profound effect on mammary cell function and tissue development. Treatment of rabbit mammary glands with FIL, or milk fractions containing FIL, by intraductal injection not only inhibited the rate of milk secretion [33] but also down-regulated prolactin binding (C.N. Bennett and C.H. Knight, unpublished work), and decreased cellular differentiation [33]. This suggested that a change in autocrine feedback by FIL, by modulating sensitivity to circulating hormones, may account for the secondary (in chronological terms) differentiative response to changes in milking frequency demonstrated in lactating goats as local changes in key enzyme activities [34,35] and abundance of lipogenic enzyme and milk protein mRNAs ([5]; J.M. Bryson and C.J. Wilde, unpublished work). Autocrine modulation of endocrine control is supported by observations *in vivo*: thrice- instead of twice-daily milking of lactating goats for 4 weeks increased total prolactin binding; conversely, incomplete milking decreased prolactin binding [36].

The ability of FIL to regulate mammary cell differentiation has been confirmed in primary cell cultures. Cell differentiation, measured by the induction of milk protein synthesis and lipogenic enzyme activities, was inhibited in mouse mammary epithelial cells cultured with lactogenic hormones on floating collagen gels [37]. Similarly, treatment of goat mammosphere cultures with purified goat FIL for 3 days decreased the abundance of mRNAs encoding α_{S1}-casein and α-lactalbumin (L.M.B. Finch, J.M. Bryson and C.J. Wilde, unpublished work).

Feedback regulation of mammary cell number

The ability of FIL to down-regulate prolactin receptors may, in addition, regulate the size of the secretory cell population. Prolactin appears to act as a cell-survival factor in rodent mammary tissue, inhibiting the induction of programmed cell death and the decline in tissue DNA content during mammary involution [38]. Conversely, DNA laddering, the classic indicator of programmed cell death, was induced within 48 h in the mammary tissue of lactating rats made prolactin-deficient by bromocriptine treatment [39]. This increase in DNA laddering was prevented by prolactin replacement after 24 h of hormone depletion. Whether prolactin, modulated locally by FIL, performs a similar role in ruminant mammary tissue is not known. Ultimately, however, the effect of milking frequency on milk yield is sustained by a change in mammary cell number [34]. In glands of lactating goats milked thrice- instead of twice-daily, this was achieved in part by ipsilateral stimulation of cell proliferation [34]. On the other hand, a significant effect on cell number was realized only in late lactation, when cell numbers had decreased in both twice- and thrice-milked glands with stage of lactation. Therefore the response was seen not as a net increase in cell number but as decreased cell loss. There is now evidence that goat mammary cell loss after peak lactation occurs by apoptosis. DNA laddering, indicative of apoptosis, has been observed in lactating ruminant mammary tissue [40], as well as in rodent tissue after peak lactation [41]. Moreover, apoptosis can be stimulated by a mechanism sensitive to milk stasis in both rodent and ruminant glands [40,42]. Therefore local control of mammary cell number by milking frequency could plausibly be attributed in part to the regulation of mammary apoptosis, and be mediated by a milk-borne factor such as FIL through its ability to modulate local sensitivity to systemic cell-survival factors. Another candidate regulator is an insulin-like growth factor binding protein (IGFBP) similar to IGFBP-5, which is induced with apoptosis during mammary involution [39,43,44]. The IGFBP would be expected to neutralize IGF-I, a mammary mitogen [45] and a cell-survival factor in a number of tissues [46–48].

A note of caution is appropriate. As discussed elsewhere [8], developmental mechanisms influenced by the acute chemical regulation of milk secretion are not necessarily the same as those induced chronically by milk stasis. The former may indeed influence mammary apoptosis, but the proven ability of the latter to do so may be as much to do with the physical effect of milk stasis on mammary gland distension. Indeed, experiments in lactating goats suggest that it is mammary distension that precipitates tissue involution and, presumably, the cell death associated with it [49]. The circumstances of cell death during lactation and involution differ in significant respects. Milk stasis causes loss of alveolar structure and basement membrane integrity [41], induced by extracellular protease activities [50–52]. In contrast, mouse mammary cell death during lactation occurs without any gross disruption of the epithelium, and is not co-ordinated at an alveolar level, i.e. it cannot be attributed to localized milk stasis. Instead, apoptotic cells in lactating mouse mammary tissue lie adjacent to apparently healthy, actively secreting epithelial cells [41]. If, therefore, cell survival in lactation is indeed regulated by the frequency of milk removal, the mechanism may perhaps be quite different from that of milk stasis, with the former influencing the susceptibility of individual cells to apoptosis through locally active chemical factors, and the latter inducing cell death through mechanical deformation of the mammary epithelium.

Again, however, a note of caution is necessary. The hierarchy of endocrine and local control mechanisms, and the relative importance of chemical feedback and mammary distension, may differ between species, depending upon such factors as physiological range of suckling or milking interval, gland anatomy and the intracellular half-life of endocrine or autocrine signals [8]. Acute regulation of milk supply by FIL may be common to most, if not all, mammals: FIL-like activity has been detected in species as evolutionarily divergent as the dairy cow [12,13] and the tammar wallaby [2]. Chronic regulation involved in arresting secretion may, however, differ between species, in some cases (the goat, for example) being induced primarily by gland distension, but in others, such as the rodent, being more dependent on galactopoietic hormone withdrawal, either systemically or at the tissue level through local receptor down-regulation.

Conclusion

This chapter describes the sequential changes in milk secretion and mammary development elicited by the frequency and completeness of milk removal, and the evidence that this regulation involves chemical feedback by a novel protein in milk. Clearly, feedback inhibition does not act in isolation, and further study is needed to establish how autocrine control by FIL is integrated with the systemic endocrine control of lactation, and how it interacts with other local mechanisms (chemical and physical) that influence mammary function. Nevertheless, autocrine control arguably provides a coherent explanation for one of the established phenomena in lactation, that of matching milk supply to demand. Moreover, the detection of FIL-like activity in ruminants, humans and the tammar wallaby suggests that this mechanism is conserved among mammals. Thus the apparently unique lactational strategy of the macropod marsupials may eventually be seen as an example of autocrine control *par excellence*.

This work was funded by the Scottish Office Agriculture, Environment and Fisheries Department.

References

1.   Nicholas, K.R. (1988) Biochem. Biophys. Res. Commun. **154**, 529–536
2.   Nicholas, K.R., Wilde, C.J., Bird, P.H., Hendry, K.A.K., Tregenza, K. and Warner, B. (1995) in Intercellular Signalling in the Mammary Gland (Wilde, C.J., Peaker, M. and Knight, C.H., eds.), pp. 153–170, Plenum Press, New York
3.   Peaker, M. (1995) in Intercellular Signalling in the Mammary Gland (Wilde, C.J., Peaker, M. and Knight, C.H., eds.), pp. 193–202, Plenum Press, New York

4. Knight, C.H. and Wilde, C.J. (1993) Livestock Prod. Sci. **35**, 3–19
5. Travers, M.T. and Barber, M.C. (1993) Comp. Biochem. Physiol. **105B**, 123–128
6. Peaker, M. and Neville, M.C. (1991) J. Endocrinol. **131**, 1–3
7. Grosvenor, C.E., Picciano M.F. and Baumrucker, C.R. (1992) Endocr. Rev. **14**, 710–728
8. Peaker, M., Wilde, C.J. and Knight, C.H. (1997) Biochem. Soc. Symp. **63**, 71–79
9. Dils, R.R. and Forsyth, I.A. (1981) Methods Enzymol. **72**, 724–742
10. Wilde, C.J., Daly, A., Calvert, D.T. and Peaker, M. (1987) Biochem. J. **242**, 285–288
11. Wilde, C.J., Addey, C.V.P., Boddy, L.M. and Peaker, M. (1995) Biochem. J. **305**, 51–58
12. Addey, C.V.P., Peaker, M. and Wilde, C.J. (1991) U.K. Patent GB 2 238 052
13. Addey, C.V.P., Peaker, M. and Wilde, C.J. (1995) U.S. Patent SN 08/395,535
14. Rennison, M.E., Kerr, M., Addey, C.V.P., Handel, S.E., Turner, M.D., Wilde, C.J. and Burgoyne, R.D. (1993) J. Cell Sci. **106**, 641–648
15. Barcellos-Hoff, M.H., Aggeler, J., Ram, T.G. and Bissell, M.J. (1989) Development **105**, 223–235
16. Hurley, W.L., Blatchford, D.R., Hendry, K.A.K. and Wilde, C.J. (1994) In Vitro Cell. Dev. Biol. **30A**, 529–538
17. Wilde, C.J., Addey, C.V.P., Casey, M.J., Blatchford, D.R. and Peaker, M. (1988) Q. J. Exp. Physiol. **73**, 391–397
18. Hawkins, R.A. and Williamson, D.H. (1972) Biochem. J. **129**, 1171–1173
19. Heesom, K.J., Souza, P.F.A., Ilic, V. and Williamson, D.H. (1992) Biochem. J. **281**, 273–278
20. Williamson, D.H., Ilic, V. and Lund P. (1995) in Intercellular Signalling in the Mammary Gland (Wilde, C.J., Peaker, M. and Knight, C.H., eds.), pp. 239–251, Plenum Press, New York
21. Knight, C.H. and Dewhurst, R.D. (1994) J. Dairy Res. **61**, 167–177
22. Knight, C.H. and Dewhurst, R.D. (1994) J. Dairy Res. **61**, 441–449
23. Knight, C.H. (1995) in Intercellular Signalling in the Mammary Gland (Wilde, C.J., Peaker, M. and Knight, C.H., eds.), pp. 1–11, Plenum Press, New York
24. Wilde, C.J., Knight, C.H. and Peaker, M. (1996) in Progress in Dairy Science (Phillips, C.J.C., ed.), pp. 311–332, CAB International, Wallingford
25. Wilde, C.J., Addey, C.V.P. and Peaker, M. (1996) J. Physiol. (London) **491**, 465–469
26. Turner, M.D., Rennison, M.E., Handel, S.E., Wilde, C.J. and Burgoyne, R.D. (1992) J. Cell Biol. **117**, 269–278
27. Lippincott-Schwartz, J., Juan, L., Bonifacino, J.S. and Klausner, R.D. (1989) Cell **56**, 801–813
28. Orci, L., Tagaya, M. Amherdt, M., Perrelet, A., Donaldson, J.G., Lippincott-Schwartz, J., Klausner, R. and Rothman, J.E. (1991) Cell **64**, 1183–1195
29. Stewart, G.M., Addey, C.V.P., Knight, C.H. and Wilde, C.J. (1988) J. Endocrinol. **118**, R1–R3
30. Wilde, C.J., Addey, C.V.P. and Knight, C.H. (1989) Biochim. Biophys. Acta **992**, 315–319
31. Wileman, T., Kane, L.P., Carson, G.R. and Terhorst, C. (1991) J. Biol. Chem. **266**, 4500–4507
32. Bennett, C.N., Knight, C.H. and Wilde, C.J. (1991) J. Endocrinol. **127** (Suppl.), 141
33. Wilde, C.J., Calvert, D.T. and Peaker, M. (1988) Biochem. Soc. Trans. **15**, 916–917
34. Wilde, C.J., Henderson, A.J., Knight, C.H., Blatchford, D.R., Faulkner, A. and Vernon, R.G. (1987) J. Anim. Sci. **64**, 533–539
35. Wilde, C.J. and Knight, C.H. (1990) J. Dairy Res. **57**, 441–447
36. McKinnon, J., Knight, C.H., Flint, D.J. and Wilde, C.J. (1988) J. Endocrinol. **119** (Suppl.), 167
37. Wilde, C.J., Blatchford, D.R. and Peaker, M. (1991) Exp. Physiol. **76**, 379–387
38. Sheffield, L.G. and Kotolski, L.C. (1992) FASEB J. **6**, A1184
39. Travers, M.T., Barber, M.C., Tonner, E., Quarrie, L.H., Wilde, C.J. and Flint, D.J. (1996) Endocrinology **137**, 1530–1539

40.	Quarrie, L.H., Addey, C.V.P. and Wilde, C.J. (1994) Biochem. Soc. Trans. **22**, 178S

41.	Quarrie, L.H., Addey, C.V.P. and Wilde, C.J. (1995) Cell Tissue Res. **281**, 413–419

42.	Quarrie, L.H., Addey, C.V.P. and Wilde, C.J. (1995) in Intercellular Signalling in the Mammary Gland (Wilde, C.J., Peaker, M. and Knight, C.H., eds.), pp. 95–96, Plenum Press, New York

43.	Guenette, R.S. and Tenniswood, M. (1995) J. Cell. Biochem. Suppl. **19B**, 280

44.	Tonner, E., Beattie, J. and Flint, D.J. (1995) in Intercellular Signalling in the Mammary Gland (Wilde, C.J., Peaker, M. and Knight, C.H., eds.), pp. 103–104, Plenum Press, New York

45.	McGrath, M.F., Collier, R.J., Clemmons, D.R., Busby, W.H., Sweeney, C.A. and Krivi, G.G. (1991) Endocrinology **129**, 671–678

46.	Rodriguez-Tarduchy, G., Collins, M.K.L., Garcia, I. and Lopez-Rivas, A. (1992) J. Immunol. **149**, 535–540

47.	Drago, J., Murphy, M., Carroll, S.M., Harvey, R.P. and Bartlett, P.F. (1991) Proc. Natl. Acad. Sci. U.S.A. **88**, 2199–2203

48.	Sell, C., Baserga, R. and Rubin, R. (1995) Cancer Res. **55**, 303–306

49.	Peaker, M. (1980) J. Physiol. (London) **301**, 415–418

50.	Talhouk, R.S., Chin, J.R., Unemori, E.N., Werb, Z. and Bissell, M.J. (1991) Development **112**, 439–449

51.	Talhouk, R.S., Bissell, M.J. and Werb, Z. (1992) J. Cell Biol. **118**, 1271–1282

52.	Strange, R., Li, F., Saurer, S., Burkhardt, A. and Friis, R.R. (1992) Development **115**, 49–58

Biochem. Soc. Symp. **63**, 91–100
Printed in Great Britain

8

Role of calcium in the pathway for milk protein secretion and possible relevance for mammary gland physiology

**Robert D. Burgoyne*, Jennifer S. Duncan
and Allan W. Sudlow**

The Physiological Laboratory, University of Liverpool, Crown Street,
Liverpool L69 3BX, U.K.

Abstract

In an attempt to define control points within the secretory pathway for casein synthesis and secretion, we have examined the role of both cytosolic and intra-organelle Ca^{2+} in the control of casein synthesis, phosphorylation and secretion. In addition, the possible role of cell volume changes in stretch-activation of Ca^{2+} signals was examined. Examination of the kinetics of casein secretion from freshly isolated lactating mouse mammary acini showed that a portion of the newly synthesized casein was secreted in a constitutive manner. A further portion remained within the cells, and this was released following elevation of the intracellular free calcium concentration ($[Ca^{2+}]_i$) using iono-mycin, indicating the presence of a Ca^{2+}-regulated pathway for casein release. An increase in $[Ca^{2+}]_i$ occurred in response to hypotonic challenge to induce cell swelling, and this involved both Ca^{2+} entry and Ca^{2+} mobilization from intracellular stores. Experiments examining the effects of depletion of intra-organelle Ca^{2+} indicated that intra-organelle Ca^{2+} was required for maintained casein phosphorylation, but not its secretion. Depletion of Ca^{2+} from the endo-plasmic reticulum led to a marked inhibition of casein synthesis. The possible significance of these control mechanisms for the physiology of the mammary gland is discussed.

---

* To whom correspondence should be addressed.

Introduction

Proteins destined to be secreted are synthesized on and translocated into the endoplasmic reticulum (ER), post-translationally modified and packed in the Golgi complex, and transported to the cell surface in secretory vesicles. The exocytotic fusion of the vesicle with the plasma membrane to release the secretory proteins can occur in a constitutive manner immediately after the newly synthesized vesicles reach the plasma membrane, or in a regulated manner [1]. In regulated exocytosis, a distinct population of secretory vesicles remains within the cell until the appropriate external and intracellular signals are received, when exocytosis then proceeds [2]. In many specialized secretory cell types, regulated exocytosis is triggered by a rise in the intracellular free Ca^{2+} concentration ($[Ca^{2+}]_i$) following cell activation.

During lactation, mammary epithelial cells synthesize and secrete large amounts of milk constituents, including the milk proteins, which are mainly the caseins. Considerable information is available on the factors that regulate the differentiation of mammary epithelial cells prior to lactation and the onset of tissue-specific expression of genes encoding milk proteins [3,4]. In addition, the mechanisms underlying the milk-ejection reflex, by which oxytocin stimulates the contraction of myoepithelial cells surrounding the epithelial cell acini leading to expulsion of milk from the lumen of the mammary acini and passage through the mammary gland ductal system, are well known [5]. In contrast, much less is known about the acute regulation of milk protein synthesis and secretion from lactating mammary epithelial cells. There is clear evidence for the local control of milk secretion [6] and marked differences in milk protein gene expression between distended and empty mammary alveoli [7], suggesting that regulatory mechanisms for the acute control of epithelial cell function do exist. Feedback control of milk protein synthesis and secretion may, at least in part, be due to the actions of a secreted milk protein known as the feedback inhibitor of lactation (FIL) [8–11], which appears to function by disrupting aspects of vesicular traffic, leading to inhibition of casein synthesis and secretion [11]. We explore here the potential role of cytoplasmic and intra-organelle Ca^{2+} in the regulation of the secretory pathway in lactating mouse mammary epithelial cells in an attempt to identify control points in the secretory pathway of mammary cells that could be of physiological relevance for the regulation of mammary gland function.

Cytoplasmic Ca^{2+} in the control of exocytosis in lactating mammary cells

We used freshly isolated acini from lactating mouse mammary gland to examine the kinetics of casein synthesis and secretion [12]. From examination of [^{35}S]methionine labelling it was found that the caseins were the predominant newly synthesized proteins present in the cells (around 80% of labelled protein), as well as being the major proteins secreted into the cell medium. Secretion of [^{35}S]methionine-labelled protein into the medium was detectable after a lag period of around 45–60 min and continued thereafter in an essentially linear fashion for at least 5 h [12,13]. This release of labelled protein was due to secretion and not cell damage, as it was both temperature-dependent and dependent upon microtubule integrity, being almost completely abolished by treatment with the anti-microtubule agent nocodazole [13]. The kinetics observed were consistent with those expected for constitutive secretion, with a transit time for newly synthesized protein through the secretory pathway from the ER to the cell surface of 45–60 min. In pulse–chase experiments, however, the data were not consistent with a purely constitutive route for casein secretion. In these experiments cells were pulse-labelled with [35S]methionine, the [35S]methionine removed and secretion of prelabelled protein followed over time. During the chase period, secretion was complete within 1 h, but only 30–40% of total newly synthesized protein was secreted, leaving a considerable proportion of newly synthesized casein still within the cells [12].

In order to determine whether additional casein secretion could be elicited, after the burst of constitutive secretion, by activation of second messenger pathways, the acini were treated with cyclic nucleotide analogues, phorbol esters to activate protein kinase C, or the Ca^{2+} ionophore ionomycin to elevate $[Ca^{2+}]_i$. Neither cyclic nucleotide analogues nor the phorbol ester PMA had any effect on secretion, but additional secretion was elicited by ionomycin in the presence but not the absence of external Ca^{2+}. The data demonstrated, therefore, the presence of a Ca^{2+}-regulated pathway for casein secretion which could be triggered after constitutive secretion was complete [12]. It should also be noted that the well known electron microscopical appearance of lactating mammary epithelial cells, with many secretory vesicles being present, is typical of a regulated secretory cell with stored secretory vesicles [14]. It appears, therefore, that casein secretion occurs by both constitutive and regulated exocytotic pathways. The constitutive pathway is distinct from the regulated pathway in mammary cells, since it is unaffected by intracellular chelation of Ca^{2+} using the membrane-permeant chelator BAPTA-AM [bis-(o-aminophenoxy)ethane-N,N,N',N'-tetra-acetic acid] [12]. Direct demonstration of Ca^{2+}-regulated exocytosis and a Ca^{2+}-independent pathway for exocytosis also came from an alternative approach using digitonin-permeabilized mammary acini, which allowed direct control of $[Ca^{2+}]_i$ [15]. The presence of Ca^{2+}-regulated exocytosis responsive to ionomycin has also been demonstrated in polarized mammary cells differentiated in Engelbreth–-Holm–Swarm (EHS)-matrix cultures [16].

Regulation of $[Ca^{2+}]_i$ in lactating mammary cells: role of cell swelling

Since lactating mouse mammary epithelial cells appear to be able to store casein-containing secretory vesicles and to release caseins following elevation of $[Ca^{2+}]_i$ with a Ca^{2+} ionophore, it seemed likely that this forms part of a physiological control mechanism for casein secretion. The question that arises, therefore, is what physiological regulator leads to elevated $[Ca^{2+}]_i$ in lactating mammary cells and activates casein secretion? Neither prolactin nor oxytocin had any stimulatory effect on the secretion of [35S]methionine-labelled casein from isolated mouse acini [14]. In contrast, Da Costa et al. [17] reported that oxytocin stimulated the release of lipid and protein from rat mammary gland slices. This effect may not have been due to stimulation of casein exocytosis, however, but instead to myoepithelial cell contraction in response to oxytocin expelling already secreted proteins from the alveolar lumen in the slices. Similarly, the reported small effects of prolactin on protein secretion from rabbit mammary gland fragments [18] has been suggested [17] to occur in a similar way due to contaminating oxytocin in the high amount of prolactin used in that study [18].

Lactating mammary cells have been shown to possess $Ins(1,4,5)P_3$-sensitive cytosolic Ca^{2+} stores [19,20], which opens up the possibility of hormonal regulation of $[Ca^{2+}]$ via these stores. Experimental manipulation of intracellular Ca^{2+} stores in mammary cells to mobilize their Ca^{2+} content, however, produces only a small and transient rise in $[Ca^{2+}]_i$ which is insufficient to activate casein exocytosis [21]. So far, no receptor agonists have been convincingly identified that directly stimulate Ca^{2+}-regulated secretion of casein from lactating mammary cells.

In many cell types, cell swelling or mechanical stimulation leads to activation of stretch-activated plasma membrane channels and Ca^{2+} entry, resulting in increased $[Ca^{2+}]_i$ [22]. Following the let-down reflex and the emptying of the aveolar lumen, the mammary epithelial cells have a columnar morphology and, as milk constituents are secreted into the lumen, the alveolus becomes distended and the epithelial cells become stretched and flattened [5]. Finally, myoepithelial cell contraction leads to emptying of the alveolar lumen and would also result in mechanical stimulation of the epithelial cells. We have, therefore, examined the possibility that lactating mammary cells would respond to cell volume changes or membrane stretching with a $[Ca^{2+}]_i$ elevation [22a].

Cell swelling can be conveniently achieved by experimental dilution of cells into a hypotonic medium. In order to determine the effect of this experimental manipulation, lactating mammary acini were loaded with the fluorescent Ca^{2+} indicator fura 2 and $[Ca^{2+}]_i$ was monitored over time. Dilution of the acini suspension with water to produce cell swelling led to a marked and rapid rise in $[Ca^{2+}]_i$, as seen in other epithelial cell types [22], with an initial transient peak declining to a new sustained plateau of elevated $[Ca^{2+}]_i$ (Fig. 1). This effect was due to hyposmotic effects rather than to ionic dilution, as dilution with sucrose did not affect $[Ca^{2+}]_i$ (Fig. 1). In contrast, cell shrinkage caused by dilution into hypertonic medium did not elicit any changes in $[Ca^{2+}]_i$. The hyposmotically induced $[Ca^{2+}]_i$ elevation was substantially reduced by pretreatment with gadolinium, which is a blocker of non-specific cation channels, and abolished by removal of external Ca^{2+}, but the initial transient was unaffected by prior emptying of internal Ca^{2+} stores using the ER Ca^{2+}-ATPase inhibitor thapsigargin [22a]. These data suggest, therefore, that cell swelling initially activated a pathway for the entry of external Ca^{2+} into the lactating acini, and may also have resulted in subsequent mobilization of Ca^{2+} from intracellular Ca^{2+} stores. It had previously been shown that mechanical stimulation of undifferentiated mammary cells in culture leads to an increase in

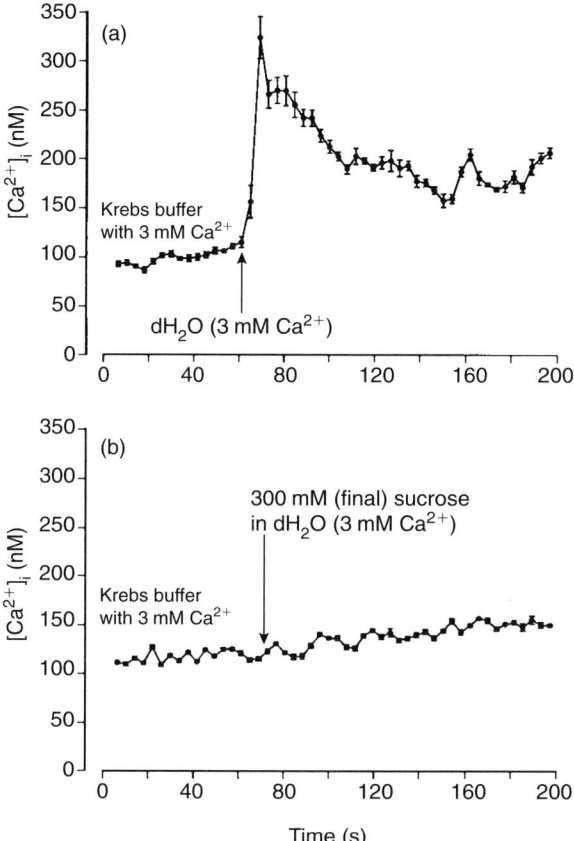

Fig. 1. Changes in [Ca^{2+}]$_i$ induced by cell swelling in lactating mammary acini. Isolated acini from lactating mouse mammary gland were loaded with the fluorescent Ca^{2+} indicator fura 2 to allow monitoring of [Ca^{2+}]$_i$. Hypotonic dilution of the cells (a) led to a rise in [Ca^{2+}]$_i$ comprising an initial transient peak and a sustained plateau of increased [Ca^{2+}]$_i$. Ionic dilution did not affect [Ca^{2+}]$_i$ (b). dH$_2$O, distilled water.

[Ca^{2+}]$_i$ [23]. The exact identity of the cells studied was unclear. In addition, the mechanisms involved differed from those involved in the [Ca^{2+}]$_i$ elevation in lactating acini, since the [Ca^{2+}]$_i$ rise was mostly due to release from internal Ca^{2+} stores and was propagated by ATP release. In contrast, we found that ATP had no effect on [Ca^{2+}]$_i$ in lactating acini.

It is not known whether cell volume/shape changes *in vivo* result in [Ca^{2+}]$_i$ elevations in mammary epithelial cells. This pathway could, however, be involved in the regulation of mammary epithelial cell function, and could possibly contribute to the differential regulation of gene expression in distended compared with empty acini [7] or to the mechanisms by which distension leads to the inhibition of protein synthesis and apoptosis during involution ([8]; see conclusions below).

Role of intra-organelle Ca²⁺ in the secretory pathway in lactating mammary cells

From experimental data on many cell types, it is known that Ca^{2+} is present at high concentrations within the lumen of the ER and the cisternae of the Golgi complex, as well as in various types of secretory vesicles (Fig. 2). Intra-organelle Ca^{2+} appears to have various roles in the secretory pathway, based on information from cell types in which this has been manipulated. Depletion of organelle Ca^{2+} leads to inhibition of protein synthesis [24], accelerated degradation of proteins in the ER [25], increased secretion of normally retained ER proteins [26] and reduced processing and secretion of α_1-antitrypsin in HepG2 cells [24]. These effects have been demonstrated by removal of extracellular Ca^{2+}, inhibition of ER Ca^{2+}-ATPases or treatment with Ca^{2+} ionophores in the absence of external Ca^{2+}. It is believed that Ca^{2+} within the ER and Golgi is important in the folding and stability of newly synthesized proteins and protein–protein interactions within these organelles that affect the traffic of secretory proteins.

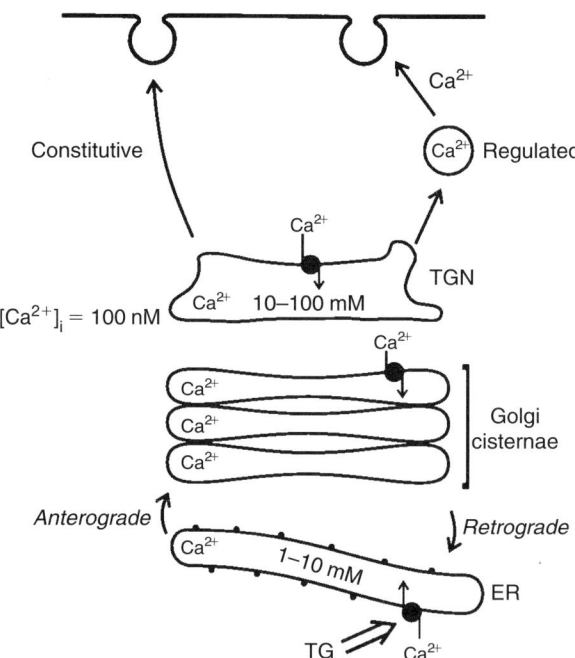

Fig. 2. General distribution of Ca²⁺ within cells. This schematic diagram is meant to show representative values of Ca^{2+} concentration in the cytoplasm and within intracellular organelles, based on data from a range of cell types. The Ca^{2+} concentration is high within the ER, Golgi cisternae and the *trans*-Golgi network (TGN). The Ca^{2+}-ATPase of the ER is sensitive to the inhibitor thapsigargin (TG). The sensitivity of the Golgi Ca^{2+}-ATPase and its distribution are unknown.

We have examined the importance of intra-organelle Ca^{2+} in lactating mammary epithelial cells [21]. Ca^{2+} within the ER was depleted by treatment with the Ca^{2+}-ATPase inhibitors thapsigargin or 2,5-di-(t-butyl)-1,4-benzohydroquinone (tBHQ). In other experiments all organelle Ca^{2+} was depleted by treating cells with ionomycin and extracellular EGTA, which would also deplete cytosolic Ca^{2+}. All of these treatments led to transient elevations of $[Ca^{2+}]_i$ which returned to or below normal resting levels within minutes.

Depletion of ER Ca^{2+} by thapsigargin or tBHQ treatment inhibited protein synthesis in lactating mammary cells (Fig. 3), as previously seen in other cell types [24]; this was likely to be due to an inhibition of translation initiation, as shown by a loss of polysomes analysed following sucrose-gradient fraction-

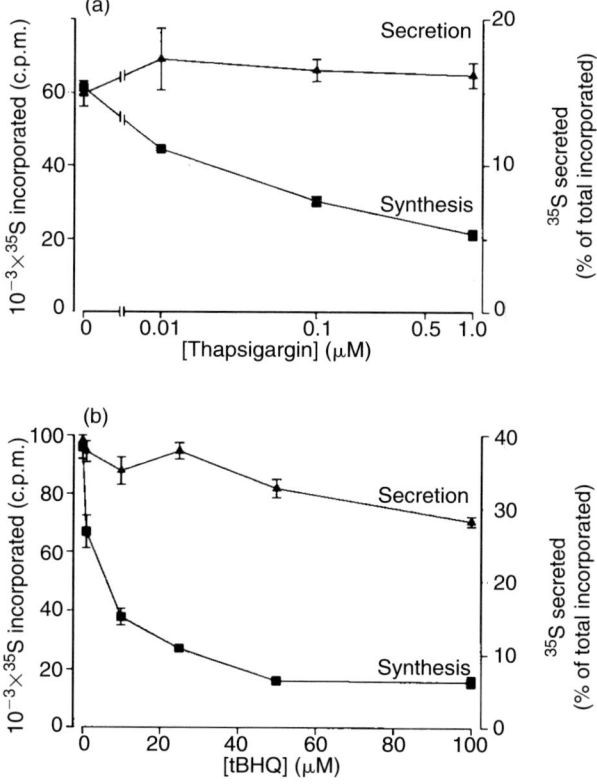

Fig. 3. Effects of thapsigargin and tBHQ on protein synthesis and secretion from lactating mammary acini. For the assay of the effects of thapsigargin (a) or tBHQ (b) on protein synthesis, isolated acini were incubated with the indicated concentrations of the drug and the extent of incorporation of [^{35}S]methionine into newly synthesized proteins over a 1 h period was determined. For the assay of the effects on protein secretion, the isolated acini were first pulse-labelled with [^{35}S]methionine for 1 h and then incubated with the indicated concentrations of the drugs during a subsequent 1 h chase period. Reproduced from [21], with permission.

ation [21]. Using pulse–chase protocols, the effect of Ca^{2+} depletion on casein phosphorylation and casein secretion was examined. Treatment with ionomycin/EGTA had no effect on an early stage of casein phosphorylation (over the first 30 min), but resulted in partial inhibition of a later phase (> 30 min) of casein phosphorylation. In contrast, the extent and time course of casein secretion was unaffected by thapsigargin, tBHQ or ionomycin/EGTA. These results indicate that Ca^{2+} is required for maintained casein synthesis and phosphorylation (the latter being consistent with previous data on the Ca^{2+}-dependency of casein kinases [27]), but not the transit through the secretory pathway of previously synthesized caseins [21].

Conclusions

Three major points emerge from the results described here. First, lactating mammary epithelial cells possess both a constitutive exocytotic mechanism for the release of casein and also a Ca^{2+}-regulated mechanism, indicating that the complete secretion of caseins into the alveolar lumen would require a signal leading to an increase in $[Ca^{2+}]_i$. Secondly, swelling (stretch) of lactating mammary cells activates a process leading to a Ca^{2+} signal comprising initial transient Ca^{2+} entry and also Ca^{2+} mobilization from intracellular stores. Thirdly, Ca^{2+} depletion from intracellular organelles has no effect on the transit of casein through the secretory pathway, but results in partial inhibition of a late phase of protein phosphorylation and a marked inhibition of casein synthesis. We do not currently have any direct evidence for the physiological relevance of these three potential control mechanisms for mammary cell function. It is not clear what signal would be responsible for Ca^{2+}-regulated secretion, and the only candidate signal that we have identified, stretch-induced Ca^{2+} entry, has not been directly linked to casein secretion. It has been suggested that hormones acting via mobilization of ER Ca^{2+} stores could regulate protein synthesis [28], and this possibility now exists also for lactating mammary cells, but no evidence for receptor-agonist-generated Ca^{2+} mobilization in lactating mammary cells is available.

Near to the end of lactation, the failure of milk withdrawal due to cessation of suckling leads to inhibition of milk protein synthesis and eventually cell death by apoptosis during the process of involution [8]. This may be mediated in part by the secreted milk protein FIL [8–11], but it has also been suggested that alveolar distension may generate signals leading to these events [29]. The results from our studies described here suggest one speculative mechanism for these events. This proposal is that distension of the alveoli due to milk accumulation in the lumen would lead to a stretch-activated response, with the generation of a Ca^{2+} signal such as that described here. If part of that signal involved emptying of the ER Ca^{2+} store, a consequence would be the inhibition of casein synthesis that is not maintained when the ER Ca^{2+} is depleted. The Ca^{2+} signal generated by prolonged distension of the aveoli would therefore play a role in the events leading to involution. While no direct evidence for this idea exists, it does lead to an additional testable question. Does the stretch-activated increase in $[Ca^{2+}]_i$ trigger the apoptosis of mammary cells which normally follows the inhibition of casein synthesis during the early stages of involution? The significance of stretch-activated changes in $[Ca^{2+}]_i$ in mammary cells for the control of casein synthesis and events leading to apoptosis and involution will be a fruitful area for future studies.

The work described here was supported by a BBSRC Link Award to R.D.B. and a Wellcome Trust Veterinary Clinical Training Award to J.S.D.

References

1. Burgess, T.L. and Kelly, R.B. (1987) Annu. Rev. Cell Biol. **3**, 243–293
2. Burgoyne, R.D. and Morgan, A. (1993) Biochem. J. **293**, 305–316
3. Burgoyne, R.D. and Wilde, C.J. (1994) Cell. Signalling **6**, 607–616
4. Groner, B. and Gouilleux, F. (1995) Curr. Opin. Genet. Dev. **5**, 587–594
5. Cowie, A.T. and Tindal, J.S. (1971) The Physiology of Lactation, Edward Arnold, London
6. Wilde, C.J., Knight, C.A., Addey, C.V.P., Blatchford, D.R., Travis, M., Bennett, C.N. and Peaker, M. (1990) Protoplasma **159**, 112–117
7. Faerman, A., Barash, I., Puzis, R., Nathan, M., Hurwitz, D.R. amd Shani, M. (1995) J. Histochem. Cytochem. **43**, 461–470
8. Peaker, M., Wilde, C.J. and Knight, C.H. (1997) Biochem. Soc. Symp. **63**, 71–79
9. Wilde, C.J., Addey, C.V.P., Bryson, J.M., Finch, L.M.B., Knight, C.H. and Peaker, M. (1997) Biochem. Soc. Symp. **63**, 81–90
10. Wilde, C.J., Addey, C.V.P., Boddy, L.M. and Peaker, M. (1995) Biochem. J. **305**, 51–58
11. Rennison, M.E., Kerr, M., Addey, C.V.P., Handel, S.E., Turner, M.D., Wilde, C.J. and Burgoyne, R.D. (1993) J. Cell Sci. **106**, 641–648
12. Turner, M.D., Rennison, M.E., Handel, S.E., Wilde, C.J. and Burgoyne, R.D. (1992) J. Cell Biol. **117**, 269–278
13. Rennison, M.E., Handel, S.E., Wilde, C.J. and Burgoyne, R.D. (1992) J. Cell Sci. **102**, 239–247
14. Burgoyne, R.D., Handel, S.E., Sudlow, A.W., et al. (Wilde, C.J., Peaker, M. and Knight, C.H., eds.), pp. 253–263, Plenum, New York
15. Turner, M.D., Wilde, C.J. and Burgoyne, R.D. (1992) Biochem. J. **286**, 13–15
16. Blatchford, D.R., Hendry, K.A.K., Turner, M.D., Burgoyne, R.D. and Wilde, C.J. (1995) Epithelial Cell Biol. **4**, 8–16
17. Da Costa, T.H.M., Taylor, K., Ilic, V. and Williamson, D.H. (1995) Biochem. J. **308**, 975–981
18. Ollivier-Bousquet, M. (1978) Cell Tissue Res. **187**, 25–43
19. Enomoto, K.-I., Furuya, K., Yamagishi, S. and Maeno, T. (1993) Cell Biochem. Funct. **11**, 55–62
20. Yoshimoto, A., Nakanishi, K., Anzai, T. and Komine, S. (1990) Cell Biochem. Funct. **8**, 191–198
21. Duncan, J.S. and Burgoyne, R.D. (1996) Biochem. J. **317**, 487–493
22. Hoffman, E.K. and Dunham, P.B. (1995) Int. Rev. Cytol. **161**, 173–262
22a. Sudlow, A.W. and Burgoyne, R.D. (1997) Pflugers Arch. **433**, 609–616
23. Enomoto, K., Furuya, K., Yamagishi, S., Oka, T. and Maeno, T. (1994) Pflugers Arch. **427**, 533–542
24. Wong, M.L., Brostrom, M.A., Kuznetsov, G., Gmitter-Yellen, D. and Brostrom, C.O. (1993) Biochem. J. **289**, 71–79

25. Wileman, T., Kane, L.P., Carson, G.R. and Terhorst, C. (1991) J. Biol. Chem. **266**, 4500–4507

26. Booth, C. and Koch, G.L.E. (1989) Cell **59**, 729–737

27. West, D.W. and Clegg, R.W. (1983) Eur. J. Biochem. **137**, 215–220

28. Brostrom, C.O. and Brostrom, M.A. (1990) Annu. Rev. Physiol. **52**, 577–590

29. Peaker, M. (1980) J. Physiol. (London) **301**, 415–428

Biochem. Soc. Symp. **63**, 101–113
Printed in Great Britain

9

Composite response elements mediate hormonal and developmental regulation of milk protein gene expression

Jeffrey M. Rosen*, Cynthia Zahnow, Alexander Kazansky
and Brian Raught

Department of Cell Biology, Baylor College of Medicine, Houston,
TX 77030-3498, U.S.A.

Abstract

Our laboratory has been studying the mechanisms by which hormones regulate the expression of differentiated function in the normal mammary gland and how these regulatory mechanisms have deviated in breast cancer. Two rat milk protein genes, encoding β-casein and whey acidic protein, have been employed as molecular markers of mammary epithelial cell differentiation. Composite response elements containing multiple binding sites for several transcription factors mediate the hormonal and developmental regulation of milk protein gene expression. In the whey protein gene promoters, these include binding sites for nuclear factor (NF)-I, as well as the glucocorticoid receptor (GR) and signal transducers and activators of transcription (Stat5). In the casein promoters, these include binding sites for Stat5, Yin Yang 1 (YY1), GR and the CCAAT/enhancer binding protein (C/EBP). The C/EBP family of DNA binding proteins may play a pivotal role in maintaining the balance between cell proliferation and terminal differentiation in mammary epithelial cells. During normal mammary gland development, expression of LIP (liver-enriched inhibitory protein, a dominant-negative isoform of C/EBPβ) is hormonally regulated and correlates with cell proliferation during pregnancy. LIP can form heterodimers with other C/EBP family members and suppress their transcriptional activity. In contrast, C/EBPα is predominantly expressed during lactation following terminal differentiation. Elevated LIP levels have been detected in mouse, rat and human breast tumours of different aetiologies. This provides a mechanism, therefore, to block terminal differentiation and facilitate continued proliferation.

* To whom correspondence should be addressed.

Introduction

An understanding of the mechanisms regulating the development of the normal mammary gland is required if we are to fully understand the aberrant regulatory mechanisms responsible for breast cancer. Previous studies in our laboratory have been directed at defining the mechanisms by which hormones regulate lactation; specifically, how peptide and steroid hormones act in a synergistic manner to regulate the expression of milk protein genes. Recent studies from several laboratories, including our own, have led to the identification of the important elements required for mammary-specific gene expression, and have provided new insights into the mechanism of synergy of prolactin and glucocorticoids in regulating milk protein gene expression (reviewed in [1]).

Composite response elements have been identified which have a modular structure that is conserved in most mammals. These elements are sometimes duplicated in the 5' flanking regions of the milk protein genes. In the casein promoters, these include binding sites for signal transducers and activators of transcription (Stat)5, Yin Yang 1 (YY1), CCAAT/enhancer binding protein (C/EBP) and the glucocorticoid receptor (GR) [2]. In the whey acidic protein (WAP) gene promoters, these include binding sites for nuclear factor (NF)-I, as well as the GR and Stat5 [3]. Thus tissue-specific expression does not appear to be mediated by the presence of a single factor, but instead requires co-operative interactions between several factors. These are mediated by both protein–DNA and protein–protein interactions. For example, direct protein–protein interactions have been demonstrated between the GR and both C/EBPα [4] and Stat5 (B. Groner, personal communication). Signal transduction pathways regulated by both peptide and steroid hormones play a critical role in transcription factor activation. Appropriate cell-specific regulation appears to require the interaction of both activators and repressors.

The following models have been proposed to explain the different kinetics of activation and the synergistic effects of glucocorticoids and prolactin on β-casein and WAP gene expression. For β-casein, glucocorticoids alter the ratio of the C/EBPβ liver-enriched inhibitory protein (LIP) and liver-enriched activating protein (LAP) isoforms [2], a slow process that requires ongoing protein synthesis. In contrast, prolactin rapidly activates Janus kinase 2 (JAK2) and Stat5 tyrosine phosphorylation, resulting in nuclear translocation and DNA binding. Direct C/EBP–GR and possibly Stat5–GR interactions facilitate the displacement of YY1 and hence transcriptional activation (Fig. 1).

For WAP, glucocorticoids rapidly induce changes in chromatin structure at the distal enhancer, facilitating the binding of NF-I [5]. Prolactin activation of Stat5 leads to a further enhancement of gene expression, and may again involve the direct interaction of Stat5 with the GR. These simplified models do not take into account the fact that additional positive (such as Ets/WAP and Oct-1/β-casein) and negative (single-stranded DNA binding proteins/β-casein) factors are also involved in the transcriptional regulation of these genes (reviewed in [6]). While less is known concerning the specific targets for insulin regulation of casein gene expression, this is most likely mediated through

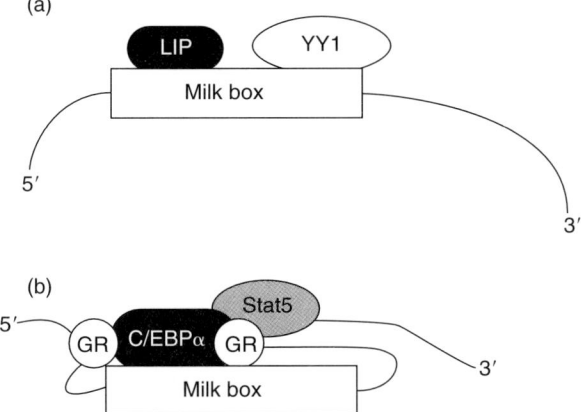

Fig. 1. Hormonal activation of casein gene expression. (a) A simplified model of the β-casein promoter 'milk box' region and its interaction with the transcription factors LIP and YY1, which repress transcription. (b) Activation of the β-casein promoter by glucocorticoids and prolactin results in a glucocorticoid-dependent switch in the C/EBPβ isoforms from LIP to LAP, followed by the induction of C/EBPα during lactation. Prolactin activation of Stat5 results in protein–DNA as well as protein–protein interactions between C/EBPα and the GR, between Stat5 and GR and possibly between C/EBPα and Stat5, leading to displacement of YY1 and gene activation.

insulin receptor substrate (IRS)-1 and IRS-2 protein scaffolding [7]. Cytokine activation of IRS-1/2 can also occur via JAK kinase activation [7].

Our recent studies have been focused primarily on investigating the regulation of three of these transcription factors and their isoforms, NF-I, Stat5 and C/EBP, during normal mammary gland development and in breast cancer. These will be summarized briefly below.

NF-I

In order to localize regulatory regions important for the hormonal and tissue-specific expression of the rat WAP gene, DNase I-hypersensitive sites were mapped in the 5' flanking region of the rat WAP transgene that demonstrated copy-number-dependent expression in transgenic mice [3]. Two mammary-specific DNase I-hypersensitive sites were identified in lactating mice, and the region containing the distal site between 830 and 720 bp 5' to the transcription start site was shown to be critical for expression in transgenic mice. Detailed analysis of this region, including genomic and *in vitro* DNase I and footprinting and dimethyl sulphate interference analyses, indicated that it contains several binding sites for the transcription factor NF-I [3].

The NF-I gene family consists of four highly related genes in mammals [8]. While the N-terminal DNA binding and dimerization domain is well conserved between all NF-I proteins, the C-terminal sequences diverge substantially. Alternative splicing leads to alterations in the C-terminal domain, possibly affecting the regulatory properties of different NF-I isoforms. At least 12 different NF-I isoforms have been identified, and further diversity exists because of the possibility of heterodimerization. Some of these NF-I isoforms contain a carboxyproline-rich *trans*-activation domain [8]. This *trans*-activation domain has considerable identity with the repeated C-terminal domain in RNA polymerase II [9].

There are now several examples of tissue-specific NF-I isoforms, and of co-operative interaction of these isoforms with nuclear hormone receptors in composite response elements, e.g. in the c-*fos* vitamin D response element [10] and the mouse mammary tumour virus long terminal repeat [11]. Both NF-I and C/EBPs are often found in composite response elements [12]. It has been suggested that NF-I might act to tether nuclear receptors via a combination of protein–protein and protein–DNA interactions. NF-I DNA binding activity has been shown to be responsive to cell–substratum interactions in mammary epithelial cells. Unlike with Stat5, this regulation appears to be independent of lactogenic hormones [13]. NF-I has also been shown recently to interfere with transformation induced by a number of different nuclear oncogenes [14] and to increase cell adhesion in chick embryo fibroblasts.

Surrounding the NF-I binding sites in the WAP distal promoter region, several specific GR binding sites have also been identified using *in vitro* DNase I footprinting with baculovirus-expressed GR [15]. This region was able to confer dexamethasone inducibility to a heterologous reporter gene in transient co-transfection experiments with GR in CVI cells [15]. Furthermore, glucocorticoid-induced changes in transgene expression were correlated with the appearance of DNase I-hypersensitive sites. Immediately downstream from the GR and NF-I binding sites is a consensus Stat5 binding site similar to that identified in the β-casein promoter.

To determine the functional importance of these sites, point mutations were introduced into the NF-I and mammary-gland-specific factor (MGF)/Stat5 binding sites and several independent lines of transgenic mice were analysed [5]. Transgene expression was totally abrogated when the palindromic NF-I site or both NF-I binding sites were mutated, and mutation of the MGF/Stat5 binding site reduced transgene expression by approx. 90% per gene copy. These results indicated that the regulation of WAP gene expression is determined by co-operative interactions among several transcription factors whose binding sites comprise a composite response element, and that NF-I plays a critical role in the regulation of WAP gene expression.

Gel-mobility-shift experiments have also suggested the existence of mammary-specific NF-I isoforms binding to the composite sites in the WAP distal enhancer [3]. Using reverse transcription–PCR and two consensus NF-I oligonucleotides, we have cloned a 1.6 kb cDNA from RNA isolated from the mammary gland of rats at day 10 of lactation (S.-J. Chen and J.M. Rosen, unpublished work). This cDNA clone is currently being used to screen a cDNA library prepared from the same RNA to identify any mammary-specific NF-I isoforms.

Stat5

Studies of the prolactin regulation of milk protein gene expression have led to the identification of a new member of the Stat family of transcription factors, originally designated as MGF but now known as Stat5, a ubiquitous factor that plays a critical role in cytokine regulation in a variety of different tissues and cell types [6,16,17]. Stat5 has now been shown to be a target for at least a dozen cytokines and several receptor tyrosine kinases, such as that for epidermal growth factor. Prolactin regulation of milk protein gene expression occurs in part through activation of the recently defined JAK/Stat pathway [6]. Prolactin receptor signalling can also be mediated through a number of different signalling pathways, including the activation of the mitogen-activated protein (MAP) kinase and Src pathways [18,19]. The JAK2 non-receptor tyrosine kinase has been demonstrated to be essential for prolactin activation of β-casein gene expression [20]. There is also recent evidence that autocrine and paracrine effects of prolactin may play important roles in regulating the growth of both rodent and human breast cancer cells [21–24]. Some of these effects of prolactin are mediated by activation of the JAK/Stat pathway.

The β-casein promoter contains the principal Stat5 response element that is now employed by many workers interested in cytokine action. Two different Stat5 genes, 5a and 5b, have been identified. The Stat5a and Stat5b gene products have similar but non-identical tissue distributions [25–27]. Both Stat5 isoforms are regulated by prolactin and many other cytokines, but functional differences between Stat5a and Stat5b remain to be established. In addition, alternatively spliced forms for both Stat5a and Stat5b have been described, both of which generate C-terminally truncated proteins that appear to function as dominant-negative isoforms [26,27]. The role of these different splice forms in normal mammary gland development and breast cancer has yet to be determined. However, elevated levels of members of the Stat family have been reported in nuclear extracts of breast carcinomas [28]. It is conceivable that both ligand-dependent and -independent mechanisms of Stat5 activation may, therefore, play an important role in breast cancer.

Two rat Stat5a isoforms (Stat5a1 and Stat5a2) resulting from alternative splicing were cloned and characterized in our laboratory [26]. A closely related rat Stat5b cDNA has also been isolated in collaboration with Dr. Li Yu-Lee at Baylor, and an alternatively spliced isoform of Stat5b, designated Stat5bΔ40C, containing a C-terminal truncation similar to that observed in Stat5a2, has been reported [27] (Fig. 2). Preliminary Northern blot (A. Kazansky and J.M. Rosen, unpublished work) and electrophoretic mobility shift assay (W. Doppler, personal communication) experiments have suggested that the levels of these alternatively spliced Stat5 isoforms may change during the transition from late pregnancy to early lactation. Co-transfection studies in COS cells have also indicated that these C-terminally truncated Stat5 isoforms display increased DNA binding to the β-casein γ-interferon-activated sequence (GAS) site, possibly due to a decreased dissociation rate. In addition, these C-terminally truncated isoforms display markedly reduced transactivation of β-casein

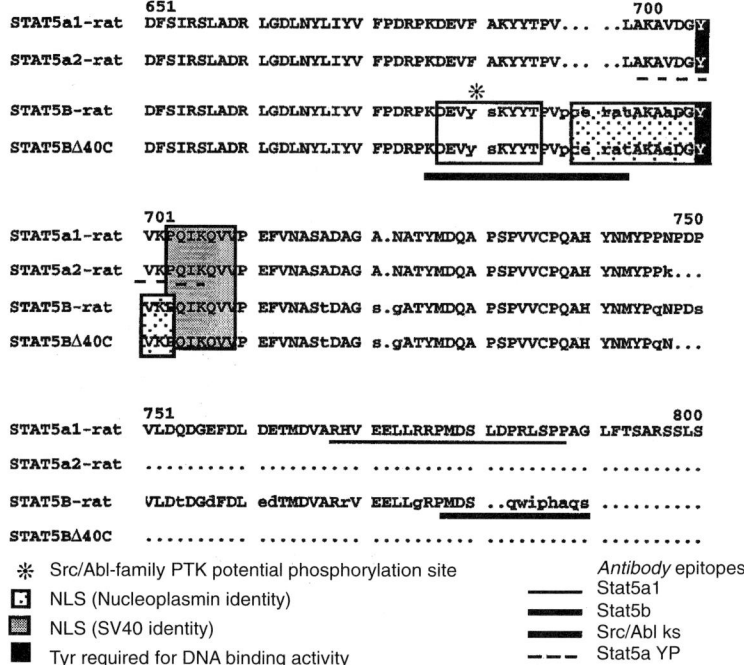

Fig. 2. Putative different functional domains in rat Stat5a and Stat5b. Sequences in the C-terminal regions of rat Stat5a and Stat5b are shown that may be responsible for differences in their nuclear localization and activation. The location of the C-terminal truncations present in the alternatively spliced isoforms of Stat5a and Stat5b is also shown. The underlined regions represent peptide epitopes used to generate specific antisera. Abbreviations: PTK, protein tyrosine kinase; NLS, nuclear localization sequence; SV40, simian virus 40.

promoter–reporter constructs (S. Lindsey and J.M. Rosen, unpublished work), and thus may be acting as dominant-negative isoforms.

A specific polyclonal antiserum to the C-terminal region of Stat5a1 was generated, and has been employed to study prolactin regulation not only in mammary epithelial cells but also in NB2 T-cells [29] and ovarian granulosa cells [30] in collaboration with Dr. Li Yu-Lee and Dr. JoAnne Richards at Baylor. This specific antibody was used to study Stat5a1 regulation during mammary gland development and its induction by prolactin in COS cells, and for immunohistochemical localization of Stat5a1. These studies indicated that Stat5a1 was expressed throughout mammary gland development, and that its expression was not correlated with maximal casein gene expression. Furthermore, studies on the activation of Stat5a1 in COS and HC11 cells have demonstrated a rapid and transient activation by prolactin that is not correlated with the long-term activation of casein gene expression.

Recently, we have also generated polyclonal antibodies that recognize the specific peptide containing the phosphotyrosine (equivalent to Tyr-694 in sheep Stat5) required for Stat5 dimer formation and DNA binding, as well as antibodies to a unique sequence in Stat5b that we suggest may be a potential *src/abl* kinase site (Fig. 2). We hypothesize that this latter region may be an important determinant of the difference in the regulation and function of Stat5a and Stat5b. Using these antibodies, we have observed a difference in the kinetics of tyrosine phosphorylation of Stat5a and Stat5b in preliminary co-transfection experiments performed in COS cells (A. Kazansky and J.M. Rosen, unpublished work). Thus Stat5a is maximally tyrosine phosphorylated within 30 min following prolactin addition, decreasing at 4.5 h and to a much greater extent at 13.5 h, while Stat5b increases in its PY-20 and *src/abl* kinase site antibody reactivity during this period. Phosphorylation on additional tyrosine(s) of Stat5b appears to occur during these later times. Thus the phosphorylation status of the two Stat5 isoforms is different, possibly reflecting different kinase as well as phosphatase susceptibilities. It is conceivable that the differential activation of Stat5b compared with Stat5a may result in differential gene activation, giving rise to a proliferative or a terminally differentiated state respectively.

C/EBP

The C/EBPs are members of the leucine zipper class of sequence-specific, bZIP DNA binding proteins [31]. Several C/EBP family members (C/EBPα, β, δ and γ) have been described that are encoded by separate, intron-free genes and which share a conserved C-terminal DNA binding domain and basic leucine zipper dimerization domain, but differ in their N-terminal *trans*-activation domains [32]. The gene encoding C/EBPβ is transcribed into a single mRNA. Translation of this mRNA occurs from three different in-frame AUG codons via a leaky ribosome scanning mechanism, resulting in the synthesis of three proteins: two LAPs (LAP1, 39 kDa; LAP2, 36 kDa) and LIP (20 kDa) (Fig. 3) [33]. As with all C/EBP family members, LAP and LIP are capable of forming homo- or hetero-dimers with each other. LAP and LIP share the same DNA binding and dimerization domains, but LIP lacks the *trans*-activating N-terminus, rendering it able to antagonize the transcriptional activating potential of LAP by competing for the DNA binding site or by its interaction in a LAP/LIP heterodimer [33]. Thus the LAP/LIP ratio may be an important indicator of C/EBPβ transcriptional activity [33].

The LAP/LIP ratio is most likely regulated at the translational level by the mRNA 5' cap binding protein [i.e. the eukaryotic translation initiation factor 4E (eIF4E)]. Thus the C/EBPβ mRNA provides a unique system with which to study eukaryotic translational control. RNAs encoding proteins involved in cell cycle progression, such as growth factors, oncogenes and *trans*-acting factors, possess long 5' untranslated regions with extensive secondary structure [34]. The C/EBPβ mRNA is one such molecule, and is, therefore, translated inefficiently. Initiation is the rate-limiting step in translation, and eIF4E is present at limiting concentrations in the cell [35]. In quiescent cells, much of the eIF4E pool is complexed with one of a family of cytoplasmic inhibitors, the eIF4E binding proteins [36]. Mitogenic stimulation leads to

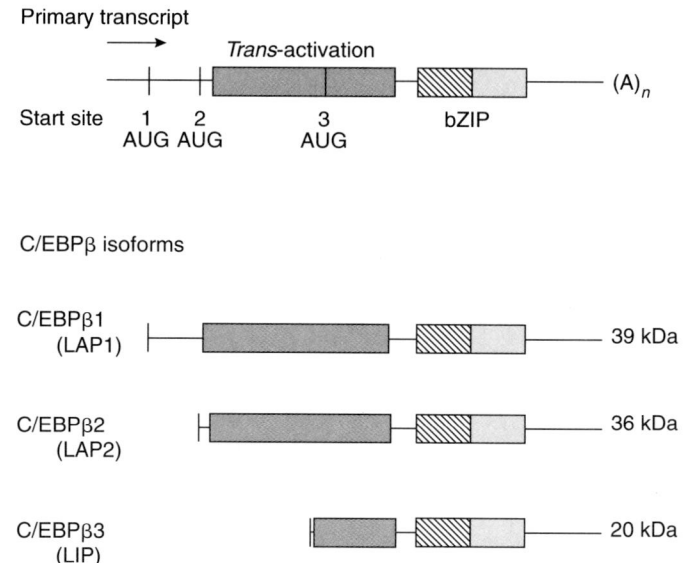

Primary transcript

Trans-activation

Start site   1   2   3   bZIP
             AUG AUG   AUG

(A)ₙ

C/EBPβ isoforms

C/EBPβ1
(LAP1)   39 kDa

C/EBPβ2
(LAP2)   36 kDa

C/EBPβ3
(LIP)   20 kDa

Fig. 3. Leaky ribosome scanning on a single mRNA generates three C/EBPβ isoforms. Diagrammatic representation of C/EBPβ mRNA with its three potential translation start sites (AUG). Sites number 1, 2 and 3 have relationships with the Kozak consensus sequences of 5/9, 6/9 and 9/9 respectively. The location of the *trans*-activation and DNA binding and dimerization domains (bZIP) are shown. Adapted from [53].

phosphorylation of eIF4E and of its binding proteins, which disrupts these complexes and increases the pool of active eIF4E. Increased eIF4E enhances the translation rate of inefficiently translated mRNAs [37].

RNA secondary structure causes significant ribosome stalling, so in unstimulated cells the few ribosomes that scan through to the C/EBPβ translation start sites are predicted to recognize the first two (at nucleotides 439 and 502) much more frequently than the third (at position 895). Thus in unstimulated cells the LAPs are predicted to be synthesized at a constitutive low level, and little LIP would be produced. In mitogenically stimulated cells, containing a much larger eIF4E pool, many more ribosomes should scan the C/EBPβ mRNA. The secondary structure of the C/EBPβ mRNA should thus be decreased significantly, and many more ribosomes should scan through the 5′ untranslated region. The LAP translation start sites are weak (5/9 and 6/9 nt match) as compared with the Kozak consensus sequence. However, the LIP start site conforms perfectly to this consensus [38]. Ribosomes unencumbered by secondary structure may often skip the imperfect Kozak sequences and recognize the LIP start site. Therefore the LAP/LIP ratio is predicted to be much lower in stimulated cells.

The C/EBP family is involved in the transcriptional regulation of genes important in the differentiation of many cell types, including myocytes, myelomonocytes, hepatocytes, adipocytes, ovarian follicles, intestinal epithelium and mammary epithelial cells [2,39,40]. C/EBP transcriptional activity can be modulated by the level of expression of the various C/EBP proteins and their respective isoforms. Differences in dimerization ratios due to an abundance or lack of a specific isoform may alter C/EBP DNA binding affinities or *trans*-activating potential.

C/EBPα, β, and δ expression is differentially regulated throughout the development of several different tissues. A regulated pattern of C/EBP isoform expression occurs during mouse 3T3-L1 cell differentiation. C/EBPβ and C/EBPδ are expressed during the early phase of 3T3-L1 differentiation into adipocytes. This expression declines and is replaced by high levels of C/EBPα as the cells progress towards terminal differentiation [32]. This temporal pattern of expression supports the hypothesis that C/EBPβ and C/EBPδ can induce C/EBPα expression, which then contributes to terminal cell differentiation by arresting adipocyte proliferation [32,41]. The inhibition of cell proliferation by C/EBPα occurs in many cell types, and does not appear to require the presence of p53 or retinoblastoma protein (Rb) [42]. Overexpression of dominant-negative isoforms of C/EBP, such as LIP [40] or CHOP/GADD153 (growth arrest and DNA damage inducible gene 153) [43], will prevent adipogenesis.

Cellular proliferation of HepG2 hepatoma cells is also blocked by LAP [44]. LAP arrests the cell cycle before the G1/S boundary in hepatoma cells, and this effect can be antagonized by LIP. During rat postnatal development, the levels of LAP in liver nuclei rise much more than those of LIP [33]. It has been suggested that the LAP/LIP ratio is more important for the regulation of gene expression than are the levels of LAP alone [33]. If so, perhaps LIP levels modulate the effect of LAP on the cell cycle and LIP expression in the hepatoma cells is not sufficient to antagonize LAP's inhibition of proliferation.

C/EBPβ activity is regulated not only by changes in expression level but also by post-translational modifications. The cell type and developmental specificity of C/EBPβ-regulated gene expression and *trans*-activation appears to be a result of interactions with multiple signal transduction pathways. Activation of these pathways by external stimuli can lead to phosphorylation and resultant increases in the *trans*-activating potential of C/EBPβ. Several protein kinases, including Ca^{2+}/calmodulin-dependent protein kinase [45], protein kinase C [46] and MAP kinase [47], have been shown to phosphorylate Ser/Thr residues at several different positions, resulting in increased C/EBPβ activity.

Recently, it has been suggested that C/EBPβ contains two conserved regions which can interact with both the *trans*-activation and DNA binding domains to repress DNA binding and transcriptional activity [48,49]. These inhibitory regions are positioned between the activation and DNA binding domains (Fig. 4). Studies have demonstrated that phosphorylation within an inhibitory region prevents intramolecular interaction with these domains and permits C/EBPβ *trans*-activation. Several phosphorylation sites are located within these inhibitory regions and may contribute to C/EBPβ *trans*-activation through modification of protein conformation [49]. Interestingly, it has also been demonstrated that these inhibitory regions are capable of forming intermolecular interactions with each other [49]. Examination of these inter-

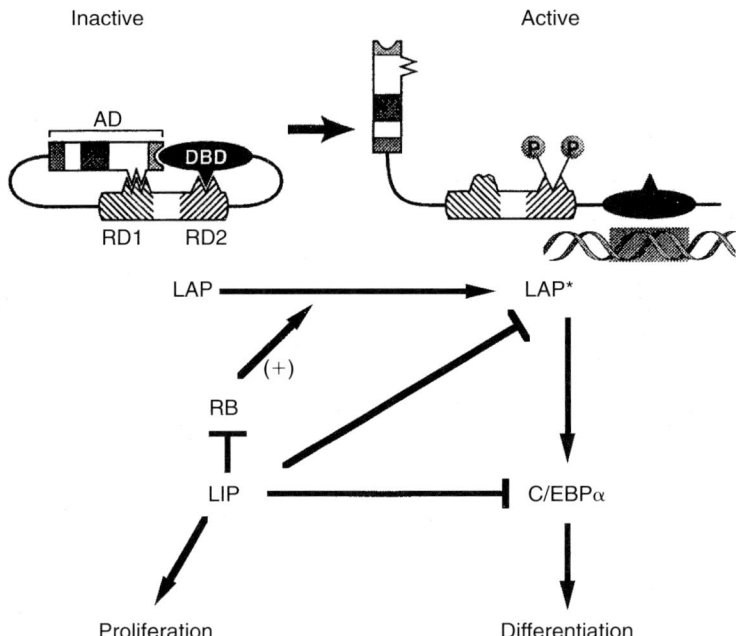

**Fig. 4. LIP expression can influence hormonally regulated prolifera-
tion or terminal differentiation.** The transient interaction of the
hypophosphorylated form of Rb with LAP results in a conformational change in
LAP similar to that observed following increased phosphorylation (adapted
from [49]). This can lead to increased transcriptional activation of C/EBPβ-
responsive genes, including C/EBPα, resulting in withdrawal from the cell cycle
and terminal differentiation. Leaky ribosome scanning in breast cancer cells
results in increased translation of the LIP isoform of C/EBPβ. This dominant-
negative isoform can inhibit both LAP and C/EBPα, as well as interacting
directly with Rb, preventing terminal differentiation and favouring proliferation.
Abbreviations: AD, *trans*-activation domain; DBD, DNA binding domain; RD,
regulatory domain.

actions may provide valuable information to further our understanding of
LIP's antagonistic effect on the transcriptional activity of C/EBP family members.

Traditionally, C/EBP family members have been described as DNA
binding proteins which regulate the transcription of genes involved in cellular
differentiation. It has now become apparent that C/EBPβ is additionally able
to interact with proteins involved in cell cycle control. Rb, a regulator of cell
cycle progression, is important for cellular differentiation and tumour suppression. During G0 and G1 of the cell cycle, hypophosphorylated Rb prevents cell
growth by blocking progression through the cell cycle. Hyperphosphorylation
of Rb during mid-G1 permits cell growth and induces proliferation. All three
C/EBPβ isoforms have been observed to interact directly with the simian virus
40 T antigen domain of hypophosphorylated Rb in differentiating or differentiated cells [50]. Two regions of C/EBPβ have been identified to interact with

Rb. One of these regions, in the N-terminus, is found in both LAP isoforms and is 54% similar to the sequence used by the transcription factor, E2F-1, to interact with Rb [50]. An additional binding region is located in the C-terminus and is present in the LIP and LAP isoforms. Transient interaction with Rb increases the DNA binding activity and *trans*-activation potential of the C/EBPβ isoforms, which may in turn activate the transcription of genes involved in cellular differentiation, such as C/EBPα [50].

Elevations in LIP expression should interfere with the activation of LAP by Rb and may antagonize the ability of LAP to transcriptionally regulate genes involved in cellular differentiation. The net result of increased LIP levels might, therefore, include an inhibition of cellular differentiation resulting in excessive proliferation and tumour growth. We propose, therefore, that the interaction of the C/EBPβ LAP isoforms with Rb is a switch to promote cellular differentiation, and that this may be blocked by increased LIP expression in breast cancer (Fig. 4). A decrease in the expression of C/EBPα, as well as rearrangements in the genes for the various C/EBP family members, has also been associated with tumour development in a number of other cell types [51,52].

Coupled with recent observations on the interaction of the hypophosphorylated form of Rb with C/EBPβ, this has led us to propose a hypothesis to explain why hormones that are responsible for hormone-dependent terminal differentiation in the normal mammary gland may elicit hormone-dependent growth in some breast cancers (Fig. 4). Thus, in breast cancer, LIP expression may be elevated as a function of leaky ribosome scanning. This most probably results from altered phosphorylation of translation initiation factors as a consequence of growth factor or oncogene activation of signal transduction pathways in breast cancer cells. At the same time overexpression of eIF4E, which has also been reported to increase levels of cyclin D1, may result in increased proliferation [37]. LIP expression will result in heterodimer formation with LAP (and C/EBPα), inhibit C/EBPα induction and prevent terminal differentiation (Fig. 4). This provides a mechanism to block terminal differentiation and facilitate continued proliferation. This model is consistent with the observation that LIP expression is detected in breast tumours, especially more aggressive tumours that are oestrogen- and progesterone-receptor-negative (C. Zahnow, B. Raught, A. James and J.M. Rosen, unpublished work).

The preceding studies are consistent with the general hypothesis that aberrant hormonal regulation of specific transcription factor isoforms can result in continued proliferation and failure to undergo terminal differentiation and apoptosis of breast epithelial cells. An understanding of the mechanisms regulating the expression and function of these different isoforms in normal mammary gland development will, therefore, be important for the understanding the aetiology of, and developing new treatments for, breast cancer.

These studies were supported by a grant from the National Institutes of Health (CA16303).

References

1. Rosen, J.M., Li, S., Raught, B. and Hadsell, D. (1996) Am. J. Clin. Nutr. **63**, 6275–6325
2. Raught, B., Liao, W.S.-L. and Rosen, J.M. (1995) Mol. Endocrinol. **9**, 1223–1232
3. Li, S. and Rosen, J.M. (1994) J. Biol. Chem. **269**, 14235–14243
4. Nishio, Y., Isshiki, H., Kishimoto, T. and Akira, S. (1993) Mol. Cell. Biol. **13**, 1854–1862
5. Li, S. and Rosen, J.M. (1995) Mol. Cell. Biol. **15**, 2063–2070
6. Groner, B. and Gouilleux, F. (1995) Curr. Opin. Genet. Dev. **5**, 587–594
7. Waters, S.B. and Pessin, J.E. (1996) Trends Cell Biol. **6**, 1–4
8. Santoro, C., Mermod, N., Andrews, P.C. and Tjian, R. (1988) Nature (London) **334**, 218–224
9. Xiao, H., Lis, J.T., Liao, H., Greenblatt, J. and Friesen, J.D. (1994) Nucleic Acids Res. **22**, 1966–1973
10. Candeliere, G.A., Jurutka, P.W., Haussler, M.R. and St-Arnaud, R. (1996) Mol. Cell. Biol. **16**, 584–591
11. Chávez, S., Candau, R., Truss, M. and Beato, M. (1995) Mol. Cell. Biol. **15**, 6987–6998
12. Kel, O.V., Romaschenko, A.G., Kel, A.E., Wingender, E. and Kolchanov, N.A. (1995) Nucleic Acids Res. **23**, 4097–4103
13. Streuli, C.H., Edwards, G.W., Delcommenne, M., Whitelaw, C.B.A., Burdon, T.G., Schindler, C. and Watson, C.J. (1995) J. Biol. Chem. **270**, 21639–21644
14. Schuur, E.R., Kruse, U., Iacovoni, J.S. and Vogt, P.K. (1995) Cell Growth Differ. **6**, 219–227
15. Li, S. and Rosen, J.M. (1994) Mol. Endocrinol. **8**, 1328–1335
16. Wakao, H., Gouilleux, F. and Groner, B. (1994) EMBO J. **13**, 2182–2191
17. Ihle, J.N. (1996) Nature (London) **377**, 591–594
18. Erwin, R.A., Kirken, R.A., Malabarba, M.G., Farrar, W.L. and Rui, H. (1995) Endocrinology **136**, 3512–3518
19. Berlanga, J.J., Vara, J.A.F., Martin-Pérez, J. and Garcia-Ruiz, J.P. (1995) Mol. Endocrinol. **9**, 1461–1467
20. Rui, H., Lebrun, J.-J., Kirken, R.A., Kelly, P.A. and Farrar, W.L. (1994) Endocrinology **135**, 1299–1306
21. Mershon, J., Sall, W., Mitchner, N. and Ben-Jonathan, N. (1995) Endocrinology **136**, 3619–3623
22. Fuh, G. and Wells, J.A. (1995) J. Biol. Chem. **270**, 13133–13137
23. Clevanger, C.V., Chang, W.-P., Ngo, W., Pasha, T.L.M., Montone, K.T. and Tomaszewski, J.E. (1995) Am. J. Pathol. **146**, 695–705
24. Ginsburg, E. and Vonderhaar, B. (1995) Cancer Res. **55**, 2591–2595
25. Mui, A.L.-F., Wakao, H., O'Farrel, A.M., Harada, N. and Miyajima, A. (1995) EMBO J. **14**, 1166–1176
26. Kazansky, A.V., Raught, B., Lindsey, S.M., Wang, Y.-f. and Rosen, J.M. (1995) Mol. Endocrinol. **9**, 1598–1609
27. Ripperger, J.A., Fritz, S., Richter, K., Hocke, G.M., Lottspeich, F. and Fey, G.H. (1995) J. Biol. Chem. **270**, 29998–30006
28. Watson, C.J. and Miller, W.R. (1995) Br. J. Cancer **71**, 840–844
29. Wang, Y.-F. and Yu-Lee, L.-Y. (1996) Mol. Cell Endocrinol. **121**, 19–28
30. Dajee, M., Kazansky, A.V., Raught, B., Hocke, G.M., Fey, G.H. and Richards, J.S. (1996) Mol. Endocrinol. **10**, 171–184
31. Lamb, P. and McKnight, S.L. (1991) Trends Biochem. Sci. **16**, 417–422
32. Cao, Z., Umek, R.M. and McKnight, S.L. (1991) Genes Dev. **5**, 1538–1552
33. Descombes, P. and Schibler, U. (1991) Cell **67**, 569–579
34. Sonenberg, N. (1996) in Translational Control (Hersey, J.W.B., Mathews, M.B. and Sonenberg, N., eds.), pp. 245–269, Cold Spring Harbor Laboratory Press, Cold Spring Harbor
35. Hiremath, L.S., Webb, N.R. and Rhoads, R.E. (1985) J. Biol. Chem. **260**, 7843–7849

36. Pause, A., Belsham, G.J., Gingras, A.-C., Donze, O., Lin, T.-A., Lawrence, J.C.J. and Sonenberg, N. (1994) Nature (London) **371**, 762–767
37. Rosenwald, I.B., Lazaris-Karatzas, A., Sonenberg, N. and Schmidt, E.V. (1993) Mol. Cell. Biol. **13**, 7358–7363
38. Kozak, M. (1992) Annu. Rev. Cell Biol. **8**, 197–225
39. Doppler, W., Welte, T. and Philipp, S. (1995) J. Biol. Chem. **270**, 17962–17969
40. Yeh, W.-C., Cao, Z., Classon, M. and McKnight, S.L. (1995) Genes Dev. **9**, 168–181
41. Umek, R.M., Friedman, A.D. and McKnight, S.L. (1991) Science **243**, 1689–1694
42. Hendricks-Taylor, L.R. and Darlington, G.J. (1995) Nucleic Acids Res. **23**, 4726–4733
43. Batchvarova, N., Wang, X.-Z. and Ron, D. (1995) EMBO J. **14**, 4654–4661
44. Buck, M., Turler, H. and Chokjier, M. (1994) EMBO J. **13**, 851–860
45. Wegner, M., Cao, Z. and Rosenfeld, M.G. (1992) Science **256**, 370–373
46. Trautwein, C., Caelles, C., van der Geer, P., Hunter, T., Karin, M. and Chojkier, M. (1993) Nature (London) **364**, 544–547
47. Nakajima, T., Kinoshita, S., Sasagawa, T., Sasaki, K., Naruto, M., Kishimoto, T. and Akira, S. (1993) Proc. Natl. Acad. Sci. U.S.A. **90**, 2207–2211
48. Kowenz-Leutz, E., Twamley, G., Ansieau, S. and Leutz, A. (1994) Genes Dev. **8**, 2781–2791
49. Williams, S.C., Baer, M., Dillner, A.J. and Johnson, P.F. (1995) EMBO J. **14**, 3170–3183
50. Chen, P.L., Riley, D.J., Chen-Kiang, S. and Lee, W.-H. (1996) Proc. Natl. Acad. Sci. U.S.A. **93**, 465–469
51. Flodby, P., Liao, D.-Z., Blanck, A., Xanthopoulos, K.G.H. and Hallstrom, P. (1995) Mol. Carcinog. **12**, 103–109
52. Inaba, T., Roberts, W.M., Shapiro, L.H., Jolly, K.W., Raimondi, S.C., Smith, S.D. and Look, A.T. (1992) Science **257**, 531–534
53. Hsu, W. and Chen-Kiang, S. (1993) Mol. Cell. Biol. **13**, 2515–2523

Biochem. Soc. Symp. **63**, 115–131
Printed in Great Britain

10

Regulation of gene expression in mammary epithelial cells by cellular confluence and sequence-specific DNA binding factors

Soner Altiok and Bernd Groner*

Institute for Experimental Cancer Research, Tumor Biology Center,
Breisacher Str. 117, D-79106 Freiburg, Germany

Abstract

Milk protein gene expression in mammary epithelial cells is regulated by interactions of the cells with each other and with extracellular-matrix components, and by the lactogenic hormones. Cell–cell and cell–extracellular-matrix interactions confer a state of competence to HC11 mammary epithelial cells. Cellular confluence and matrix deposition are prerequisites for the lactogenic hormone induction of, for example, β-casein synthesis. We have studied how these cellular interactions influence transcription factor activity. Proximal and distal regulatory elements have been identified in the DNA of the β-casein gene promoter that confer transcriptional induction to the lactogenic hormones in competent cells. A region located between positions –221 and –170 of the rat β-casein promoter contains overlapping binding sites for DNA binding factors with positive and negative regulatory activity. A construct containing 221 nt of 5′ promoter sequences linked to a chloramphenicol acetyltransferase (CAT) reporter gene and transfected into HC11 cells has low constitutive expression and is strongly inducible. Deletion of the sequences to –183 results in an increase in both constitutive and induced expression. Mutations in or deletion of the region from –183 to –170 abolish promoter activity. A sequence-specific single-stranded DNA binding transcriptional repressor (STR), composed of two proteins, binds to the upper strand of the –194 to –163 fragment and negatively regulates transcription. STR also recognizes the 5′ untranslated region of the β-casein mRNA and is sequestered into the cytoplasm by RNA after lactogenic hormone induction. Sequestration by RNA allows an activator to bind to

* To whom correspondence should be addressed.

the fragment −183 to −170. This activator has been identified as SARP, a sequence-specific single-stranded DNA activator region binding protein. The binding site of SARP is found both in the upper and the lower strands of this fragment. SARP has no affinity for RNA. It enhances transcription of a promoter construct containing rat β-casein promoter sequences from −183 to −1 and of a heterologous promoter containing multimerized copies of the −194 to −163 fragment in a lactogenic-hormone-independent manner. Mutations between positions −183 and −170, which result in a loss of promoter activity, also prevent SARP from binding to the DNA. Confluence of HC11 cells up-regulates the DNA binding activity of SARP. High SARP activity is also detected in mammary gland cells of lactating mice and is regulated by suckling. Withdrawal of pups from their lactating mothers results in a rapid decrease of SARP activity. We have purified SARP from the lactating mammary tissue of sheep and have identified proteins of 28 and 35 kDa.

Introduction

Expression of the β-casein gene in HC11 mammary epithelial cells [1] is regulated by sequential events governing the growth and differentiation status of the cells. HC11 cells grown to confluence in the presence of epidermal growth factor (EGF) assume a pre-differentiated state. They can be induced to synthesize β-casein upon treatment with the lactogenic hormones glucocorticoids, insulin and prolactin [2–4]. HC11 cells have been shown to deposit components of the extracellular matrix during their growth phase. In particular, the synthesis and proper assembly of laminin in response to EGF seems to be a prerequisite for the response to the lactogenic hormones [5]. The molecular mechanisms relating matrix deposition and confluence to transcription factor activity have not been defined.

The regulatory sequences of the rat β-casein gene promoter involved in the lactogenic hormone response have been characterized. A total of 221 nucleotides of promoter sequences upstream of the transcription initiation site are sufficient for induction [6]. Three regions within the rat β-casein gene promoter have been identified which contribute to the regulation. The binding site for the mammary gland factor (MGF/Stat5) is located between positions −100 and −85. This factor confers the prolactin signal. It is phosphorylated on tyrosine upon prolactin receptor activation and assumes DNA binding activity upon phosphorylation. It is a member of the signal transducer and activator of transcription (Stat) gene family [7–10], and has been designated Stat5 [11,12]. A repressor element between positions −150 and −110, adjacent to the MGF/Stat5 binding site, suppresses transcription in uninduced HC11 cells. This element is counteracted by the lactogenic hormone activation of MGF/Stat5. Competition for overlapping DNA binding sites between MGF/Stat5 and a repressor complex including the Yin Yang 1 (YY1) factor has been shown [7,13]. A third regulatory region is positioned between nucleotides −170 and −221 and has both negative and positive regulatory functions [6]. A sequence-specific single-stranded DNA binding transcriptional repressor (STR), composed of two proteins, p35 and p54, represses transcription by binding to the upper strand [6]. STR also has binding activity for RNA and a binding site is found in the 5' untranslated region (UTR) of the β-casein mRNA. STR is sequestered into the cytoplasm by binding to the β-casein mRNA during lactation in the mouse mammary gland and upon lactogenic hormone treatment of HC11 cells. This leads to a decrease in nuclear STR. Interaction of STR with RNA may also influence post-transcriptional utilization of mRNA [14].

The promoter region between −183 and −170 does not only have a repressor function in uninduced cells. It also comprises a positively acting element which functions independently of the lactogenic hormones. A single-stranded DNA activator region binding protein (SARP), found in the nuclear extracts of various cell lines, recognizes a sequence element in both the upper and the lower strands of the region between positions −194 and −163. Mutations in the region −183 to −170 result in a loss of SARP binding and of promoter activity. The DNA binding activity of SARP is up-regulated by confluence. SARP can also interact with double-stranded DNA in a sequence-specific manner. In contrast to STR, SARP does not have RNA binding activity. Binding of STR and SARP to the upper strand seems to be mutually exclusive. The interaction of SARP with upper-strand DNA can only be detected if STR is RNA-bound, i.e. during lactation in the mouse mammary gland or after lactogenic hormone treatment in HC11 cells. Our data suggest that SARP is an enhancer binding protein which mediates the positive effect of cell confluence on β-casein gene transcription.

Materials and methods

Cell culture

HC11 mammary epithelial cells were grown in RPMI 1640 medium containing 10% (v/v) heat-inactivated fetal calf serum, 5 μg/ml bovine insulin, 10 ng/ml murine EGF, 50 μg/ml gentamicin and 2 mM glutamine. Cells were maintained for 4 days at confluence in growth medium containing EGF, before induction with the lactogenic hormones. The hormone induction was for 2 days in RPMI 1640 medium without EGF, but either with 5 μg/ml insulin alone (uninduced) or with insulin, 5 μg/ml ovine prolactin and 0.1 μM dexamethasone (induced).

Plasmid preparation

The β-casein promoter constructs pbc(−344/−1)CAT (where CAT is chloramphenicol acetyltransferse) and pbc(−183/−1)CAT have been described previously [14,15]. For preparation of the 4xbc(−194/−163)CAT plasmid, the upper- and lower-strand oligonucleotides containing the sequences of the β-casein promoter between positions −194 and −163 were annealed. An *Xba*I restriction site in the 5' end and *Bgl*II and *Pst*I restriction sites at the 3' end were included. Gel-purified double-stranded oligonucleotides were inserted between the *Pst*I and *Xba*I sites of the pUC18 plasmid. Plasmids containing the insert were digested either with *Bgl*II or with *Bam*HI and ligated (head to tail). After repeating the last step, a fragment containing four copies of the −194 to −163 sequence was obtained after *Hin*dIII and *Eco*RI digestion, and inserted into the PBLCAT2 vector. The sequences of the plasmids were verified by DNA sequencing.

Transfection and CAT activity measurements

HC11 cells were transfected with 10 µg of reporter plasmid and 1 µg of the pSV2neo plasmid by the calcium phosphate precipitation technique [15]. Resistant colonies were pooled after selection with 0.2 µg/ml G418 and used for hormone induction and CAT activity determinations as described [15].

Nuclear extract preparation and gel-retardation experiments

Nuclear extracts were prepared from cell lines and mouse organs. Bandshift experiments were carried out as described [6].

Protein purification

Mammary gland tissue obtained from sheep lactating for 4 days was frozen in liquid nitrogen and stored at $-70°C$. All following procedures were carried out at $4°C$ as previously described [7,8]. The tissue was thawed in buffer H [10 mM Hepes/NaOH, pH 7.5, 10 mM NaCl, 0.1 mM EDTA, 0.1 mM EGTA, 1 mM dithiothreitol (DTT), 0.7 mM spermidine, 0.15 mM spermine and 0.2 mM PMSF] and disrupted in a Waring blender. The homogenate was filtered through cheesecloth to remove connective tissue and further dissociated using a Potter homogenizer. After homogenization, 0.1 vol. of buffer D [20 mM Hepes/NaOH, pH 7.5, 50 mM NaCl, 2 mM EDTA, 1 mM DTT, 10% (v/v) glycerol, 0.1% Nonidet P-40 and 0.2 mM PMSF], but containing 1 M NaCl, was added to raise the NaCl concentration to 0.1 M. The nuclei were collected by centrifugation at 1800 g and washed with buffer H containing 0.1 M KCl instead of NaCl. The nuclear pellet was resuspended in extraction buffer [20 mM Hepes/NaOH, pH 7.5, 0.4 M NaCl, 0.2 mM EDTA, 2 mM EGTA, 1 mM DTT, 0.75 mM spermidine, 0.15 mM spermine, 25% (v/v) glycerol and 0.2 mM PMSF] and incubated on ice for 45 min with gentle agitation. The nuclei were removed by centrifugation at 2000 g for 20 min and the supernatant was dialysed against buffer D after addition of Nonidet P-40 to a final concentration of 0.1% (v/v). Dialysed nuclear proteins were loaded on to a Red-A resin (Amicon) column pre-equilibrated with buffer D. The column was washed with 3 vol. of buffer D containing 0.3 M NaCl and subsequently with the same volume of buffer D containing 0.05 M KSCN. Proteins were eluted with a linear gradient of 0.05 mM–1 M KSCN. Binding to the upper strand of the –194/–163 fragment of the rat β-casein promoter was monitored by a bandshift assay. The STR components p54 and p35 were eluted between 0.35 and 0.4 M and between 0.5 and 0.65 M KSCN respectively. SARP was eluted at approx. 0.6 M KSCN. The active fractions for each protein were pooled separately, dialysed against buffer E [10 mM Tris/HCl, pH 7.5, 0.05 M NaCl, 0.1 mM EDTA, 1 mM DTT, 5% (v/v) glycerol, 0.1 % Nonidet P-40 and 0.2 mM PMSF] and loaded on to a pre-equilibrated DNA affinity column. The affinity column consisted of Sepharose 4B-CNBr (Pharmacia) coupled to a DNA oligonucleotide (the upper strand of the rat β-casein promoter between positions –194 and –163) and was prepared as described by Eisenberg et al. [16].

The column was washed with 5 column vol. of buffer E containing 0.25 M NaCl. p54, p35 and SARP were eluted with 0.6 M NaCl. Proteins found in the flow-through and the 0.25 M and 0.6 M NaCl eluates were separated on an SDS/10%-polyacrylamide gel and visualized by silver staining.

Results

A lactogenic-hormone-independent enhancer element is located between positions −183 and −170 of the rat β-casein promoter

The region of the β-casein gene promoter located between positions −221 and −170 contains elements with negative and positive regulatory functions [4,6,14]. Deletion of the nucleotides from −344 to −183 results in a 50-fold increase in the basal activity of the rat β-casein promoter. Further deletions or mutations in the sequences between −183 and −170 abolish the inducibility and the high basal expression. This is most probably due to the disruption of an activator element. The negative element in this region has been shown to bind an STR. This binding site overlaps with the positive regulatory element [6].

We further investigated the function of the positive regulatory element located between positions −183 and −170. This element is essential for the activity of the β-casein promoter. The increase in the basal activity upon deletion of sequences upstream of position −183 indicates that the element functions independently of lactogenic hormones. The basal and induced activities of pbc(−344/−1)CAT and pbc(−183/−1)CAT were compared in growing and confluent HC11 cells after stable transfection. Very low levels of expression of the construct pbc(−344/−1)CAT were observed in exponentially growing HC11 cells (Fig. 1a). Lactogenic hormone treatment increased the activity of this promoter about 95-fold. In accordance with our earlier results, the induction was restricted to confluent cells and could not be observed in growing cells. The basal and lactogenic-hormone-induced CAT activities of the pbc(−183/−1) CAT construct in growing cells were much higher than those of the pbc(−344/−1)CAT construct (40-fold, uninduced; 90-fold, induced). Confluence also enhanced the lactogenic hormone inducibility of pbc(−183/−1)CAT, but had no influence on basal activity. These data indicate that confluence is a prerequisite for the lactogenic hormone inducibility of the −344/−1 promoter construct. They also suggest that a factor, constitutively present in HC11 cells, interacts with the positive regulatory element and that its function can be observed when the STR DNA binding site is deleted.

The presumptive constitutive enhancer function of the −194/−163 fragment was tested. Four copies of the sequence were inserted upstream of the minimal promoter sequence in the pBLCAT2 vector [17]. HC11 cells were stably transfected and CAT activities were determined in uninduced and induced cells. Insertion of the oligomerized −194/−163 fragment resulted in a 10-fold increase in CAT expression when compared with pBLCAT2 (Fig. 1b). This increase was hormone independent. The enhancer element functions in the context of a heterologous promoter, and the activation function of this region is dominant over the repression.

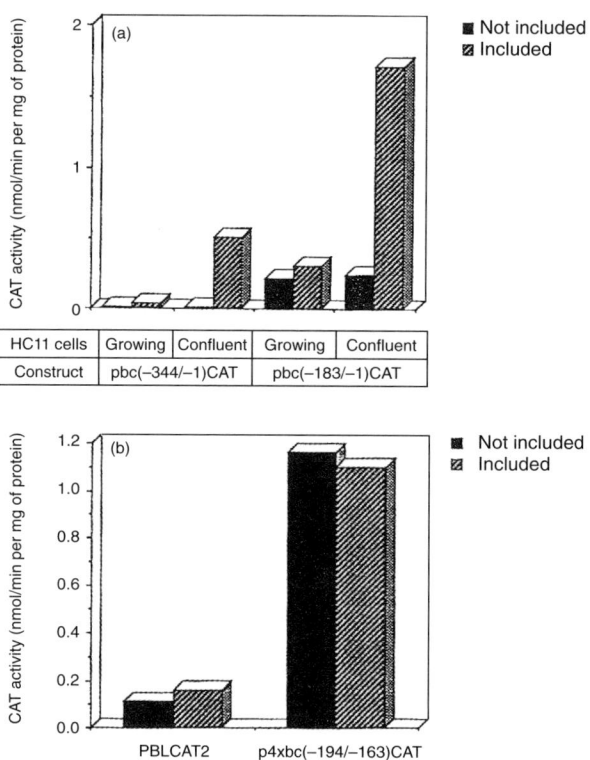

Fig. 1. The enhancer element located between positions −183 and −163 of the β-casein gene promoter is essential and functions independently of lactogenic hormones. (a) HC11 cells were stably transfected with the β-casein constructs pbc(−344/−1)CAT and pbc(−183/−1)CAT. CAT activities were determined in exponentially growing and confluent cells [15]. (b) The −194/−163 fragment of the β-casein promoter was multimerized by head-to-tail ligation and inserted in the pBLCAT2 vector [17]. Transfection experiments and hormone treatment were performed as described in the Materials and methods section. Three independent transfection experiments were carried out and similar results were obtained. The results of a representative experiment are shown.

The binding activity of an enhancer specific DNA binding factor is up-regulated by cellular confluence

Specific interactions of the enhancer element in the −194/−163 region with nuclear proteins were investigated in band-shift assays. Upper and lower strands of the −194/−163 fragment, as well as double-stranded DNA, were employed as probes. When the upper strand was used as a probe and extracts were prepared from growing HC11 cells, the STR complex was detected (Fig. 2a, lane 1). The STR complex comprises a sequence-specific single-stranded DNA binding factor composed of two proteins which has a repressive effect on

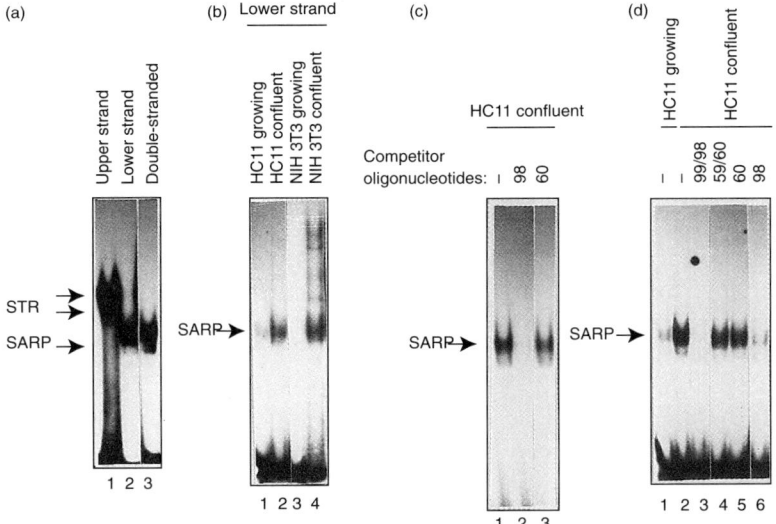

Fig. 2. Confluence regulates the binding of SARP to the −194 to −163 region of the β-casein gene promoter. Oligonucleotides representing the upper and lower strands of the rat β-casein promoter from position −194 to −163 were end-labelled and used as single-stranded or double-stranded probes in band-shift assays. (a) Nuclear extracts from growing HC11 cells were incubated with upper-strand probe (lane 1; 1 μg) or with lower-strand (lane 2; 6 μg) or double-stranded (lane 3; 6 μg) probes. (b) Nuclear extracts (4 μg) prepared from growing or confluent HC11 (lanes 1 and 2) or NIH 3T3 (lanes 3 and 4) cells were used in band-shift assays with the lower strand as a probe. (c) The wild-type (lane 2) and mutated (lane 3) lower-strand oligonucleotides (see Table 1) were added as unlabelled competitors in a 100-fold molar excess to the reaction mixture. (d) A double-stranded DNA probe corresponding to the −194/−163 fragment of the β-casein promoter was incubated with 4 μg of nuclear extracts prepared from growing (lane 1) or confluent (lanes 2–6) HC11 cells. Wild-type (lanes 3 and 6) or mutated (lanes 4 and 5) double-stranded or lower-strand oligonucleotides were used as unlabelled competitor in a 100-fold molar excess. Nuclear extract preparation and band-shift experiments were performed as described in the Materials and methods section.

transcription. This factor has been described previously by Altiok and Groner [6,14]. The same extract also yielded a specific complex with the lower strand (lane 2) or the double-stranded DNA (lane 3) as probes. Similar DNA binding activities to these probes were also observed with nuclear extracts from HeLa cells and extracts from rat tissues (brain, lung, kidney, liver and pancreas; results not shown). The protein which gives rise to this complex has been named SARP (single-stranded DNA activator region binding protein).

Confluence of HC11 cells is a prerequisite for the lactogenic hormone induction of β-casein synthesis. The molecular basis of the regulation exerted by confluence is at the transcriptional level, and it is likely that it is mediated by the activity of specific transcription factors. The increase in the basal activity of the pbc(–183/–1)CAT and p4bc(–194/–163)CAT constructs in confluent cells suggests that confluence may regulate the binding activity of SARP. To test this idea, nuclear extracts were prepared from growing, confluent and hormone-induced HC11 cells and introduced into band-shift assays. The binding of SARP to the lower-strand probe (Fig. 2b, lanes 1 and 2) and to the double-stranded probe (Fig. 2d, lanes 1 and 2) of the –194/–163 fragment was increased in extracts from confluent cells when compared with extracts from growing cells. The up-regulation of SARP DNA binding activity in confluent cells is not restricted to HC11 mammary epithelial cells. The same effect has been observed with extracts from NIH 3T3 fibroblasts (Fig. 2b, lanes 3 and 4). Lactogenic hormone treatment did not cause a further increase in the binding of SARP in HC11 or NIH 3T3 cells (results not shown).

The binding to the lower-strand and the double-stranded DNA probes is sequence-specific. Wild-type (Fig. 2c, lane 2), but not mutated (lane 3), oligonucleotides corresponding to the –194/–163 fragment of the β-casein promoter compete for binding. Binding to the double-stranded probe of this fragment was also competed by wild-type (Fig. 2d, lane 3), but not by mutated (lane 4), double-stranded oligonucleotide. The lower-strand oligonucleotide can compete for the binding of the double-stranded probe (lane 6). Mutations in the lower strand resulted in a loss of competition (lane 5). The electrophoretic mobilities and the competition specificities indicate that the lower strand and the double-stranded fragment from –194 to –163 form complexes with similar proteins.

SARP and STR bind to overlapping sequences in the upper strand of the β-casein promoter region between positions –194 and –163

STR binding activity is specific for the upper strand of the –194/–163 fragment [6]. Lactogenic hormone treatment of HC11 cells results in down-regulation of nuclear STR binding activity [6,14]. The decrease in STR binding upon lactogenic hormone treatment occurs concomitant with the appearance of a new, faster-migrating complex (Fig. 3, lanes 2 and 3). The electrophoretic mobility of this new complex is very similar to that formed by SARP with the lower-strand probe (lane 1). To investigate the sequence specificity of the binding to the upper strand, we performed competition experiments. Various oligonucleotides were used as unlabelled competitors in the band-shift assays (Table 1). The binding was competed by the wild-type sequence (lane 5), but not by a mutated oligonucleotide (lane 4). An oligonucleotide corresponding to the upper strand of the –183/–163 fragment, the region comprising the enhancer element, competed with the faster-migrating band (lane 7), but not with STR (lane 6). From these results, we conclude that SARP can bind the upper strand of the –194/–163 fragment, but only if STR binding is diminished.

Sequence similarities occur in the upper [5′ (–189) TTCACCAGCT TCTGAA (–172) 3′] and lower [5′ (–172) TTCAGAAGCTGGTGAA (–189) 3′] strands of the regulatory region of the β-casein promoter, and might be involved in the sequence-specific interaction with SARP.

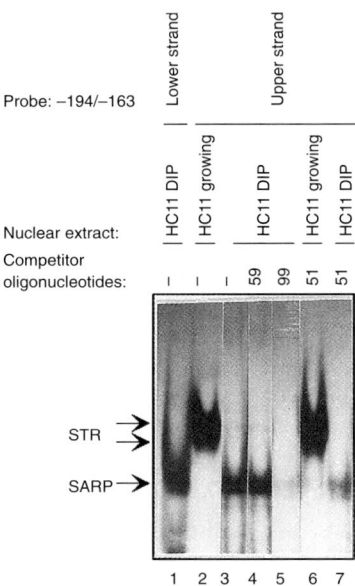

Fig. 3. SARP and STR bind mutually exclusively to the upper strand of the regulatory region from positions –194 to –163, and binding is regulated by the lactogenic hormones. Nuclear extracts from growing HCII cells (lanes 2 and 6) or from confluent, lactogenic-hormone-treated HCII cells (DIP) (lanes 3, 4, 5 and 7) were used in band-shift experiments in the presence of upper-strand (lanes 2–7) or lower-strand (lane 1) probe. Oligonucleotides shown in Table 1 were used as unlabelled competitors in a 100-fold molar excess (lanes 4–7). Nuclear extract preparation and band-shift assays were as described in the Materials and methods section.

Table 1. Oligonucleotides used in band-shift assays.

Oligonucleotide no.	Sequence
99 (–194)	5'-GTTCCTTCACCAGCTTCTGAATTGCTGCCTTG–3' (-163)
98 (–194)	5'-CAAGGCAGCAATTCAGAAGCTGGTGAAGGAAC–3' (-163)
59 (–194)	5'-GTTCATACATAAGCTTAGTATACGCTGCCTTG–3' (-163)
60 (–194)	5'-CAAGGCAGCGTATACTAAGCTTATGTATGAAC–3' (-163)
51 (–183)	5'-.........AGCTTCTGAATTGCTGCCTTG–3' (-163)
38 (–183)	5'-.........AGCTTAGTATACGCTGCCTTG–3' (-163)
5' UTR RNA	5'-UUCACCUUCGCUAUGUUCACCUUCGCUAUG–3'

SARP DNA binding activity is up-regulated in mammary gland tissue during lactation and in HCII cells upon hormone treatment

Two factors have previously been identified which are reversibly regulated during the course of pregnancy, lactation and post-lactation. MGF/Stat5 DNA binding activity is low during pregancy and post-lactation and high during lactation. This factor positively regulates milk protein gene transcription. The activity of the repressor factor STR is down-regulated in the nuclei of mammary cells during the lactation period, but is high during pregnancy and post-lactation [6,18]. We investigated the developmental regulation of SARP binding activity in the mouse mammary gland. Nuclear extracts prepared from mammary glands of pregnant, lactating and post-lactating mice were used in band-shift assays with the upper-strand probe of the −193/−163 fragment (Fig. 4). No SARP activity could be detected in mammary gland extracts at day 10 of pregnancy (lane 1). SARP activity increased with the onset of lactation (lane 2); at the same time, a decrease in STR binding was observed. The post-lactational state was analysed after removal of the pups from their mothers for 1 day. Decreased SARP activity and increased STR activity accompanied this state (lane 3). We also investigated STR and SARP binding to the upper-strand probe using nuclear extracts prepared from the mammary glands of lactating cows, rats and sheep. Low STR and high SARP binding was consistently observed (results not shown).

These results indicate that, in the mammary gland, SARP binding to the upper strand of the distal regulatory region is hormonally regulated. Suckling, and in its wake high circulating prolactin levels, are required to maintain high SARP activity during the lactation period. It seems that STR and SARP compete for binding to the distal regulatory region between positions −194 and −163. There is a positive correlation between β-casein gene expression and the binding of SARP to the distal regulatory region. Loss of promoter activity is observed upon deletion or mutation of the SARP binding site. SARP is most likely a positive regulator of β-casein transcription.

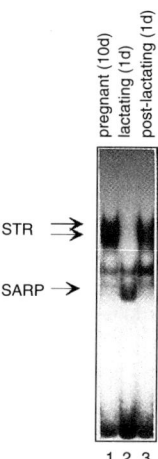

Fig. 4. SARP binding to the upper strand is increased during lactation. A probe representing the upper strand of the −194/−163 fragment was mixed with nuclear extracts prepared from the mammary glands of mice pregnant for 10 days (lane 1), of mice lactating for 1 day (lane 2) or of mice at 1 day post-lactation (lane 3). Nuclear extract preparation and mobility shift assays were performed as described in the Materials and methods section.

STR but not SARP binds to a specific RNA sequence

We have suggested that the binding of STR to β-casein mRNA and transport to the cytoplasm causes the sequestration of STR from the nucleus during the early phase of hormonal induction [6,14]. No SARP binding to the upper strand of the –194/–163 fragment could be observed when extracts from the nuclei of growing HC11 cells were tested (Fig. 2, lane 1). We investigated whether the inability of SARP to bind to the upper strand of the –194/–163 fragment is due to the high STR level in these extracts. Free STR was removed from the reaction by the addition of a specific RNA sequence. A synthetic RNA oligonucleotide (5′ UTR RNA) containing the STR binding site or total RNA prepared from different sources were used as unlabelled competitors in the band-shift experiments. Total RNA prepared from lactogenic-hormone-induced HC11 cells (Fig. 5, lane 2) and a synthetic RNA oligonucleotide containing the STR binding site present in the 5′ UTR of the vitellogenin mRNA [2] (lane 3) competed with STR binding to the upper-strand DNA probe. RNA derived from growing HC11 (lane 8) or NIH 3T3 (lane 9) cells, or tRNA (lane 10), did not compete.

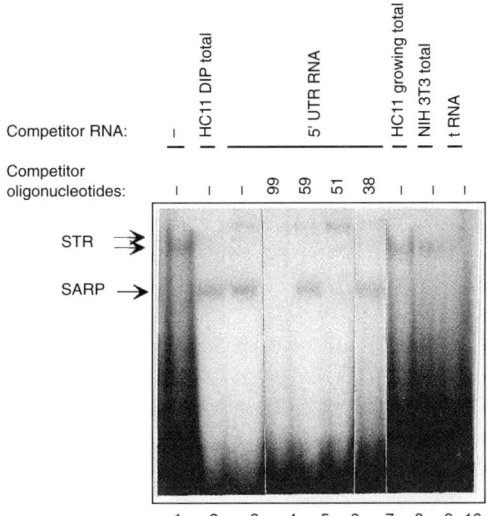

Fig. 5. Interaction of STR with RNA allows SARP to bind to the upper strand of the –194/–163 fragment. tRNA (lane 10), an RNA oligonucleotide representing the STR binding site (5′ UTR RNA; lane 3), and total RNA prepared from lactogenic-hormone-treated HC11 cells (DIP; lane 2), from exponentially growing HC11 cells (lane 8) or from NIH 3T3 cells (lane 9) were used as unlabelled competitors in band-shift experiments. DNA oligonucleotides were added to the reaction mixture together with RNA oligonucleotide (lanes 4–7) in a 100-fold molar excess. Nuclear extracts were derived from growing HC11 cells (1 μg). The sequences of the synthetic oligonucleotides are shown in Table 1. Total RNA and nuclear extract preparation from cell lines and performance of the band-shift assays were as described in the Materials and methods section.

When total RNA from induced HC11 cells or the 5′ UTR sequences of the vitellogenin mRNA were added in the competition experiments and STR binding was competed, a faster-migrating complex appeared (Fig. 5, lanes 2 and 3). The formation of this complex was competed by the wild-type sequence −194/−163 (lane 4) and by an oligonucleotide corresponding to the region −183 to −163 (lane 6), but not by their mutated sequences (lanes 5 and 7). These data indicate that the complex observed in the absence of the STR complex reflects SARP activity. SARP activity is constitutive in the nuclear extracts of HC11 cells, but is detected only if STR binding to the upper strand is quenched by titration with RNA. In contrast to STR, SARP interacts only with single-stranded DNA, not with RNA. This might result in SARP binding to the upper strand of the distal regulatory region to increase transcription as β-casein mRNA sequesters STR from the nucleus.

SARP contains a component of 28 kDa

For logistical reasons we used nuclear extracts from the mammary tissue of lactating sheep to purify SARP. Nuclear proteins were bound to a column of Red-A resin and eluted with a linear gradient from 0.05 mM to 1 M KSCN. Elution with KSCN resulted in better recovery than elution with NaCl. Band-shift assays were performed to identify the fractions containing nuclear proteins recognizing the upper and lower strands of the −194/−163 fragment. Two previously characterized components of the STR complex, p35 and p54, were detected. p35 was eluted between 0.35 and 0.4 M KSCN and p54 between 0.5 and 0.65 M KSCN (Fig. 6a). SARP was eluted at approx. 0.6 M KSCN. Lower-strand binding activity was only detected in the fractions containing SARP activity (Fig. 6b, lane 1), and not in the fractions containing p35 or p54 (results not shown).

Oligonucleotide competition experiments showed that the wild-type sequence efficiently competed with SARP binding to the upper strand (Fig. 6b, lane 3). Oligonucleotides with mutations which result in a loss of promoter activity also failed to be effective as competitors (lane 5). An oligonucleotide representing the sequence of the upper strand of the −183/−163 fragment competed with the formation of the SARP–DNA complex, but not with the formation of the p35–DNA complex (lane 4). These data are consistent with our previous observations (Fig. 3, lane 7) and confirm the identity of SARP.

SARP was purified further by single-stranded DNA affinity column chromatography. An affinity resin was prepared by coupling the oligonucleotide representing the sequence of the upper-strand positions −194 to −163 of the rat β-casein promoter to CNBr-activated Sepharose. Fractions eluted from the Red-A column at 0.6 M KSCN, which contained both p35 and SARP activity, were pooled and loaded on to the DNA affinity column. After washing with 0.25 M NaCl the upper-strand binding proteins were eluted with 0.6 M NaCl (Fig. 6c, lanes 4–6). No SARP activity was detected in band-shift assays in the flow-through fraction (lane 2) or in the 0.25 M NaCl eluate (lane 3). Proteins eluted with 0.6 M NaCl were separated by SDS/PAGE and visualized by silver staining (Fig. 6d). Above the background of other proteins, the p35 component of the STR complex and a protein of 28 kDa were the major

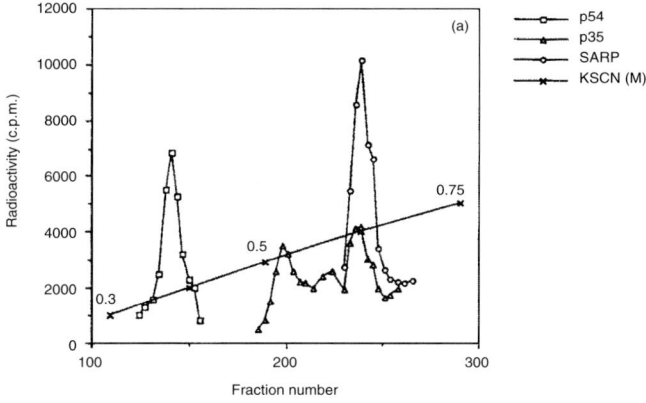

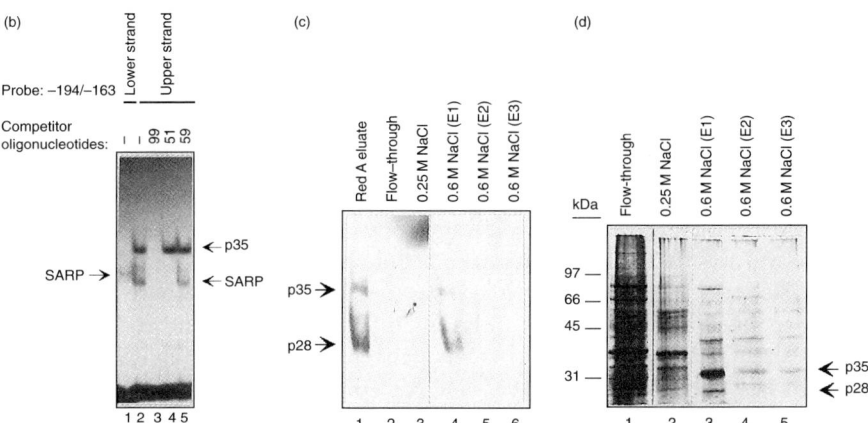

Fig. 6. STR and SARP are eluted at different salt concentrations from the Red-A–Sepharose column. (a) Nuclear extracts prepared from the mammary tissue of lactating sheep were loaded on to a Red-A–Sepharose column. Proteins were eluted with a linear gradient of KSCN from 0.05 M to 1 M. Complex-formation with an upper-strand probe was monitored in band-shift assays. The retarded bands were cut from the polyacrylamide gel and their radioactivity was quantified. (b) The fractions containing p35 and SARP were pooled and used in band-shift experiments. The lower (lane 1) and the upper (lanes 2–5) strands of the −194/−163 fragment were employed as end-labelled probes. DNA oligonucleotides, shown in Table 1, were added to the reaction mixture as unlabelled competitors in a 100-fold molar excess (lanes 3–5). (c) p35- and SARP-containing fractions were pooled, dialysed and loaded on a DNA affinity column made from single-stranded oligonucleotides corresponding to the upper strand of the −194/−163 fragment of the rat β-casein promoter (lane 1). The binding activities were eluted at 0.6 M NaCl (lanes 4–6) and detected in band-shift assays. No activity was found in the flow-through fractions (lane 2) or in the 0.25 M NaCl fractions (lane 3). (d) Fractions tested in band-shift assays in (c) were used for SDS/PAGE analysis. The protein bands were visualized by silver staining. The experiment was repeated three times. The p35 component of the STR complex and a protein of 28 kDa, which most probably corresponds to SARP, are indicated.

components detected in the 0.6 M NaCl eluate. The p35 and p28 proteins were excised from the gel and renatured. The renatured 28 kDa protein was tested in a band-shift assay, and a complex with the migration properties of SARP was detected. This strongly suggests that p28 is SARP.

Discussion

A regulatory region between positions −221 and −163 of the β-casein promoter has both negative and positive regulatory properties. STR, composed of two proteins with molecular masses of 35 kDa and 54 kDa, exerts a repressor effect on transcription through this sequence. STR interacts only with the upper strand of the −194 to −163 region and has no affinity for double-stranded DNA. STR binding activity is down-regulated in mammary gland cells of mice during lactation and in HC11 cells upon lactogenic hormone treatment [6]. STR binds with high affinity to RNA. The 5′ UTR of the β-casein mRNA contains an STR binding site. Upon lactogenic hormone treatment, the transcribed β-casein mRNA sequesters STR into the cytosol, which leads to a decrease in STR activity in the nuclei of mammary epithelial cells. Interaction of STR with RNA also influences post-transcriptional utilization of mRNA [14].

A positive regulatory element is also located between positions −183 and −170 of the β-casein promoter. Deletion or mutation of the sequence from −183 to −170 abolishes the inducibility of the promoter and the high basal expression of a reporter construct. We conclude from these results that an activator recognizes a positively acting element only when STR does not bind to its adjacent binding site. The positively acting element functions also in exponentially growing HC11 cells. The pbc(−183/−1)CAT construct exhibits high expression in exponentially growing HC11 cells, whereas a promoter construct, pbc(−344/−1)CAT, was active only in the lactogenic-hormone-induced confluent HC11 cells.

These data led us to propose the following model. A protein, SARP, which recognizes the positively acting element, is present in the nuclei of growing and hormone-induced cells. A decrease in STR binding to the promoter, caused by removal of STR from the nucleus by β-casein mRNA upon lactogenic hormone induction or by deletion of the STR binding site in the promoter, increases the transcription of the β-casein gene. This allows the binding of the activator SARP to its binding site, which overlaps with the STR binding sequence. This mechanism could strongly augment β-casein gene transcription after an initial induction of mRNA by the lactogenic hormones in the mammary gland. Overlapping sequences for competing repressors and activators have been found in the regulatory regions of several other gene promoters, e.g. the EGF [19], the immunoglobulin heavy chain [20], the β-interferon [21,22] and the skeletal actin muscle [23] genes. Competition for DNA binding between a positively and a negatively acting nuclear factor was also found in the proximal regulatory region of the β-casein gene promoter [7].

Expression of a chimaeric gene construct containing the multimerized −194/−163 fragment of the β-casein promoter is enhanced in a lactogenic-hormone-independent manner. We identified a sequence-specific DNA binding factor, SARP, which specifically recognizes DNA between positions −183 and −163 of the β-casein gene promoter. SARP has binding affinity for both single- and double-stranded DNA. The SARP binding site is found in the upper and lower strands of this region. Mutations between positions −184 and −163 which disrupt the binding of SARP to DNA also abolish promoter activity. It is conceivable that binding of SARP to double-stranded DNA in the −194/−163 region, upon removal of STR, might change the structure of the promoter and increase promoter activity. This could explain the constitutive increase in heterologous gene expression induced by the multimerized −194/−163 oligonucleotides.

Many proteins that bind to single-stranded DNA play important roles in transcriptional regulation [19,23–33]. Some of these factors, such as the oestrogen receptor [25], Myo D [31], p53 [34], transcription factor TFIIIA and FRG Y2 [35], recognize both single- and double-stranded DNA. Others only bind to DNA when it is present as a single-stranded structure, e.g. formed H-DNA [36,37], cruciform DNA [29], tetrad guanidines [38] or at the sites where bending occurs [39]. Binding of these proteins could stabilize unusual DNA structures and could influence gene expression by preventing proteins that bind to double-stranded DNA from interacting with their binding sites. The regulatory region of the β-casein gene promoter between −194 and −163 can potentially form a stable stem–loop structure with its flanking sequences (results not shown). We speculate that STR, which has no affinity for double-stranded DNA, can specifically interact with the upper strand after formation of an altered DNA structure and inhibit SARP binding. The construct containing the oligimerized −194/−163 DNA sequence of the β-casein promoter may not be able to form this special secondary DNA structure. This could be the reason why no repression of this construct by STR has been observed.

SARP and STR compete for binding to the upper strand of DNA, and binding is mutually exclusive. SARP binding to the upper strand could only be detected when nuclear extracts of lactogenic-hormone-treated HC11 cells and of mammary glands from lactating mice were analysed. In these cells, STR activity in the nucleus is down-regulated. Competition between factors that bind to single-stranded and double-stranded DNA for binding to overlapping sequences in the regulatory regions of promoters has been observed, e.g. in the regulation of the rat thyrotropin [32], low-density lipoprotein receptor [30] and growth hormone [28] genes.

SARP is expressed in different cell types, and its binding to lower-strand and double-stranded probes is increased by confluence. Cell–cell and cell–substratum interactions have been reported to influence the status of differentiation of mammary epithelial cells and milk protein gene expression. Confluence is a prerequisite for the lactogenic hormone responsiveness of HC11 cells [2], a process possibly mediated through the deposition of extracellular-matrix components [5]. Our results suggest that the up-regulation of SARP in confluent cells might contribute to the regulation β-casein gene expression and that SARP activity may mediate the effects of confluence and of the extracellular matrix on transcription.

We thank Ines Fernandez for editorial assistance before submission.

References

1. Ball, R.K., Friis, R.R., Schoenenberger, C.A., Doppler, W. and Groner, B. (1988) EMBO. J. **7**, 2089–2095
2. Taverna, D., Groner, B. and Hynes, N.E. (1991) Cell Growth Differ. **2**, 145–154
3. Venesio, T., Taverna, D., Hynes, N.E., et al. (1992) Cell Growth Differ. **3**, 63–71
4. Groner, B. and Gouilleux, F. (1995) Curr. Opin. Genet. Dev. **5**, 587–594
5. Chammas, R., Taverna, D., Cella, N., Santos, C. and Hynes, N.E. (1994) J. Cell Sci. **107**, 1031–1040
6. Altiok, S. and Groner, B. (1993) Mol. Cell. Biol. **13**, 7303–7310
7. Schmitt-Ney, M., Doppler, W., Ball, R.K. and Groner, B. (1991) Mol. Cell. Biol. **11**, 3745–3755
8. Wakao, H., Gouilleux, F. and Groner, B. (1994) EMBO J. **13**, 2182–2191
9. Gouilleux, F., Wakao, H., Mundt, M. and Groner, B. (1994) EMBO J. **13**, 4361–4369
10. Gouilleux, F., Pallard, C., Dusanter-Fourt, I., Wakao, H., Haldosen, L.-A., Norstedt, G., Levy, D. and Groner, B. (1995) EMBO J. **14**, 2005–2013
11. Ihle, J.N. (1995) Nature (London) **377**, 591–594
12. Ihle, J.N. (1996) Cell **84**, 331–334
13. Meier, V. and Groner, B. (1994) Mol. Cell. Biol. **14**, 128–137
14. Altiok, S. and Groner, B. (1994) Mol. Cell. Biol. **14**, 6004–6012
15. Doppler, W., Groner, B. and Ball, R.K. (1989) Proc. Natl. Acad. Sci. U.S.A. **86**, 104–108
16. Eisenberg, S., Francesconi, S.C., Civalier, C. and Walker, S.S. (1988) Methods Enzymol. **182**, 521–529
17. Luckow, B. and Schutz, G. (1987) Nucleic Acids Res. **15**, 5490
18. Schmitt-Ney, M., Happ, B., Ball, R.K. and Groner, B. (1992) Proc. Natl. Acad. Sci. U.S.A. **89**, 3130–3134
19. Brunel, F., Alzari, P.M., Ferrara, P. and Zakin, M.M. (1991) Nucleic Acids Res. **19**, 5237–5245
20. Lenardo, J.M., Staudt, L., Robbins, P., Khang, A., Mulligan, R.C. and Baltimore, D. (1989) Science **243**, 544–546
21. Goodburn, S. and Maniatis, T. (1988) Proc. Natl. Acad. Sci. U.S.A. **85**, 1447–1451
22. Harada, R.S., Fujita, T., Miyamoto, M., et al. (1989) Cell **58**, 729–739
23. Kamada, S. and Miwa, T. (1992) Gene **119**, 229–236
24. Jansen Durr, P., Boshart, M., Lupp, B., Bosserhoff, A., Frank, R.W. and Schutz, G. (1992) Nucleic Acids Res. **20**, 1243–1249
25. Lannigan, D.A. and Notides, A.C. (1989) Proc. Natl. Acad. Sci. U.S.A. **86**, 863–867
26. Mukherjee, R. and Chambon, P. (1990) Nucleic Acids Res. **18**, 5713–5716
27. Nordstrom, L.A., Dean, D.M. and Sanders, M.M. (1993) J. Biol. Chem. **268**, 13193–13202
28. Pan, W.T., Liu, Q.R. and Bancroft, C. (1990) J. Biol. Chem. **265**, 7022–7028
29. Quinn, J.P. and McAllister, J. (1993) Nucleic Acids Res. **21**, 1637–1641
30. Rajavashisth, T.B., Taylor, A.K., Andalibi, A., Svenson, K.L. and Lusis, A.J. (1989) Science **245**, 640–643
31. Santoro, I.M., Yi, T.M. and Walsh, K. (1991) Mol. Cell. Biol. **11**, 1944–1953

32. Shimura, H., Ikuyama, S., Shimura, Y. and Kohn, L.D. (1993) J. Biol. Chem. **268**, 24125–24137

33. Wilkison, W.O., Min, H.Y., Claffey, K.P., Satterberg, B.L. and Spiegelman, B.M. (1990) J. Biol. Chem. **265**, 477–482

34. Oberosler, P., Hloch, P., Ramsperger, U. and Stahl, H. (1993) EMBO J. **12**, 2389–2396

35. Tafuri, S.R. and Wolffe, A.P. (1993) Trends Cell Biol. **3**, 94–99

36. Hoffman, E.K., Trusko, S.P., Murphy, M. and George, D.L. (1990) Proc. Natl. Acad. Sci. U.S.A. **87**, 2705–2709

37. Pestov, D.G., Dayn, A., Siyanova, E.Y., George, D.L. and Mirkin, S.M. (1991) Nucleic Acids Res. **19**, 6527–6532

38. Walsh, K. and Gualbertos, A. (1992) J. Biol. Chem. **267**, 13714–13718

39. Kawamoto, T., Makino, K., Orita, S., Nakata, A. and Kakunaga, T. (1989) Nucleic Acids Res. **17**, 523–537

Biochem. Soc. Symp. **63**, 133–140
Printed in Great Britain

11

Gene expression in the mammary glands of transgenic animals

A.J. Clark

Division of Molecular Biology, Roslin Institute, Roslin, Midlothian EH25 9PS, Scotland, U.K.

Abstract

The gene encoding the milk protein β-lactoglobulin in sheep is expressed in the mammary gland in a tissue-specific manner during pregnancy and lactation. The unmodified sheep gene behaves appropriately in transgenic mice, and we have shown that many of the *cis*-acting elements that mediate this pattern of expression are located in the proximal 400 bp of the promotor. Using a combination of approaches we have identified a number of discrete *cis*-acting elements and their corresponding *trans*-acting factors that control the responsiveness of this gene *in vivo*. The β-lactoglobulin promoter elements can be used to target the expression of foreign genes to the mammary gland in transgenic mice. We have used this approach in basic studies of mammary gland biology and for the production of therapeutic proteins in the milk of transgenic animals. In these circumstances, however, the promoter rarely functions optimally, and it may even be silenced; consequently, we have had to develop a number of strategies to overcome this problem. Nevertheless, foreign proteins do appear to be appropriately post-translationally modified when they are expressed in the mammary gland.

Introduction

For a number of years we have been studying the control of milk protein gene expression in the mammary glands of transgenic animals. As well as advancing our understanding of the molecular mechanisms controlling these genes in the mammary gland, we have also been interested in using this technology to produce recombinant proteins in transgenic livestock. In this paper I shall provide an overview of this area of our work, as well as highlighting some of our more recent results on the basic mechanisms of gene control, strategies for improving transgene expression and the capacity for post-translational modification of foreign proteins in the mammary gland.

Control of milk protein gene expression in transgenic mice

The major protein constituents of milk are the caseins and the whey proteins. In most mammalian species there are four or five distinct caseins and, usually, two different whey proteins synthesized by the gland and secreted into milk. The genes encoding these proteins are expressed specifically and abundantly in the secretory epithelial cells of the mammary gland during pregnancy and lactation. We have been studying the regulation of the ovine β-lactoglobulin gene (the major whey protein gene in sheep milk) in cell culture and in transgenic mice

The β-lactoglobulin gene comprises seven exons and encompasses 4.9 kb of chromosomal DNA [1]. We have introduced this gene into transgenic mice and showed that it is expressed very efficiently, with the appropriate patterns of tissue-specific and developmental regulation [2,3]. Transgenic mice carrying β-lactoglobulin can express the transgene at very high levels; in some cases the foreign protein comprises nearly 50% of the total protein content of the milk, although this does not appear in any way to be detrimental to the pups. Interestingly, this very high level of β-lactoglobulin expression results in a corresponding decrease in the protein levels of the endogenous mouse milk protein, and there is no overall increase in the protein content of the milk from these animals [4]. There is thus a limit to the overall level of protein production in the mammary gland. At what level this limitation acts within the gland is not clear. The decrease in the level of the endogenous proteins is correlated with a corresponding decrease in their steady-state mRNA levels. This shows that competition at the level of transcription may occur but, so far, we have been unable to confirm this by direct measurements of transcription rates.

Resection analysis of the 5′ flanking regions of the β-lactoglobulin gene followed by testing in transgenic mice has shown that only 406 bp of the proximal promoter is required to direct tissue-specific and developmentally specific expression of this gene to the mammary gland. β-Lactoglobulin transgenes comprising this promoter region are expressed in an efficient and position-independent manner [5]. Important elements for expression lie within this region, as further resection dramatically reduces the efficiency and level of β-lactoglobulin expression in transgenic mice. Additional evidence for the importance of this promoter region comes from an analysis of the chromatin structure of the β-lactoglobulin gene. In the actively expressing gland the 400 bp β-lactoglobulin promoter region is almost precisely encompassed by a very strong DNase-hypersensitive site which, like the expression of the gene itself, is developmentally regulated [5,6]

The 406 bp minimal promoter element of the β-lactoglobulin gene has been dissected further using a combination of biochemical and functional assays. Gel-mobility-shift assays were used to identify putative transcription factors binding to this segment of DNA. Three related sites were identified which bound a common DNA binding protein termed MPBF (milk protein binding factor) that had high activity in nuclear extracts from the mammary gland [7]. Site-specific mutation of these sites followed by functional analysis in mammary gland cells in culture and in transgenic mice showed that these sites mediated, in part, the lactogenic responsiveness of the gene and were important for attaining maximal transcription *in vivo* [8,9]. These studies also showed that MPBF was similar, if not identical, to a transcription factor termed MGF (mammary-gland-specific factor) identified by B. Groner and colleagues in the rat mammary gland and now known to be a member of the Stat (signal transducers and activators of transcription) family of transcription factors [10]. MPBF/MGF is now termed Stat5. Stat proteins function as cellular signalling molecules for the cytokine family of receptors, of which both the prolactin and growth hormone receptors are members [11]. For β-lactoglobulin we have shown that the most proximal MPBF binding site is required to mediate the prolactin or growth hormone responsiveness of the β-lactoglobulin promoter in CHO cells that have been transfected with the corresponding receptor gene [12].

We have also observed a number of other transcription factors that bind to the β-lactoglobulin promoter (T. Burdon, unpublished work). In some cases, discrete mutation of these sites abolished or even eliminated expression from reporter constructs in the mouse mammary cell line HC11. However, when tested in transgenic mice the importance of such sites is unclear, and we have failed to identify discrete factor binding sites whose integrity is required for expression of β-lactoglobulin *in vivo*. It seems likely that there are no discrete sites/transcription factors that determine mammary gland specificity but, rather, that mammary-gland-specific expression is a matter of combinatorial interactions between a number of different factors and their binding sites.

Expression of foreign proteins in the mammary gland

We have used the promoter from the β-lactoglobulin gene to target expression of different human proteins, including human factor IX and human α_1-antitrypsin (α_1AT), to the mammary gland. The idea has been for these proteins to be synthesized in the gland and secreted into milk, from where they can be subsequently harvested. Of course, production on a commercial scale requires that the producer animal makes substantial quantities of milk, and we have elected to use sheep for this purpose [13]. Fusion genes were constructed in which the cDNA sequences encoding these proteins were linked to sequences derived from the β-lactoglobulin gene. Factor IX and α_1AT are both plasma proteins which are synthesized normally in the liver. Factor IX is an essential protein in the blood clotting cascade and is used in the treatment of haemophilia B, a genetic disorder which afflicts about 1 in 30000 males. α_1AT is an inhibitor of the lung protease, elastase. Reduced blood levels of this protein (in many cases caused by mutation of the α_1AT gene) can lead to the degenerative lung disorder emphysema. Large amounts of human α_1AT would be required for replacement therapy, and these cannot be supplied by conventional plasma fractionation. The general protease activities of α_1AT may also be useful in ameliorating the tissue degeneration that is associated with cystic fibrosis.

The β-lactoglobulin–α_1AT and β-lactoglobulin–factor-IX fusion genes were introduced into sheep and a number of transgenic lines were established. Expression of the transgenes was analysed at both the RNA and protein levels [14,15]. Expression of both α_1AT and factor IX transgenes was detected specifically in the mammary gland, and the human protein products were shown to be secreted into the milk. In both cases, however, the levels of the human protein were rather low, and certainly insufficient for commercial exploitation.

Enhancing transgene expression

The early experiments with transgenic sheep demonstrated the feasibility of producing human therapeutic proteins in the milk of transgenic animals. Nevertheless, there was a clear requirement to improve the level of expression of the transgenes so that commercial levels of protein production could be obtained. Over the years we have innovated a number of strategies to improve transgene expression for this purpose. Because of the limitations of working with large animals, we have made substantial use of transgenic mice. In this regard we have been particularly encouraged by the efficient and appropriate expression of the sheep β-lactoglobulin gene in mice, reflecting the common mechanisms of milk protein gene control among the different mammalian species.

The DNA sequences encoding a particular protein of interest may only be available as cDNA sequences. This may reflect the original cloning experiment or the fact that many of the candidate genes are encoded by very large genes (for example, the factor VIII gene is about 180 kb in length [16]). As such, cDNA segments lack introns and, although no specific role in controlling gene expression has been ascribed to them, their absence is a common feature of many poorly expressing transgenes.

In a large study we compared the expression levels of a number of different transgenes either containing or lacking introns [17]. The results were quite clear in that the transgenes containing most or all of their natural introns were expressed much more efficiently than their intronless counterparts, and this was consistent with observations from a number of other laboratories [18,19]. For example, constructs comprising the β-lactoglobulin sequences fused to the cDNA sequences encoding human α_1AT were poorly expressed, if at all. By contrast, a construct comprising the same β-lactoglobulin promoter elements used in the cDNA constructs but fused to a genomic minigene encoding human α_1AT was expressed much more efficiently [20]. Indeed, mice expressing 7–8 mg of the human protein/ml were produced. Using an anti-elastase assay (elastase is the natural substrate for α_1AT), this protein was shown to have full biological activity.

Given the successful outcome in transgenic mice, it was decided to introduce the same transgene into sheep. This was done as a collaborative project with PPL Therapeutics Ltd., a company established specifically to develop transgenic technology for human pharmaceutical protein production. A number of sheep carrying this construct were generated. When the founder females were reproductively mature they were mated, and milk was collected from them soon after the birth of their lambs and analysed for the presence of human α_1AT. The milk of all three of the founder females contained the human protein; most importantly, one of these animals was shown to produce exceedingly high levels of the human protein – more than 30 mg/ml [21]. A transgenic flock of human α_1AT sheep has now been established which stably express high levels of this protein in their milk. Recently PPL Therapeutics has completed the construction of a plant to purify and produce this protein from the milk of the sheep, and phase I clinical trials are anticipated shortly.

Poorly expressed transgenes, such as those lacking the appropriate introns, appear to be greatly influenced by effects exerted at the site of transgene integration; so-called 'position effects', which reduce or even silence gene expression. We have reasoned, therefore, that engineering the site of integration rather than the construct itself might provide a strategy for rescuing poorly expressed genes. For targeting expression to the mammary gland, the vicinity of an actively expressed milk protein gene could constitute a position that would rescue the expression of otherwise poorly expressed constructs. Gene targeting by homologous recombination in embryonic stem cells [22] would, in principle, enable the insertion of constructs adjacent to endogenous, highly expressed milk protein genes. Gene targeting is limited, however, to mice, since no proven embryonic stem cells have yet been described in livestock species. We have favoured an alternative approach that involves the co-injection of two different DNA constructs into pro-nuclei, since this can result in their co-integration at a single site. Since the β-lactoglobulin gene is very efficiently expressed (presumably containing all the sequences required to overcome chromosomal position effects), we chose to co-inject this gene with the poorly expressed cDNA-derived constructs [23].

In the first series of experiments the unmodified β-lactoglobulin gene was co-injected with β-lactoglobulin–cDNA constructs encoding either human α_1AT or human factor IX. The frequency of co-integration was quite high, and in both experiments more than 50% of the founder mice had integrated both β-lactoglobulin and the β-lactoglobulin–cDNA construct at a single locus. When the β-lactoglobulin–cDNA constructs were injected alone they were expressed very poorly, if at all [17]. By contrast, most of the transgenic lines carrying these constructs co-integrated with β-lactoglobulin expressed them, although a considerable variation in expression levels was observed between the various lines generated [23]. This 'rescue' effect appears to require the expression of the β-lactoglobulin gene, since only in the mouse lines expressing the β-lactoglobulin gene is expression of the second transgene observed. Similarly, co-integration with a transcriptionally inactivated β-lactoglobulin gene does not lead to rescue of the second gene, although a translationally inactivated β-lactoglobulin will function in this regard [24].

It is axiomatic that efficient expression requires that the transgene mRNA be correctly processed. This may not always be the case when 'abnormal' genes (e.g. cDNAs) are targeted to a cell type in which they are not normally expressed (e.g. both factor IX and α_1AT are expressed normally in hepatocytes, not mammary epithelial cells). In our attempts to express factor IX in the mammary gland we have shown that this can be a significant problem. Thus, using the rescue strategy described above, we produced transgenic mice that expressed high levels of the transgene mRNA in the mammary gland. We were only able to detect low levels of the protein in the milk, however [23]. Close inspection of β-lactoglobulin–factor-IX mRNA showed that it was about 400 nt smaller than predicted from the structure of the transgene. Cloning and sequencing studies demonstrated that this resulted from a specific cryptic RNA splice that removed the C-terminal sequences encoding factor IX from the mRNA [25]. Both transgenic mice and transgenic sheep carrying factor IX cDNA constructs suffered from this problem, leading to a low level of factor IX production in the milk. Removal of the cryptic acceptor site, which is located in the 3' untranslated region of the factor IX sequences, resolves this problem. By using a combination of transgene rescue and a corrected factor IX cDNA transgene, we have generated transgenic mice producing more than 120 μg of human factor IX/ml in their milk (this is more than 20-fold higher than the normal concentration of factor IX in human plasma).

Post-translational modifications in the mammary gland

The strategy of producing human therapeutic proteins in the milk of transgenic animals requires that the mammary gland carries out the appropriate post-translational modifications of the various target proteins. This is clearly essential if the ensuing products are to have the necessary biological activity, stability and lack of immunogenicity required of a therapeutic agent. At the outset of this work little was known concerning the capacity of the secretory epithelial cells of the mammary gland in this regard.

Factor IX requires the γ-carboxylation of a cluster of 12 Glu residues near the N-terminus for full biological activity [26]. This domain serves to bind Ca^{2+}, which is an essential cofactor for factor IX activity. In our studies on the expression of factor IX in the mammary glands of transgenic mice, we have used a monoclonal antibody specific for this Ca^{2+} binding γ-carboxyglutamic acid domain to purify the factor IX produced in the milk [24]. This resulted in recovery of about half the factor IX from the starting material, all of which was shown to be fully active in a clotting assay. This also demonstrates that the factor IX propeptide is correctly processed in the mammary gland, since this is a prerequisite for biological activity. The mammary gland thus appears to be capable of carrying out the γ-carboxylation of factor IX quite efficiently. This is particularly gratifying, since this post-translational modification has not been reported for any of the endogenous proteins made in the gland. Another γ-carboxylated protein, protein C, has been obtained from the milk of transgenic animals. In transgenic mice propeptide cleavage and γ-carboxylation were incomplete, and only trace activity was detected [27]. In transgenic pigs protein C was present in milk at levels between 0.5 and 1.0 mg/ml, but this material was only 30–60% active [28]. Interestingly, preliminary results in trangenic sheep indicate that protein C expressed in milk at levels >0.1 mg/ml is active (I. Cottingham, unpublished work).

Glycosylation is also a crucial type of post-translational modification which can affect the solubility, stability, biological activity and immunogenicity of proteins. Human α_1AT has three N-linked glycosylation sites, and the glycosylation status of these is an important consideration for its pharmacokinetics. Thus glycoproteins containing high-mannose or desialylated structures may have a short half-life in the circulation due to high-mannose and asialoglycoprotein receptors in the liver. We have characterized the glycosylation status of two of the three N-linked sites in human α_1AT produced in the milk of transgenic mice. The material from transgenic mice exhibited biantennary and triantennary structures at these sites but a higher level of fucosylation than the human-plasma-derived material, although high-mannose and hybrid structures were not detected at either site [29]. In a study of human tissue type plasminogen activator produced in the milk of transgenic goats, N-acetylglucosamine and sialic acid (present in the plasma-derived protein) were detected, but N-acetylgalactosamine was also detected, which is not normally found in the native protein. Clearly there is a requirement to characterize more fully the glycosylation status of human proteins produced by this route, particularly bearing in mind that there may be significant species differences.

Concluding remarks

Transgenic mice provide a tool for the the analysis of gene expression, and we have made extensive use of them to define the requirement for specific segments and sequence elements in mediating expression of the milk protein gene β-lactoglobulin in the mammary gland. Thus the unmodified β-lactoglobulin gene is expressed efficiently and at high levels in the mammary glands of transgenic mice; we have defined the promoter segment required for this and, indeed, made a significant start to identifying the *cis* sequence elements (and the corresponding *trans*-acting factors) that function in this regard. By contrast, hybrid transgenes in which the β-lactoglobulin promoter is used to drive the expression of foreign gene sequences are expressed much less efficiently and we have had to adopt a variety of strategies to improve expression. Nevertheless, once expression of foreign proteins has been achieved, such proteins appear to be appropriately post-translationally modified even if such modifications, as is the case with γ-carboxylation, are not normally carried out in this tissue.

I thank all my colleagues and collaborators who have contributed to the work described in this presentation, in particular Tom Burdon, Anona Cranston, Ian Cottingham (PPL Therapeutics), Jerome Demmer, Jean Djiane (INRA), Nigel Jenkins (University of Kent), Pauline Kemp (University of Kent), Roberta Wallace, Christine Watson, Bruce Whitelaw and Fiona Yull. This research was supported by the Biotechnology and Biological Sciences Research Council (U.K.) and PPL Therapeutics.

References
1.   Ali, S. and Clark, A.J. (1988) J. Mol. Biol. **199**, 415–426
2.   Simons, J.P., McClenaghan, M. and Clark, A.J. (1987) Nature (London) **328**, 530–532
3.   Harris, S., McClenaghan, M., Simons, J.P., Ali, S. and Clark, A.J. (1991) Dev. Genet. **12**, 299–307
4.   McClenaghan, M., Springbett, A., Wallace, R.M., Wilde, C.J. and Clark, A.J. (1995) Biochem. J. **310**, 637–641
5.   Whitelaw, C.B.A., Harris, S., McClenaghan, M., Simons, J.P. and Clark, A.J. (1992) Biochem. J. **286**, 31–39
6.   Whitelaw, C.B.A. (1995) Biochem. Biophys. Res. Commun. **209**, 1089–1093
7.   Watson, C.J., Gordon, K.E., Robertson, M. and Clark, A.J. (1991) Nucleic Acids Res. **19**, 6603–6610
8.   Burdon, T., Demmer, J., Clark, A.J. and Watson, C.J. (1994) FEBS Lett. **350**, 177–182
9.   Burdon, T., Maitland, A., Demmer, J., Clark, A.J., Wallace, R. and Watson, C.J. (1994) Mol. Endocrinol. **8**, 1528–1536
10. Wakao, H., Gouilleux, F. and Groner, B. (1994) EMBO J. **9**, 2182–2192
11. Bazan, J.F. (1990) Proc. Natl. Acad. Sci. U.S.A. **87**, 6934–6938
12. Demmer, J., Burdon, T., Djiane, J., Watson, C.J. and Clark, A.J. (1995) Mol. Cell. Endocrinol. **107**, 113–121
13. Clark, A.J., Simons, J.P., Wilmut, I. and Lathe, R. (1987) Trends Biotechnol. **5**, 20–24
14. Clark, A.J., Bessos, H., Bishop, J.O., et al. (1989) Bio/Technology **7**, 487–492
15. McClenaghan, M., Archibald, A.L., Harris, S., Simons, J.P., Whitelaw, C.B.A., Wilmut, I. and Clark, A.J. (1991) J. Anim. Biotechnol. **2**, 161–176
16. Gitschier, J., Wood, W.I., Goralka, T.M., et al. (1984) Nature (London) **312**, 326–330
17. Whitelaw, C.B.A., Archibald, A.L., Harris, S., McClenaghan, M., Simons, J.P. and Clark, A.J. (1991) Transgenic Res. **1**, 3–13
18. Brinster, R.L., Allen, J.M., Behringer, R.R., Gelinas, R.E. and Palmiter, R.D. (1988) Proc. Natl. Acad. Sci. U.S.A. **85**, 836–840
19. Choi, T., Huang, M., Gorman, C. and Jaenisch, R. (1991) Mol. Cell. Biol. **11**, 3070–3074
20. Archibald, A.L., McClenaghan, M., Hornsey, V., Simons, J.P. and Clark, A.J. (1990) Proc. Natl. Acad. Sci. U.S.A. **87**, 5178–5182
21. Wright, G., Carver, A., Cottom, D., et al. (1991) Bio/Technology **9**, 830–834
22. Capecchi, M.R. (1989) Science **244**, 1288–1292
23. Clark, A.J., Cowper, A., Wallace, R., Wright, G. and Simons, J.P. (1992) Bio/Technology **10**, 1450–1454
24. Yull, F., Binas, B., Harold, G., Wallace, R. and Clark, A.J. (1996) Transgenic Res. **6**, 11–17
25. Yull, F., Harold, G., Cowper, A., Percy, J., Cottingham, I. and Clark, A.J. (1995) Proc. Natl. Acad. Sci. U.S.A. **92**, 10899–10903
26. Anson, D.S., Austen, D.E.G. and Brownlee, G.G. (1985) Nature (London) **315**, 683–685
27. Drohan, H., Zhang, D., Paleyanda, R.K., et al. (1994) Transgenic Res. **3**, 355–364
28. Velander, W.H., Johnson, J.L., Page, R.L., et al. (1992) Proc. Natl. Acad. Sci. U.S.A. **89**, 12003–12007
29. Kemp, P., Freedman, R.A., Clark, A.J. and Jenkins, N. (1997) Proc. Jpn. Assoc. Anim. Cell. Tech., in the press

Biochem. Soc. Symp. **63**, 141–147
Printed in Great Britain

12

Production of therapeutic proteins in the milk of transgenic livestock

Alan Colman

PPL Therapeutics, Roslin, Edinburgh, Midlothian EH25 9PP, Scotland, U.K.

Abstract

With the advent of the Human Genome Project and associated developments in 'functional genomics', there are going to be increasing numbers of proteins identified and developed for clinical use. There are a number of production methods available, although only three, bacterial, yeast and mammalian cell culture, have produced recombinant proteins that have been approved for clinical use. Nevertheless other production systems are under development, and one, the production of human proteins in the milk of transgenic livestock, is showing great promise, with two proteins now in clinical trials. This chapter will compare and contrast the various competing technologies and will then concentrate on factors influencing the choice and use of the transgenic system.

Introduction

Recombinant proteins now account for over £3 billion in sales of drugs for human use. In order to meet such a large and growing market, a variety of production technologies have and are being developed. To date, the majority of recombinant proteins on the market are produced in bacterial, yeast or mammalian cell culture. However, a number of additional technologies are jostling for a place at the table. In this chapter, I will first review the perceived advantages and disadvantages of the competing methods, before concentrating in detail on the production of human recombinant proteins in the milk of transgenic livestock. This relatively new method, while it has yet to boast any sales for clinical use, is now generating products that have entered clinical trials, a mandatory step before such products can be approved.

Production of recombinant proteins for therapeutic use

The choice of production system for a given therapeutic protein is a complex one. The following factors have to be considered: running costs of production, running costs of purification, production scale, production and purification yields, capital equipment costs, time-scale of production, ease of scale-up, protein quality and complexity, regulatory issues, etc. Table 1 lists the various production systems, along with comments on their suitability.

Clearly, the nature and characteristic features of the target protein are of considerable relevance to the eventual choice of production system. Bacteria are incapable of performing various post-translational modifications which are commonplace in eukaryotic cells. These inadequacies would seem to simplify decision making where the target is, for example, a glycosylated protein. This is not always the case, however, since modifications such as glycosylation some-

Table 1. Methods of recombinant protein production for clinical use.

Method	Advantages	Disadvantages
Bacterial culture	Low cost Proven Broad application Large-scale production	Limited ability to post-translationally modify eukaryotic proteins
Yeast culture	Low cost Some successes Broadening applications Large-scale production	Limited ability to correctly post-translationally modify eukaryotic proteins
Insect cell culture	Commercially unproven Probably low cost	Limited ability to correctly post-translationally modify eukaryotic proteins
Mammalian cell culture	Proven Broad application	Expensive Low-scale production
Milk from transgenic livestock	Broad applications Low cost Commercially unproven, but proteins in clinical trials Large-scale production	May be problems with some bioactive proteins
Transgenic plants	Very low cost Negligible infection risk Large-scale production Commercially unproven	Many problems with production of complex/bioactive proteins Extraction a problem

times do not affect the bioactivity of the protein; depending on the protein and its intended therapeutic use, glycosylation may be dispensable. Thus granulo-cyte colony-stimulating factor is normally a N-glycosylated protein; neverthe-less, the preparation which is currently approved for clinical use is made in bac-teria and consequently is not glycosylated. However, there are many human proteins that require either eukaryotic modifications, such as glycosylation or γ-carboxylation, or intra- or inter-chain assembly for their bioactivity, solubil-ity or serum stability; in these cases, a higher-eukaryotic production system is needed. At the present time we believe that, in these circumstances, there are only two options: mammalian cell culture or production in the milk of trans-genic livestock. We would exclude yeast, insect and transgenic plant systems at present for the reasons summarized in Table 1. However, future refinements such as the customization of these systems with mammalian glycosyltrans-ferases may change the situation.

To date, there are numerous therapeutic recombinant proteins approved for human use that have been produced in mammalian cell culture. Examples include the blood clotting agents factors VII and VIII, tissue plasminogen acti-vator, erythropoietin, growth hormone, follicle-stimulating hormone, various interferons, etc. The preferred cell lines used are Chinese hamster ovary (CHO) and baby hamster kidney (BHK) cells. This is in contrast with the situ-ation with transgenic production systems, where no products are currently approved for use. Nevertheless, as will be described below, these systems hold out enormous promise for the future, especially in the realm of complex and/or high-volume proteins.

Production of therapeutic proteins in the milk of transgenic livestock

In 1987, John Clark and his colleagues [1] showed for the first time that the milk of transgenic animals, in this case mice, could provide a reservoir for large quantities of a foreign secretory protein. This demonstration was soon followed by the generation of transgenic sheep secreting modest quantities of the human proteins α_1-antitrypsin (α_1AT) and factor IX [2]. Table 2 displays the current situation and clearly shows that considerable quantities of a large variety of human proteins can be manufactured in the milk of sheep, pigs, goats and rabbits. These accumulating data and other considerations underpin a check list which should be appraised before a transgenic production route is chosen. The more important questions are outlined below.

Choice of protein

As indicated in Table 1, proteins that undergo post-translational modifi-cations, and/or are required at low cost in large amounts, are candidates for this technology.

Choice of promotor

A variety of milk gene promotors have been used to drive transgenic pro-tein expression in milk. These include the promotors from rabbit, cow and

Table 2. Production of potential therapeutic proteins in the milk of transgenic livestock. Abbreviations: tPA, tissue plasminogen activator; WAP, whey acidic protein; IGF, insulin-like growth factor; gDNA, genomic DNA; βLG, β-lactoglobulin.

Promoter	Protein	cDNA/gDNA	Expression level (mg/ml)	Animal	References
α$_{S1}$-Casein (bovine)	Lactoferrin	cDNA	Undisclosed	Cow	3
β-Casein (goat)	Longer-acting tPA	cDNA	2–3	Goat	4
WAP (mouse)	Longer-acting tPA	cDNA	0.003	Goat	4
WAP (mouse)	Protein C	cDNA	1	Pig	5
α$_{S1}$-Casein (bovine)	IGF	cDNA		Rabbit	6
βLG (sheep)	Factor IX	cDNA	25×10^{-6}	Sheep	2
βLG (sheep)	Protein C	cDNA	300	Sheep	*
			750	Rabbit	*
			750	Pig	*
βLG (sheep)	α$_1$AT	gDNA	35	Sheep	8
βLG (sheep)	Fibrinogen	gDNA	5	Sheep	*
βLG (sheep)	Nutritional enzyme	gDNA	>4	Sheep	*

*PPL Therapeutics, unpublished work.

sheep casein genes, the cow α-lactalbumin gene, the sheep β-lactoglobulin gene and the mouse whey acid protein gene. There is very little to choose between any of these promotors.

Choice of DNA configuration

For reasons that are not understood, it appears that genomic gene fragments express as least as well and often better than the cDNA equivalent. This situation does not seem to hold for expression in cultured cells, where cDNAs are preferred. Unfortunately, size and availability often preclude the use of genomic fragments.

Choice of integration locus

If only it were so simple! At the present time, targeted insertion is only possible in mice, using embryonic stem (ES) cells. For livestock, microinjection of DNA into the fertilized embryo is the only practical route to transgenesis. Unfortunately, this means that DNA integration is a random event, so that often the integrated transgenes are subject to chromosomal position effects that negatively affect their expression. On the other hand, this is somewhat compensated for by the fact that insertion of multiple copies is the norm via the microinjection route, whereas this would be difficult using ES cells. Some of the disadvantages of the present methods may be remedied by the use of very large DNA fragments (e.g. yeast artificial chromosomes), or by the use of nuclear transplantation, as an alternative to ES cells.

Choice of species

This is a difficult decision. Mice are usually chosen for proof of concept studies because milk can be obtained within 4 months of starting the microinjections. However, volumes of milk (and therefore amounts of protein for evaluation) are quite limited (approx. 0.4 ml), and some researchers or customers prefer the rabbit, which can deliver several hundred millilitres within 8 months of microinjection. Pigs (>150 litres), sheep (~400 litres), goats (~500 litres) and cows (~10 000 litres) give increasingly large yields of milk during an average lactation period, but the penalty is time to lactation (from microinjection), which for the pig is 15 months, for sheep and goats about 18 months, and for the cow about 32 months. The choice will therefore be influenced by the amounts of protein needed for clinical development and subsequent sales. In addition, there will be regulatory concerns regarding the presence of pathogenic agents such as prions in the production animals. While some of these concerns can be allayed by the use of validated purification methods, we have chosen to work with sheep from New Zealand and cows from the U.S.A. because no prion disease has been detected in these species within these countries.

Finally, the choice will depend on the ability of the different species to produce high-quality protein. In a comparison of mice, rabbits, pigs and sheep, all transgenic for the human anticoagulant agent protein C, we have found the sheep to be the best species in terms of its γ-carboxylation of this protein, a modification which is essential for bioactivity.

From concept to clinic: α_1AT produced in the milk of transgenic sheep

Human α_1AT is currently prepared for clinical use from human plasma. It is used in the U.S.A. and some European countries to treat congenital emphysema. However, supplies from this source are limited and many sufferers go untreated. Moreover, there is no surplus material for testing the efficacy of α_1AT on other diseases such as cystic fibrosis. We have taken the transgenic route to remedy the supply problem.

A genomic α_1AT gene was fused downstream of the ovine β-lactoglobulin promotor and injected into fertilized she ep embryos. From 112 lambs born to this experiment, five were transgenic. The oldest animal, 'Tracy', was shown to produce over 30 g of human α_1AT/litre in her milk [7]. Although she transmitted the transgene to her offspring, gene rearrangement occurred and this line was not developed for commercial purposes. Instead, a male transgenic was chosen. Transgenic female offspring from this animal produced on average 15 g/litre α_1AT [8], and a commercial process has been developed from this line. Several G1 males (production founders) have been used to collect and prepare over 10000 doses of semen. The semen is stored in liquid nitrogen and thawed aliquots are used to generate a production flock of several hundred G2 females. Milk is collected twice a day, pooled, skimmed and then frozen; pathogen testing is performed on unfrozen samples. Bulked milk is then purified through a sequence of centrifugation, precipitation, chromatography and viral filtration steps. Pure (>99.9999%) protein is then placed into vials, and it has now entered clinical trials.

Conclusions and future prospects

The α_1AT described above and a human anti-thrombin produced in goat milk are just the first of many products obtained using this production route, which we believe will enter clinical development within the next few years. Already we are developing sheep-produced human fibrinogen. This complicated protein, consisting of three pairs of different polypeptide chains, has been produced at 5 g/litre in sheep milk. The protein is fully bioactive. When production of protein in milk was first mooted as a commercial production route, a number of 'insuperable' hurdles were suggested. First, it was said that milk was too complex a medium for simple protein purification; however, we have found purification to be facile for a variety of proteins. Secondly, the pathogen load in milk and the concerns about prions were raised as impassable regulatory blocks; we have demonstrated that the purification methods used would be capable of removing prions and any viruses of concern in the highly unlikely event of them being present. Finally, it was conjectured that human glycosylated proteins made in sheep would not be identical to those made in the normal human host; this is true, and we find that the sugars added to the protein backbone by the livestock mammary gland are slightly different from those conferred by the cognate human tissue. However, the same is true for all those glycosylated proteins in clinical use made in CHO and BHK cells, and no problems have been reported. We are therefore understandably optimistic about the commercial prospects of this technology in the future.

References

1. Simons, J.P., McClenaghan, M. and Clark, A.J. (1987) Nature (London) **328**, 530–532
2. Clark, A.J., Bessos, H., Bishop, J.O., et al. (1989) Biotechnology **7**, 487–492
3. Krimpenfort, P., Rademakers, A., Eyestone, W., et al. (1991) Biotechnology **9**, 844
4. Ebert, K.M., Selgarth, J.P., DiTullio, P., et al. (1991) Biotechnology **9**, 835–838
5. Velander, W.H., Johnson, J.L., Page, R.L., et al. (1992) Proc. Natl. Acad. Sci.U.S.A. **89**, 12003–12007
6. Brem, G., Hartl, P., Besenfelder, U., Wolf, E., Zinovieva, N. and Pfaller, R. (1994) Gene **149**, 351–355
7. Wright, G., Carver, A., Cottom, D., et al. (1991) Biotechnology **9**, 830–834
8. Carver, A., Dalrymple, M.A., Wright, G., et al. (1993) Biotechnology **11**, 1263–1270

Biochem. Soc. Symp. **63**, 149–157
Printed in Great Britain

13

Oncogenic activation of Neu/ErbB-2 in a transgenic mouse model for breast cancer

William J. Muller*†§, Jason Ho*‡ and Peter M. Siegel*‡

*Institute for Molecular Biology and Biotechnology, †Department of Pathology and ‡Department of Biology, McMaster University, 1280 Main Street West, Hamilton, Ontario, Canada L8S 4K1

Abstract

Recent evidence has suggested that amplification and overexpression of *erbB-2/neu* is an important determinant in the initiation and progression of human breast cancer. Consistent with this assertion is the observation that transgenic mice that overexpress the *neu* proto-oncogene heritably develop mammary adenocarcinomas. More recently, we have demonstrated that activation of *neu* in many of these tumours occurs as a result of somatic mutations located within the transgene itself. Indeed, careful examination of the altered *neu* transcripts revealed the presence of in-frame deletions that encode aberrant Neu receptors lacking 5–12 amino acids within the extracellular domain, located adjacent to the transmembrane domain. Interestingly, the majority of the deletions analysed affect one of several conserved cysteine residues present within this region. Moreover, introduction of these activating mutations into the wild-type *neu* cDNA results in its oncogenic conversion. These observations suggest that this cysteine-rich region plays an important role in regulating the catalytic activity of Neu.

Introduction

The transgenic mouse is an important model system in the investigation of the tissue-specific transforming properties of a number of oncogenes. Because breast cancer is a prevalent and poorly understood human disease, our laboratory has been interested in using transgenic mice to directly assess the importance of certain genetic events in the genesis of human breast cancer. For example, amplification and overexpression of the *erbB-2/neu* oncogene has

§To whom correspondence should be addressed, at Institute for Molecular Biology and Biotechnology.

been implicated in the initiation and progression of a large percentage of primary breast cancers [1–4]. The *neu* oncogene encodes a receptor tyrosine kinase (RTK) belonging to the epidermal growth factor receptor (EGFR) family. In addition to *neu*, the EGFR family comprises three other closely related genes, including EGFR, *erbB-3* and *erbB-4* [5–7]. Interestingly, members of the EGFR family can interact with each other. For example, Neu is a substrate for the activated EGFR following stimulation of cells with EGF [8–10] or for activated ErbB-4 following stimulation with heregulin [11,12]. The observed tyrosine phosphorylation of Neu by EGFR is thought to be mediated by heterodimerization between Neu and EGFR family members, resulting in a high-affinity receptor for these mitogenic ligands [9,13]. In addition to activation of ErbB-2/Neu by a variety of physiological ligands, overexpression or mutation of the receptor can result in its oncogenic activation ([14]; Fig. 1).

Initial direct evidence for the involvement of Neu in the induction of mammary tumours stemmed from observations made with transgenic mice expressing a constitutively activated version of Neu [15] in the mammary epithelium [16,17]. In several of these transgenic strains, high-level expression of activated Neu resulted in the development of multifocal mammary adenocarcinomas that affected every female carrier [16]. Consistent with these observations, infection of the mammary epithelium of rats with a retroviral vector bearing the activated *neu* cDNA [15] also resulted in the rapid development of multifocal mammary tumours [18]. Taken together, these observations suggest that activated Neu can act as a potent oncogene in the mammary epithelium. However, in human breast cancer, examination of primary breast cancer samples has thus far failed to reveal a comparable transmembrane mutation in ErbB-2 [19]. However, because these studies were directed towards analyses of the transmembrane domain, it is possible that mutations in other regions of ErbB-2 may be involved in tumour progression. Given the observation that the point mutation in the transmembrane domain does not appear to occur in primary human breast cancers, we decided to test directly the oncogenic potential of wild-type Neu in the mammary epithelium. To accomplish

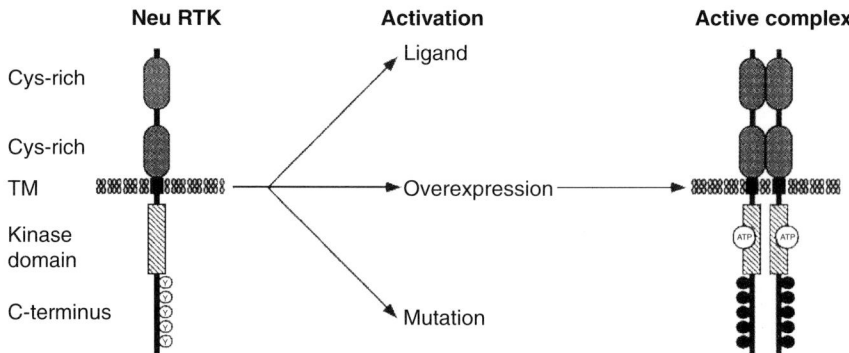

Fig. 1. Schematic representation of the various events that can activate the Neu RTK. Cys-rich, cysteine-rich regions; TM, transmembrane domain; Kinase domain, tyrosine kinase domain.

this objective, several independent strains of transgenic mice carrying a mouse mammary tumour virus (MMTV)-driven *neu* proto-oncogene have been established [20]. In contrast to transgenic mice expressing the activated version of *neu*, mammary-gland-specific expression resulted in the stochastic appearance of focal mammary tumours. Biochemical analyses of these mammary tumours revealed that tumorigenesis in these mice was correlated with increased Neu intrinsic tyrosine kinase activity and with the appearance of several tyrosine-phosphorylated proteins [20].

Because activation of the catalytic activity of Neu can occur through the mutation of a single amino acid in the transmembrane domain [15], we investigated whether this mutation could be detected during tumour progression in these transgenic strains. To this end, total RNA from both breast tumours and adjacent morphologically normal mammary epithelium was subjected to reverse transcription followed by PCR (RT-PCR). The resulting PCR products were then hybridized to oligonucleotides corresponding to either the wild-type sequence or a transmembrane point mutation in Neu. The results showed that, while there was no evidence for the presence of the point mutation, many of the PCR products derived from the Neu-induced tumours possessed deletions [21]. Significantly, sequence analyses of the altered products revealed that these deletions were located in a confined region of the extracellular domain and that they encoded functional Neu proteins due to maintenance of the protein's reading frame. Furthermore, it was demonstrated that these in-frame deletions resulted in constitutive activation of the kinase activity of Neu. The observation that the identified activating mutations reside in a region of Neu not previously known to be involved in its oncogenic activation raises the intriguing possibility that comparable mutations within the ErbB-2 protein might be functionally involved in human breast cancer.

Results and discussion

Previous studies with tumours induced by the expression of *neu* revealed that 65% of the tumours analysed displayed evidence of altered transcripts (34 samples analysed; [21]). In addition, these deletions were noted in mammary tumours arising in three independent transgenic strains expressing the MMTV–*neu* fusion gene [21]. Because the initial riboprobe used in these analyses spans both the extracellular and intracellular regions, it was unclear whether these additional deletions were present in the same extracellular location observed for those characterized by sequence analyses [21]. To test this possibility, separate riboprobes specific for either the extracellular and transmembrane (Fig. 2a) or intracellular (Fig. 2b) regions were generated. These riboprobes were hybridized to RNA derived from tumours that exhibited evidence of deletions with the full-length riboprobe and subjected to RNase protection analyses. As shown in Fig. 2, the results of these RNase protection analyses revealed that these deletions were occurring exclusively in the extracellular domain (Fig. 2a). In contrast, no altered transcripts corresponding to the intracellular domain were detected (Fig. 2b). As observed previously [21], these mammary tumours also expressed comparable levels of wild-type *neu*

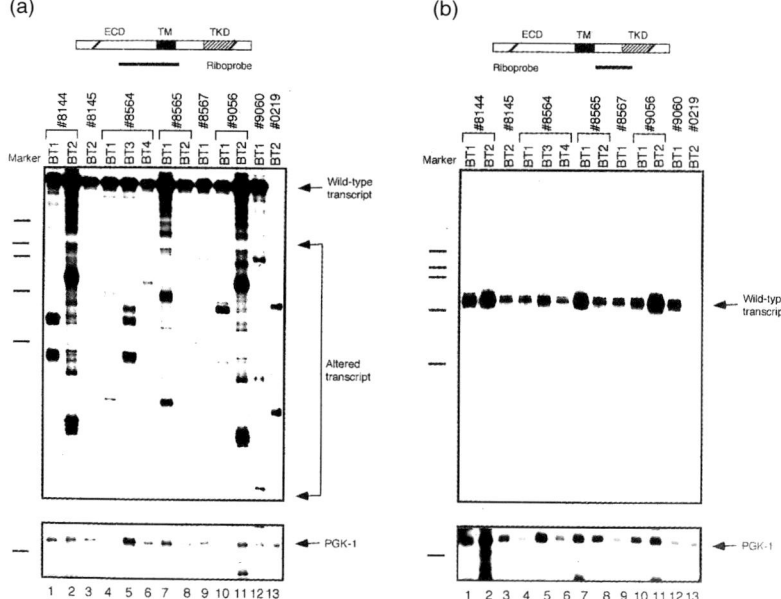

Fig. 2. RNase protection analyses map the remaining deletions to the extracellular juxtamembrane domain. (a) Total RNA from mammary tumour tissue (BT) from the N#202 (#8144, #8145, #8564, #8565, #8567, #9056 and #9060) and N#732 (#0219) transgenic lines were subjected to RNase protection analysis using the riboprobe illustrated in the diagram (ECD, extracellular domain; TM, transmembrane domain; TKD, tyrosine kinase domain). The riboprobe spans nucleotides 1684–2092 of the *neu* cDNA [15] and was released by a *Sma*I/*Bst*11071 digest. The 408 nt wild-type protected fragment is indicated by the top arrow. The bracket indicates the protected fragments corresponding to the altered *neu* transcripts. Migration of DNA markers is indicated on the left (top to bottom: 310, 281, 271, 234, 194 and 118 nt). In the lower panel, an antisense internal control probe, directed against the phosphoglycerate kinase gene, was included to control for equal loading of RNA. The 124 nt protected fragment is indicated by PGK-1. (b) The same tumour samples analysed in (a) were again subjected to RNase protection analysis using a riboprobe to the intracellular juxtamembrane domain, as indicated by the diagram. The riboprobe spans nucleotides 2092–2332 of the *neu* cDNA [15] and was excised as a *Bst*11071/*Xba*I fragment. The 240 nt wild-type protected fragment is indicated by the arrow. The migration of DNA markers is indicated on the left (sizes as described in a). In the lower panel, the PGK-1 internal control riboprobe (described in a) was included to control for equal loading of RNA.

transgene product (Fig. 2). These data argue that the observed activating mutations appear to be localized exclusively in the extracellular domain of Neu.

To define precisely the boundaries of these deletions, several of the representative altered transcripts were subjected to RT-PCR, and the PCR products were inserted into plasmid vectors and subjected to DNA sequence analyses.

For each matched pair of samples, several independent subclones were analysed. The results of these and other previously published alterations are summarized in Fig. 3(a). These PCR products contained deletions ranging from 15 to 36 bp (5–12 amino acids). In addition, one of the alterations (Neu8564) contained a 9-base insertion (Fig. 3a). Significantly, in both insertion and deletion mutants the reading frame of the Neu protein was conserved. The finding that the observed alterations preserved the reading frame of the Neu protein suggested that these alterations may be directly involved in the activation of the intrinsic catalytic domain of Neu. Indeed, previous observa-

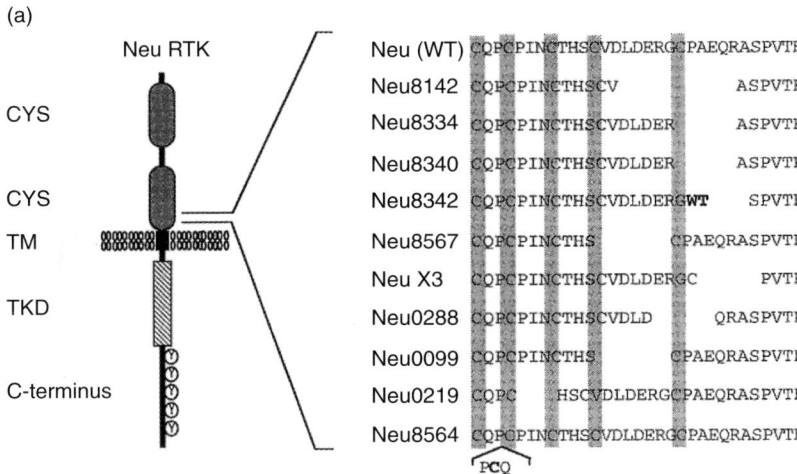

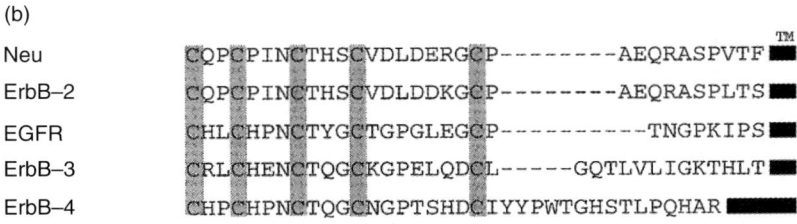

Fig. 3. The cysteine-rich region of Neu containing the identified deletions displays identity among other members of the EGFR family. (a) Protein sequence alignment of the deletions within Neu that have been cloned and sequenced [21]. The abbreviations to the left are defined in the legend to Fig. 1. WT, wild type. (b) Protein sequence alignment of the four members of the EGFR family. Both the rat (Neu) and human (ErbB-2) sequences are included for Neu/ErbB-2, while the human sequence alone is presented for EGFR, ErbB-3 and ErbB-4. The dashes have been included for maximal alignment. The black box represents the position of the transmembrane domain (TM). Reproduced with permission from Siegel, P.M. and Muller, W.J. (1996) Proc. Natl. Acad. Sci. U.S.A. **93**, 8878–8883, ©1996, National Academy of Sciences, U.S.A.

tions have demonstrated that insertion of several of these deletions into an otherwise wild-type *neu* cDNA resulted in its oncogenic activation [21]. To confirm that the other deletion and insertion mutants behaved in a similar manner, three of the deletion mutants and the single insertion mutant were placed into a wild-type *neu* expression cassette and tested for their capacity to transform Rat-1 fibroblasts. Consistent with previous observations [21], expression of these altered Neu receptors was capable of transforming Rat-1 fibroblasts, whereas expression of the wild-type *neu* cDNA was not.

Because the transforming activity of Neu is closely correlated with its activation of intrinsic tyrosine kinase activity [22–24], we also measured the state of tyrosine phosphorylation of Neu in cell lines transformed by these altered cDNAs. The results showed that tyrosine-phosphorylated Neu was detected in cell lines expressing these altered *neu* cDNAs, but was not detected in cell lines expressing elevated levels of wild-type Neu [21]. Thus the increase in the levels of tyrosine-phosphorylated Neu in these cell lines probably reflects the catalytic activation of these altered receptors. The above observations suggest that activation of the Neu tyrosine kinase is a pivotal step in the initiation of mammary tumorigenesis and occurs primarily through somatic mutations in this transgenic mouse model of human breast cancer. The observation that the identified mutations are located in a region of Neu previously not known to be involved in its oncogenic activation raises the intriguing possibility that comparable mutations might be detected in human breast cancers.

It is striking that the mutations we have detected reside in a relatively narrow region of Neu located outside the transmembrane domain (Fig. 3a). In fact, this region in Neu appears to be conserved among the other members of the EGFR family, including EGFR, ErbB-3 and ErbB-4 (Fig. 3b). Specifically, this region in all four known family members contains five cysteine residues that are perfectly conserved (Fig. 3b). Moreover, the amino acids located adjacent to these cysteine residues exhibit a high degree of similarity (Fig. 3b). Interestingly, with the exception of the deletion detected in Neu X3, the deletions that have been sequenced thus far have resulted in the removal or alteration of at least one of the conserved cysteine residues (Fig. 3b). Furthermore, in the mutant Neu molecule possessing the three-amino-acid insertion, one of the inserted amino acids is a cysteine residue. These data suggest that the balance of cysteine residues within this region of Neu may play an important role in activation of the receptor.

Although these observations suggest that these cysteine residues may be involved in the oncogenic activation of the Neu receptor, the precise molecular mechanism by which this occurs remains to be addressed. In this regard, it has been reported that transforming Neu mutants possessing the point mutation in the transmembrane domain demonstrate an increased propensity to homo-dimerize [25–27]. Indeed, immunoprecipitation analyses of this mutant Neu receptor under both reducing and non-reducing conditions revealed that the activated Neu species could be detected as a multimeric complex under non-reducing conditions, which was converted into a monomeric species under reducing conditions [25]. In contrast, the wild-type Neu receptor remained as a monomer species under both reducing and non-reducing conditions. These observations suggest that receptor dimerization is occurring through the formation of disulphide bonds.

Given that many of the deletion and insertion mutations affect different cysteine residues, it is conceivable that, as with the transmembrane point mutation, alteration of these cysteine residues in the mutants promotes receptor dimerization through the formation of cysteine disulphide bonds. Indeed, we have recently demonstrated that these altered receptors dimerize in a manner that is dependent on the formation of disulphide bonds (P.M. Siegel and W.J. Muller, unpublished work). It is possible that these deletions and insertions of cysteine residues disrupt the normal cysteine pairing that occurs in the wild-type receptor. As a consequence, the unpaired cysteine residue would be free to participate in disulphide bond formation with another altered receptor.

Consistent with this proposed model, it has recently been demonstrated that, in inherited forms of endocrine neoplasia type 2A, a single mutation in a cysteine residue located in the cysteine-rich juxtatransmembrane domain of the Ret RTK is responsible for its oncogenic activation. Similar to the Neu deletion mutants, the generation of this cysteine imbalance results in the constitutive dimerization of the Ret RTK in a manner that is dependent on the formation of disulphide bonds [28,29]. In addition to these studies, dimerization of the haemapoetic/cytokine receptor superfamily is thought to involve cysteine disulphide bonding. For example, replacement of specific amino acids with cysteine residues in the juxtatransmembrane domain of either the thrombopoietin receptor or the erythropoietin receptor results in the formation of disulphide-linked dimers that constitutively activate these receptors [30–32]. In addition, it has recently been demonstrated that disruption of disulphide bonding by the administration of reducing agents to the external media of cultured cells can interfere with signalling from the thrombopoietin receptor by preventing its dimerization [30]. Indeed, we have recently demonstrated that addition of 2-mercaptoethanol to the external media of cells can interfere with the transforming potential of these altered Neu receptors in a dose-dependent manner (P.M. Siegel and W.J. Muller, unpublished work). Taken together, these observations suggest that this mode of receptor dimerization may be shared by other receptor systems.

Future objectives

The data generated thus far suggest that the occurrence of these deletions within Neu in this transgenic mouse model is probably directly involved in the induction of mammary tumours expressing the MMTV/wild-type *neu* fusion gene. To directly assess the significance of these activating mutations in Neu, we have recently established transgenic mice that express certain of these activated *neu* alleles under the transcriptional control of the MMTV promoter. Although we are still in the early stages of characterization of these lines, preliminary observations suggest that, in contrast with the parental strains expressing the wild-type *neu* gene, these mice develop multifocal mammary tumours with a relatively shorter latency period (P.M. Siegel and W.J. Muller, unpublished work). However, unlike the transgenic mice expressing the transmembrane point mutation, which exhibit a rapid-progression phenotype [16], these mice possess preneoplastic lesions. One potential explanation for these observations is that, in the latter strains, the level of Neu-associated tyrosine kinase activity is below a certain threshold required for the rapid transformation of the mammary epithelial cell, whereas the rapid-progression strains exceed this critical threshold. Future experiments with these various strains should allow this hypothesis to be rigorously tested.

The frequent occurrence of activating mutations in the juxtatransmembrane domain of Neu raises the possibility that comparable mutations in ErbB-2 might also be involved in the genesis of human breast cancer. We are currently examining human breast cancer biopsies for the occurrence of these mutations to test this hypothesis. Given that activating mutations in Ret RTK can result in the hereditary predisposition to development of endocrine neoplasias, it is conceivable that a comparable germ-line mutation in ErbB-2 may in part be responsible the development of hereditary breast and ovarian cancers. In this regard, it should be noted that ErbB-2 is closely linked to the hereditary breast and ovarian cancer gene *BRCA1*.

Finally, the observation that the region that is deleted in Neu appears to be highly conserved among the different EGFR family members (Fig. 3b) raises the possibility that mutational activation of these other members may also be involved in the genesis of human breast cancer. Indeed, there is considerable evidence to suggest that these other EGFR family members are overexpressed in human breast cancer [6,7]. Although no direct evidence exists for mutational activation of these EGFR family members in human cancers, it has recently been demonstrated that the *Caenorhabditis elegans* EGFR homologue, LET-23, can be activated by mutation of a single cysteine residue in the extreme N-terminus of the protein [33]. Given the potential of the various EGFR family members to heterodimerize, it is conceivable that mutational activation of any one of the EGFR family can activate the other family members. Future studies should allow these issues to be addressed.

References

1.   King, C.R., Kraus, M.H. and Aaronson, S.A. (1985) Science **229**, 974–976
2.   Slamon, D.J., Clark, G.M., Wong, S.G., Levin, W.J., Ullrich, A. and McGuire, W.L. (1987) Science **235**, 177–182
3.   Slamon, D.J., Godolphin, W., Jones, L.A., et al. (1989) Science **244**, 707–712
4.   van de Vijer, M., Peyerse, J., Mooi, W.J., Wisman, P., Lomans, J., Dalesio, O. and Nusse, R. (1988) N. Engl. J. Med. **319**, 1239–1245
5.   Ullrich, A., Coussens, L., Hayflick, J.S., et al. (1984) Nature (London) **309**, 418–425
6.   Kraus, M.H., Issing, I., Miki, T., Popescu, N.C. and Aaronson, S.A. (1989) Proc. Natl. Acad. Sci. U.S.A. **86**, 9193–9197
7.   Plowman, G., Whitney, G., Neubauer, M., Green, J., McDonald, V., Todaro, G. and Shoyab, M. (1990) Proc. Natl. Acad. Sci. U.S.A. **87**, 4905–4909
8.   Stern, D.F. and Kamps, M.P. (1988) EMBO J. **7**, 995–1001
9.   Wada, T., Qian, X. and Greene, M.I. (1990) Cell **61**, 1339–1347
10.   Qian, X., Decker, S.J. and Greene, M.I. (1992) Proc. Natl. Acad. Sci. U.S.A. **89**, 1330–1334
11.   Riese, II, D.J., van Raaji, T.M., Plowman, G.D., Andrews, G.C. and Stern, D.F. (1995) Mol. Cell. Biol. **15**, 5770–5776

12. Beerli, R.R., Graus-Porta, D., Woods-Cook, K., Chen, X., Yarden, Y. and Hynes, N.E. (1995) Mol. Cell. Biol. **15**, 6496–6505

13. Goldman, R., Ben Levy, R., Peles, E. and Yarden, Y. (1990) Biochemistry **29**, 11024–11028

14. Hynes, N.E. and Stern, D.F. (1994) Biochim. Biophys. Acta **1198**, 165–184

15. Bargmann, C.I., Hung, M.-C. and Weinberg, R.A. (1986) Cell **45**, 649–657

16. Muller, W.J., Sinn, E., Wallace, R., Pattengale, P.K. and Leder, P. (1988) Cell **54**, 105–115

17. Bouchard, L., Lamarre, L., Tremblay, P.J. and Jolicoeur, P. (1989) Cell **57**, 931–936

18. Wang, B., Kennan, W.J., Yasukawa-Barnes, J., Lindstrom, M.J. and Gould, M.N. (1991) Cancer Res. **51**, 5649–5654

19. Lemoine, N.R., Staddon. S., Dickson, C., Barnes, D.M. and Gullick, W.J. (1990) Oncogene **5**, 237–239

20. Guy, C.T., Webster, M.A., Schaller, M., Parsons, T.J., Cardiff, R.D. and Muller, W.J. (1992) Proc. Natl. Acad. Sci. U.S.A. **89**, 10578–10582

21. Siegel, P.M., Dankort, D.L., Hardy, W.R. and Muller, W.J. (1994) Mol. Cell. Biol. **14**, 7068–7077

22. Bargmann, C.I. and Weinberg, R.A. (1988) Proc. Natl. Acad. Sci. U.S.A. **85**, 5394–5398

23. Stern, D.F., Kamps. M.P. and Cao, H. (1988) Mol. Cell. Biol. **8**, 3969–3973

24. Weiner, D.B., Kokai, Y., Wada, T., Cohen, J.A., Williams, W.V. and Greene, M.I. (1989) Oncogene **4**, 1175–1183

25. Weiner, D.B., Liu, J., Cohen, J.A., Williams, W.V. and Greene, M.I. (1989) Nature (London) **339**, 230–231

26. Brandt-Rauf, P.W., Rackovsky, S. and Pincus, M.R. (1990) Proc. Natl. Acad. Sci. U.S.A. **87**, 8660–8664

27. Cao, H., Bangalore, L., Bormann, B.J. and Stern, D.F. (1992) EMBO J. **11**, 923–932

28. Santoro, M., Carlomagno, F., Romano, A., et al. (1995) Science **267**, 381–383

29. Asai, N., Iwashita, T., Matsuyama, M. and Takahashi, M. (1995) Mol. Cell. Biol. **15**, 1613–1619

30. Alexander, W.S., Metcalf, D. and Dunn, A.R. (1995) EMBO J. **14**, 5569–5578

31. Watowich, S.S., Yoshimura, A., Longmore, G.D., Hilton, D.J., Yoshimura, Y. and Lodish, H.F. (1992) Proc. Natl. Acad. Sci. U.S.A. **89**, 2140–2144

32. Watowich, S.S., Hilton, D.J. and Lodish, H.F. (1994) Mol. Cell. Biol. **14**, 3535–3549

33. Katz, W.S., Lesa, G.M., Yannoukakos, D., Clandinin, T.R., Schlessinger, J. and Sternberg, P.W. (1996) Mol. Cell. Biol. **16**, 529–537

Biochem. Soc. Symp. **63**, 159–165
Printed in Great Britain

14

Use of mouse mammary tumour virus (MMTV)/*neu* transgenic mice to identify genes collaborating with the c-*erbB-2* oncogene in mammary tumour development

Paul Jolicoeur*†§|, Louise Bouchard*, Alain Guimond*, Michel Ste-Marie*, Zaher Hanna*‡ and Anne Dievart*

*Laboratory of Molecular Biology, Clinical Research Institute of Montreal, 110 Pine Avenue West, Montreal, Quebec H2W 1R7, †Department of Microbiology and Immunology and ‡Department of Medicine, Université de Montréal, Montreal, Quebec H3C 3J7, and §Department of Experimental Medicine, McGill University, Montreal, Quebec H3G 1A4, Canada

Abstract

Mouse mammary tumour virus (MMTV)/*neu* transgenic mice develop clonal or oligoclonal mammary tumours stochastically. The pathology of these tumours is very similar to that of human breast tumours. Moreover, these mouse tumours metastasize in the lungs. We present evidence that this mouse model of human breast tumours can be instrumental in identifying novel genes of two distinct classes (activated oncogenes or tumour suppressor genes) which may collaborate with the c-*erbB-2*/*neu* transgenic oncogene.

Introduction

Breast cancers are frequent, constitute a high percentage of tumours in women and remain a significant daily clinical problem. Fortunately, over the last decade, a better understanding of the molecular events occurring in these tumours has emerged. Some oncogenes, such as *myc*, *erbB-2* and H-*ras* have been identified as being activated or overexpressed in these tumours. Among

---

|To whom correspondence should be addressed, at Laboratory of Molecular Biology, Clinical Research Institute of Montreal.

these, the *erbB-2/neu* gene is of special interest, as its overexpression is relatively frequent [1–3], particularly in comedo-type adenocarcinoma ([4], and references therein). Moreover, its amplification has been correlated in numerous (although not all [5]) studies with a more aggressive phenotype and a poorer prognosis [1–3]. The gene encodes a growth factor receptor transmembrane tyrosine kinase [6,7]. It was found to be activated in a carcinogen-induced rat neuroblastoma tumour by a point mutation in the transmembrane domain leading to the constitutive activation of its tyrosine kinase. This mutant allele can transform fibroblasts *in vitro* [8,9].

In addition to activated oncogenes, a few tumour suppressor genes have also been reported to be involved in human breast tumours, as documented by their inactivation in a variable percentage of cases. To date, p53 is the tumour suppressor gene found most frequently to be inactivated in human breast cancers [10–14]. The gene encoding retinoblastoma protein (Rb) has been found to be implicated at a lower frequency [15]. More recently, the *BRCA1* [16] and *BRCA2* [17,18] genes have been identified in a high proportion of familial breast cancers. Evidence of frequent loss of heterozygosity (interpreted as the loss or the inactivation of tumour suppressor genes) in breast tumours strongly suggests that several other, as yet unidentified, tumour suppressor genes are involved in breast tumour development.

Because of the difficulty of studying the molecular events occurring in human breast cancers, animal models of mammary tumours have been developed. Our laboratory has constructed one of these models in the mouse, by expressing the activated c-*erbB-2/neu* oncogene under the control of promoter of the mouse mammary tumour virus (MMTV) long terminal repeat [19]. Here we discuss some of the features of this model and show how it can be used to identify genes that potentially collaborate with the c-*erbB-2/neu* oncogene in oncogenesis.

Results

The MMTV/*neu* transgenic mouse model

MMTV/*neu* mice [19] harbour a transgene composed of a full-length *neu* cDNA, mutated (Val-664→Glu) in the transmembrane coding region, under the regulation of the MMTV promoter. A simian virus 40 poly(A) addition signal has been ligated at the 3' end. This DNA was inoculated in C57BL/6 × C3H F2 1-day mouse embryos to generate transgenic mice (MMTV/*neu*). These mice have been backcrossed in a Balb/c background for several generations. The MMTV/*neu* mice are predisposed to tumour formation. They develop mammary tumours stochastically at high frequency after a relatively long latency, depending on the transgenic line. Over the years, we have found that mice from one line (MN-10) exhibited this phenotype after a longer latency period than we used to detect a few years ago, for reasons that are not clear. Surprisingly, the stochastic appearance of these tumours was different from the rapid onset of mammary tumours observed by Muller et al. [20] in other transgenic mice expressing a very similar transgene. We have discussed previously the potential reasons for these apparently contrasting results [19].

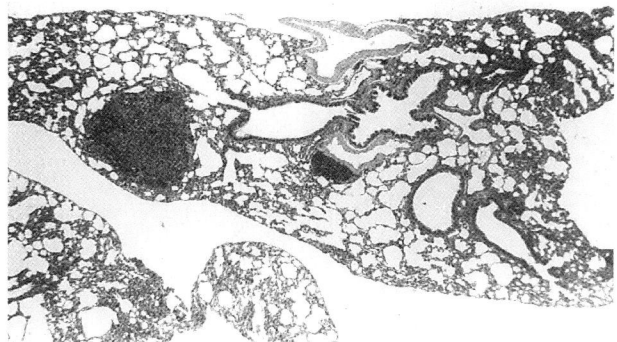

Fig. 1. Metastasis observed in the lung of a MMTV/*neu* transgenic mouse carrying large mammary tumours.

Tumours arising in MMTV/*neu* transgenic mice are malignant, as they grow in nude mice. Interestingly, pathological examination of these tumours revealed that they were mostly adenocarcinoma, often of the ductal type, sometimes harbouring calcifications and exhibiting necrosis. This phenotype is most similar to the comedo-type ductal carcinoma seen in human breast tumours. To our knowledge, this type of pathology has not been seen before in other models of mouse mammary tumours. Moreover, these tumours infiltrated local lymph nodes and metastasized to the lungs relatively frequently (Fig. 1), as do the human tumours, again a feature not often seen in other mouse mammary tumours.

Mammary tumours in MMTV/*neu* transgenic mice are clonal or oligoclonal

The stochastic appearance of these tumours and the long latency period required before their development strongly suggested that they may be clonal or oligoclonal. To determine whether this was indeed the case, we decided to tag these tumours with MMTV proviruses. To do so, newborn MMTV/*neu* transgenic mice were foster-nursed to C3H/OuJ lactating mice, which produce infectious MMTV in milk. The MMTV-infected MMTV/*neu* transgenic female were observed for spontaneous tumour development and a few mammary tumours were collected. Tumour DNAs were extracted and analysed by the Southern blotting procedure, using an MMTV-specific viral probe. As shown in Fig. 2, in addition to germ-line and transgene-specific fragments, each tumour analysed harboured discrete, newly acquired, viral fragments of distinct length in each tumour. This type of pattern is typical of clonal or oligoclonal tumours.

The clonality of tumours arising in MMTV/*neu* transgenic mice strongly suggested that the c-*erbB-2/neu* oncogene was not sufficient to induce the full malignant phenotype, and that additional genetic events were required for the development of these malignant tumours.

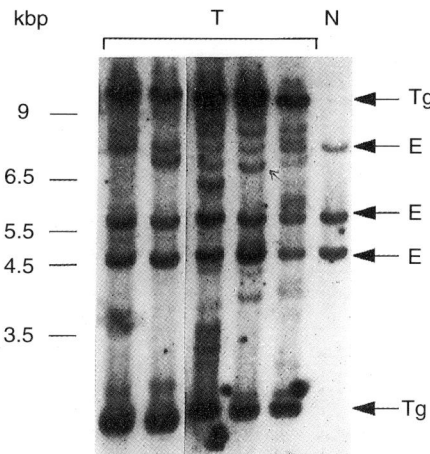

Fig. 2. Clonality of mammary tumours arising in MMTV/*neu* transgenic mice. *Eco*RV-digested DNAs from independent mammary tumours (T) arising in MMTV-infected MMTV/*neu* transgenic mice were subjected to Southern blot analysis, using a ^{32}P-labelled MMTV-specific probe. Lanes T, tumour DNAs; lane N, DNA from normal control mouse. Note the discrete MMTV-specific fragments unique to each tumour. Arrows show transgenic-specific (Tg) or viral endogenous (E) fragments.

Search for tumour suppressor genes involved in tumour development in MMTV/*neu* transgenic mice

Among the genetic events that may occur during the development of mammary tumours in MMTV/*neu* transgenic mice is the inactivation of tumour suppressor genes. As discussed above, one way to identify and map tumour suppressor genes is through the loss of heterozygosity (LOH). LOH is generally interpreted as the loss of one allele of a tumour suppressor gene and inactivation by mutation of the remaining allele. Dietrich et al. [21] have shown that LOH can be fully exploited in mouse tumours arising in F1 inbred mice. The microsatellite PCR technique indeed now allows the detection of specific alleles derived from distinct parental inbred mouse strains.

To determine whether such an approach could be fruitful, the MMTV/*neu* transgenic mice (bred on a Balb/c background) were crossed with C57BL/6 mice. The F1 MMTV/*neu* transgenic females were allowed to become pregnant and observed for the appearance of mammary tumours, which were collected. Tumour DNAs were isolated and subjected to PCR microsatellite detection, essentially as described [21,22].

To validate the assay, we first used the D14–34, D14–37 and D14–60 primers [22], in the region of the well-known Rb tumour suppressor gene. Although a small number of tumours were used in this preliminary test, it was possible to detect LOH in about 10% of the tumours (Table 1). This initial result suggests that this approach may be useful to identify and map novel tumour suppressor genes in this system.

Table 1. LOH on chromosome 14 in mammary tumours arising in MMTV/neu transgenic mice.

Primer	LOH
D14–34	4/40 (10%)
D14–37	1/10 (10%)
D14–60	1/8 (12%)

Search for novel activated oncogenes in tumours arising in MMTV/neu transgenic mice

The activation of novel oncogenes may be among the additional genetic events that are required for the development of malignant tumours in MMTV/*neu* transgenic mice. The provirus insertional mutagenesis approach has been very powerful in identifying novel oncogenes involved in tumours of various cell types [23,24]. This approach has also been used for mammary tumours, resulting in the identification of quite interesting genes by this method (Table 2).

We used this approach to identify novel oncogene(s) that may collaborate with the c-*erbB-2*/*neu* oncogene in MMTV/*neu* transgenic mice. Newborn MMTV/*neu* transgenic mice were first infected with MMTV by foster-nursing to C3H/OuJ mice. Female transgenic mice were observed for the development of mammary tumours while being allowed to become pregnant. Mammary tumours were collected, and their DNAs were extracted and analysed by the Southern procedure using genomic probes free of reiterated sequences derived from various provirus insertion sites. One probe identified rearrangement in two out of 24 tumours (10%), therefore constituting a common provirus insertion site, which was designated *Mis-7* (Fig. 3). Identification and characterization of the gene potentially mutated by this insertion is under way.

Table 2. Genes identified by MMTV provirus insertional mutagenesis in mouse mammary tumours.

Genes	Refs.
Wnt-1/INT1	[25,26]
FGF3/INT2	[27,28]
Wnt-3/INT4	[29]
FGF4/HST-1/k-FGF	[30,31]
INT6	[32]
INT3 (NOTCH-related)	[33,34]
FGF8/AIGF	[35]
(INT-H, INT-P, INT41)	[36–38]

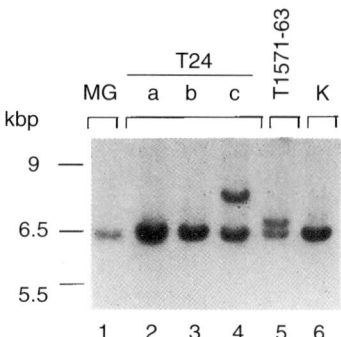

Fig. 3. Rearrangement of the *Mis-7* locus as detected by Southern blot analysis of DNA from mammary tumours arising in MMTV-infected MMTV/*neu* transgenic mice. *Eco*RV-digested DNAs (20 μg) were from three individual tumours in mouse T24 (lanes 2–4), from one tumour in mouse T1571-63 (lane 5) and from control Balb/c mammary gland (MG; lane 1) or kidney (K; lane 6). A ^{32}P-labelled *Mis-7*-specific probe was used. Note the rearrangement in lanes 4 and 5.

Discussion

The *erbB-2/neu* oncogene is frequently involved in the formation of human breast tumours. The MMTV/*neu* transgenic mice described here appear to represent a very good animal model for this specific set of human tumours overexpressing the *erbB-2* gene, as the animal mammary tumours are pathologically very similar to the human tumours, especially the comedo-type adenocarcinoma. In these human tumours overexpressing the *erbB-2* oncogene, other genetic events are likely to contribute to the tumour phenotype. We show here that this is also likely to be the case in the MMTV/*neu* transgenic mice. For this reason, this mouse model is likely to be instrumental in identifying some of these genetic events that appear to collaborate with the c-*erbB-2/neu* oncogene. These fall into two broad categories: the activation of oncogenes and the inactivation of tumour suppressor genes. Our preliminary data indicate that these MMTV/*neu* transgenic mice are amenable to searching for both classes of events. Given the histological similarity between the mouse and the human tumours, it is likely that the genes identified in the MMTV/*neu* transgenic tumours would also play a role in human breast tumours, at least those overexpressing *erbB-2*.

This work was supported by a grant from the Canadian Breast Cancer Research Initiative (National Cancer Institute of Canada) to P.J.

References

1.   Varley, J.M., Swallow, J.E., Brammar, W.J., Whittaker, J.L. and Walker, R.A. (1987) Oncogene 1, 423–430

2. Berger, M.S., Locher, G.W., Saurer, S., Gullick, W.J., Waterfield, M.D., Groner, B. and Hynes, N.E. (1988) Cancer Res. **48**, 1238–1243
3. Slamon, D.J., Clark, G.M., Wong, S.G., Levin, W.J., Ullrich, A. and McGuire, W.L. (1987) Science **235**, 177–182
4. van de Vijver, M.J., Peterse, J.L., Mooi, W.J., Wisman, P., Lomans, J., Dalesio, O. and Nusse, R. (1988) N. Engl. J. Med. **319**, 1239–1245
5. Ali, I.U., Campbell, G., Lidereau, R. and Callahan, R. (1988) Science **240**, 1795–1796
6. Stern, D.F., Heffernan, P.A. and Weinberg, R.A. (1986) Mol. Cell. Biol. **6**, 1729–1740
7. Bargmann, C.I., Hung, M.C. and Weinberg, R.A. (1986) Nature (London) **319**, 226–230
8. Bargmann, C.I., Hung, M.C. and Weinberg, R.A. (1986) Cell **45**, 649–657
9. Hung, M.C., Schechter, A.L., Chevray, P.Y., Stern, D.F. and Weinberg, R.A. (1986) Proc. Natl. Acad. Sci. U.S.A. **83**, 261–264
10. Prosser, J., Thompson, A.M., Cranston, G. and Evans, H.J. (1990) Oncogene **5**, 1573–1579
11. Runnebaum, I.B., Nagarajan, M., Bowman, M., Soto, D. and Sukumar, S. (1991) Proc. Natl. Acad. Sci. U.S.A. **88**, 10657–10661
12. Davidoff, A.M., Humphrey, P.A., Iglehart, J.D. and Marks, J.R. (1991) Proc. Natl. Acad. Sci. U.S.A. **88**, 5006–5010
13. Deng, G., Chen, L.C., Schott, D.R., Thor, A., Bhargava, V., Ljung, B.M. and Chew, K.S. (1994) Cancer Res. **54**, 499–505
14. Callahan, R. (1992) J. Natl. Cancer Inst. **84**, 826–827
15. van de Vijver, M.J. and Nusse, R. (1991) Biochim. Biophys. Acta **1072**, 33–50
16. Miki, Y., Swensen, J., Shattuck-Eidens, D., et al. (1994) Science **266**, 66–71
17. Wooster, R., Neuhausen, S.L., Mangion, J., et al. (1994) Science **265**, 2088–2090
18. Wooster, R., Bignell, G., Lancaster, J., et al. (1995) Nature (London) **378**, 789–792
19. Bouchard, L., Lamarre, L., Tremblay, P.J. and Jolicoeur, P. (1989) Cell **57**, 931–936
20. Muller, W.J., Sinn, E., Pattengale, P.K., Wallace, R. and Leder, P. (1988) Cell **54**, 105–115
21. Dietrich, W.F., Radany, E.H., Smith, J.S., Bishop, J.M., Hanahan, D. and Lander, E.S. (1994) Proc. Natl. Acad. Sci. U.S.A. **91**, 9451–9455
22. Dietrich, W.F., Miller, J.C., Steen, R.G., et al. (1994) Nature Genet. **5**, 220–245
23. Peters, G. (1990) Cell Growth Differ. **1**, 503–510
24. van Lohuizen, M. and Berns, A. (1990) Biochim. Biophys. Acta **1032**, 213–235
25. Nusse, R. and Varmus, H.E. (1982) Cell **31**, 99–109
26. Nusse, R., van Ooyen, A., Cox, D., Fung, Y.K. and Varmus, H. (1984) Nature (London) **307**, 131–136
27. Dickson, C., Smith, R., Brookes, S. and Peters, G. (1984) Cell **37**, 529–536
28. Peters, G., Brookes, S., Smith, R. and Dickson, C. (1983) Cell **33**, 369–377
29. Roelink, H., Wagenaar, E., Lopes da Silva, S. and Nusse, R. (1990) Proc. Natl. Acad. Sci. U.S.A. **87**, 4519–4523
30. Shackleford, G.M., MacArthur, C.A., Kwan, H.C. and Varmus, H.E. (1993) Proc. Natl. Acad. Sci. U.S.A. **90**, 740–744
31. Peters, G., Brookes, S., Smith, R., Placzek, M. and Dickson, C. (1989) Proc. Natl. Acad. Sci. U.S.A. **86**, 5678–5682
32. Marchetti, A., Buttitta, F., Miyazaki, S., Gallahan, D., Smith, G.H. and Callahan, R. (1995) J. Virol. **69**, 1932–1938
33. Gallahan, D. and Callahan, R. (1987) J. Virol. **61**, 66–74
34. Robbins, J., Blondel, B.J., Gallahan, D. and Callahan, R. (1992) J. Virol. **66**, 2594–2599
35. MacArthur, C.A., Shankar, D.B. and Shackleford, G.M. (1995) J. Virol. **69**, 2501–2507
36. Gray, D.A., McGrath, C.M., Jones, R.F. and Morris, V.L. (1986) Virology **148**, 360–368
37. Schuermann, M. and Michalides, R. (1987) Virology **156**, 229–237
38. Garcia, M., Wellinger, R., Vessaz, A. and Diggelmann, H. (1986) EMBO J. **5**, 127–134

Biochem. Soc. Symp. **63**, 167–184
Printed in Great Britain

15

Induction of a variety of preneoplasias and tumours in the mammary glands of transgenic rats

Barry R. Davies*§, Joe R. Warren†, Gunter Schmidt‡ and Philip S. Rudland‡

*CRC Human Cancer Genetics Research Group, Department of Pathology, Level 3 Laboratories Block, Addenbrookes Hospital, University of Cambridge, Cambridge CB2 2QQ, U.K. †University of Wisconsin Biotechnology Center, Madison, WI, U.S.A., and ‡Department of Biochemistry, University of Liverpool, Liverpool L69 3BX, U.K.

Abstract

Although transgenic mouse models for breast cancer have frequently been reported in the literature, transgenic rat models have not been described. We have generated transgenic rats overexpressing the human transforming growth factor α (TGFα) and c-*erbB-2* genes in the mammary gland under the control of the mouse mammary tumour virus (MMTV) long terminal repeat promoter, and have analysed multiple lines of these rats to the second (F_2) generation. Female MMTV/TGFα rats frequently develop severe hyperplasias during pregnancy, and a variety of tumours of long latency. The mammary glands of MMTV/TGFα rats fail to involute fully after the completion of lactation. Expression of the TGFα transgene is highest in the hyperplasias. MMTV/c-*erbB-2* female rats develop a spectrum of benign and malignant lesions, including ductal carcinoma *in situ* and carcinomas. Expression of the c-*erbB-2* transgene is found in benign tumours such as fibroadenomas, but is highest in the carcinomas. These animals model a spectrum of lesions found in human breasts and suggest that TGFα overexpression can act at a relatively early stage in the pathogenesis of breast cancer in the rat, resulting in a predominantly hyperplastic response, whereas overexpression of c-*erbB-2* plays a role in the induction of various benign lesions and more advanced breast carcinomas.

§To whom correspondence should be addressed.

Reason for the development of transgenic rat models for breast cancer
    The introduction of foreign genetic material into mice, either by pronu-
clear microinjection into the germ-line to create transgenic mice [1–3] or by
transplantation of genetically modified mammary epithelium to create 'transgenic tissue' [4], are powerful techniques that have contributed greatly to our
understanding of the role that defined oncogenes play in the pathogenesis of
breast cancer. However, the rat has certain potential advantages over the mouse
for creating breast cancer models that accurately reflect the human disease. The
origin, spectrum of tumour types in terms of their pathology, and hormone-
sensitivity of spontaneously arising rat mammary tumours more closely
resemble human breast cancer than that in the mouse (Table 1) [5,6]. Unlike rat
and human breast cancer, many mouse mammary tumours are viral in origin,
caused by integration of mouse mammary tumour virus (MMTV). The common human benign breast tumours, such as the fibroadenoma, are also
relatively common in aging rats, but are virtually never seen in the mouse.
Mouse mammary tumours are almost all epithelial and are either malignant
from the outset or, if left long enough, become so. Moreover, mammary
tumours in the rat are generally strongly hormone-dependent with regard to
both induction and growth. Carcinogen-induced rat mammary tumours
regress after the same types of endocrine manipulations as with human cancers,
and, as in the human disease, not all rat tumours show this hormone-sensitiv-
ity. Rat mammary tumours induced by carcinogens or by implantation of
oestrogen pellets undergo regression after oophorectomy, adrenalectomy and
hyperphysectomy, and, just as in the human disease, these effects are not per-
manent and the tumours eventually resume growth [5]. By contrast, most

Table 1. Comparison of pathology of human, rat and mouse mammary tumours. Modified from [5].

Characteristic	Human	Rat	Mouse
Benign/ malignant ratio	About 1:4	Benign more common	Usually malignant
Fibroadenoma	Common	Common	Very uncommon
Carcinoma			
Spontaneous	Common	Uncommon	Common
Induced	–	Uncommon*	Common
Differentiation			
Range	Wide	Wide	Limited
Degree	Poorly differentiated	Highly differentiated	Very highly differentiated
Hormone response	Sometimes positive	Sometimes positive	Not in virus-induced tumours; only in BR6 strain

*Can be achieved by transplantation [53].

mouse tumours, virus-induced or otherwise, tend to be hormone-insensitive, with the exception of the pregnancy-dependent mammary tumour described in BR6 mice [7].

Given the structural and functional resemblance of rat mammary tumours to their human counterparts, it is not surprising that the experimental induction of rat mammary tumours by methods such as administration of carcinogens or irradiation has been carried out for many years. In contrast with these relatively crude methods of induction, the creation of transgenic rats that are predisposed to breast cancer by expressing defined oncogenes in the mammary gland enables a more defined analysis of the pathogenesis of the disease to be carried out at the molecular level.

There are two further reasons for creating transgenic rat models. First, the results obtained from expressing a defined oncogene in the mouse may be peculiar to that species and may not be representative of its function in the human disease; it is therefore useful to establish whether expression of the gene has similar phenotypic effects in a relevant alternative species. Secondly, the rat is the preferred species for the screening of new pharmaceuticals and for toxicology/carcinogenicity testing [8]. Appropriate transgenic rat models may, therefore, be of some commercial value. Given that the rat mammary gland is sensitive to both chemical and radiation-induced carcinogenesis, rats predisposed to breast cancer may be particularly useful for carcinogenicity tests.

Choice of oncogenes and design of constructs

In order to create transgenic rat models that mimic human breast cancer, we decided to target overexpression of the oncogenes transforming growth factor α (TGFα) and c-erb-B2 (HER-2) to the mammary glands.

TGFα is a mitogenic polypeptide that structually and functionally resembles epidermal growth factor (EGF) [9]. TGFα is the most abundant member of the EGF family in the mammary gland, and it stimulates the growth of fibroblastic, myoepithelial-like and epithelial cells derived from normal mammary glands and benign tumours [10]. TGFα normally binds to the EGF receptor (EGFR) and induces a mitogenic response by activating the tyrosine kinase activity of this receptor [11]. Immortalized mouse mammary epithelial cells have been shown to be susceptible to transformation by TGFα [12,13]. Moreover, overexpression of TGFα and its cognate receptor, EGFR, has been implicated in the pathogenesis of human breast cancers, and it has also been shown that TGFα can mediate the growth-stimulating effects of oestrogen in a human breast cancer cell line [14]. Minimal expression of inmmunoreactive TGFα is detectable in normal human breast tissue, but increased expression occurs in ductal hyperplasia, atypical hyperplasia and ductal carcinoma in situ [15]. Immunoreactive TGFα has also been detected in 30–70% of human breast carcinomas, and its presence correlates with tumour burden [16–18].

Transgenic mice overexpressing TGFα from various promoters have been generated and characterized. Both multiparous and virgin MMTV/TGFα mice develop cystic and solid hyperplasias and mammary carcinomas after long latencies of > 300 days [19,20]. These animals developed dramatically increased numbers of tumours of shorter latencies when treated with suboptimal doses of the chemical carcinogen dimethylbenzanthracene (DMBA) [21]. In one transgenic mouse model in which expression of TGFα was controlled by the metallothionein-1 promoter, secretory mammary adenocarcinomas and hyperplastic alveolar nodules developed [22], and in another model impeded morphogenic penetration of the ductal epithelial cells into the fat pad was reported, even though DNA synthesis was enhanced in the transgenic mammary glands [23]. Although no mammary carcinomas developed in this latter model, the same construct induced hyperplasia, secretory mammary adenomas and adenocarcinomas in multiparous females of a different genetic background [24]. These animals also exhibited a delay in involution of the mammary tissue after lactation. These results suggested that, at least in the mouse, the susceptibility of the mammary gland to TGFα-induced hyperplasia and neoplasia was specific to the strain used. Multiparous whey acidic protein promoter-driven TGFα transgenic mice also developed well differentiated secretory adenocarcinomas, with frequent induction of cyclin D1 expression, and also showed delayed or inhibited involution of the mammary gland after lactation [25].

The c-erbB-2 gene product has also been strongly implicated in the development of human breast cancer. This proto-oncogene encodes a tyrosine kinase receptor that is structurally related to the EGFR [26,27] and is the human homologue of the transforming rat oncogene neu [28], which contains a point mutation in the transmembrane domain of the protein that results in constitutive tyrosine kinase activity [29].

The level of c-erbB-2 expression in normal human breast tissue is very low [30], but in invasive breast carcinomas, expression of c-erbB-2 is observed in 20–30% of breast tumours, and in some cases is accompanied by gene amplification [31–33]. An inverse correlation has been noted between patient survival and c-erbB-2 expression, particularly in patients with no involved lymph nodes [32,33]. In addition, almost 50% of early X-ray-screened breast lesions of the ductal/lobular carcinoma in situ (cis) type express c-erbB-2 [34–36]. Its expression occurs in large-cell, especially comedo-type in situ, lesions, precursors for ductal carcinoma and often in Pagets disease of the nipple [37].

Expression of neu in the mammary glands of certain lines of transgenic mice resulted in the rapid development of multifocal mammary tumours that metastasized at high frequency [38–40], but other laboratories have reported only the stochastic development of mammary tumours with MMTV/neu [41,42]. Perhaps surprisingly, expression of non-mutated c-erbB-2 in the mouse mammary gland did not induce the development of tumours [42]. The reason for these discrepancies is unclear; perhaps the level of transgene expression or differences in the constructs are responsible.

In contrast, in a further MMTV/c-erbB-2 model, the animals died at an early age as a result of hyperplastic lesions in both the kidneys and the lungs which caused organ failure. The mammary glands of these mice were underdeveloped and lactation-deficient, although one virgin mouse developed a focal adenocarcinoma [43]. Mammary tumours expressing the neu proto-oncogene have also been shown to possess elevated c-src tyrosine kinase activity, suggesting that c-src is involved in neu-mediated signal transduction [44].

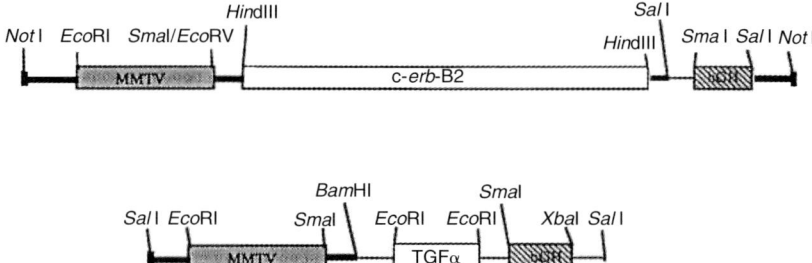

Fig. 1. Structure of the MMTV/TGFα and MMTV/c-erbB-2 transgenes. The diagram shows the structure and important restriction sites utilized in the construction of the transgenes. The MMTV LTR promoter is used to drive expression of the downstream oncogenes, and a 3′ fragment of the human growth hormone (hGH) gene ensures correct processing of the transcript. Thick and thin lines represent sequences derived from the polylinkers of plasmids pPolyIII-I and pBluescript respectively.

We decided to use the MMTV promoter linked to the Rous sarcoma virus long terminal repeat (LTR) enhancer to drive expression of TGFα and non-mutated c-erbB-2 in the mammary glands. Constructs were made by subcloning human cDNAs for TGFα or c-erbB-2 downstream of the MMTV promoter. To provide an intron to enhance expression of the cDNAs and a splice and polyadenylation signal to ensure correct processing of the transcript, a 700 bp fragment from the 3′ end of the human growth hormone gene was placed downstream of the cDNAs (Fig. 1). The completed transgenes were released from their parental plasmids by digestion with restriction enzymes, purified and microinjected into rat embryos.

Generation of transgenic rats

The generation of transgenic rats is similar, in theory, to the generation of transgenic mice. The only major difference is in the method of inducing superovulation in the animals. Outbred Sprague–Dawley female rats were induced to superovulate by continuous infusion with pituitary follicle-stimulating hormone via mini osmotic pumps [45]. Pumps were inserted intraperitoneally 2 days prior to mating. In contrast, the usual method for inducing superovulation in mice is to give a single injection of pregnant mares serum gonadotrophin (PMSG) [46]. Synchronization of ovulation was induced 48–52 h later by intraperitoneal injection of leutinizing hormone releasing hormone. Females were then mated overnight with males of proven fertility. The following day, the females were killed and embryos were collected in Dulbecco's PBS. When pronuclei were visible in the embryos, one pronucleus at a time (usually the male) was microinjected in modified M16 medium or M2 medium [46]. Embryos were then kept in modified M16 medium until they were transferred into the infundibulum of both oviducts of pseudopregnant recipients [47].

Rat embryos are far less resilient than those of the mouse; they are less elastic and spongier, making them difficult to microinject without damaging

Table 2. Generation of **MMTV/TGFα** and **MMTV/c-erb-B2** transgenic rats

Founder	Sex	Copies of transgene	Successfully mated	Mosaic or Mendelian inheritance
1. MMTV/TGFα				
TGF/1	Female	5–10	Yes	Mendelian
TGF/2	Female	1	Yes	Mosaic
TGF/3	Male	10	Yes	Mosaic
TGF/4	Male	10	Yes	Mosaic
TGF/5	Male	5–10	Yes	No transmission
TGF/6	Male	1–5	No	Unknown
2. MMTV/c-erb-B2				
ERB/1	Female	10–20	Yes	Mendelian
ERB/2	Female	1–5	Yes	Mendelian
ERB/3	Female	~50	Yes	Mendelian
ERB/4	Male	1 and > 20	Yes	Mendelian; two integration sites
ERB/5	Female	< 1	Yes	Unknown
ERB/6	Female	5–10	Yes	Mosaic
ERB/7	Male	1	Yes	Sex-linked: transgene on Y chromosome

them. Moreover, the pronuclei are more difficult to visualize than in mouse embryos. Furthermore, in our experience, oviduct transfers are less effective in the rat, with fewer resulting pregnancies and generally smaller litter sizes.

Transgenic rats were identified by Southern blot analysis of tail genomic DNA, as for trangenic mice. The animals contained from less than one up to 50 copies of the integrated transgene per haploid genome. The characteristics of the founder transgenic rats are summarized in Table 2. With the exception of one of the male MMTV/TGFα founders, all of the offspring were fertile and were mated successfully. Five of the founders transmitted the transgene in a Mendelian fashion to their offspring and four other founders transmitted the transgene at a much lower frequency; these latter founder animals were probably mosaics. No transmission was observed from one line of MMTV/TGFα transgenics, and one of the MMTV/c-erbB-2 female animals appeared to be sub-fertile, because only one litter was obtained; all the animals from this single litter were negative for the transgene. It was not possible to analyse any females from another of the MMTV/c-erbB-2 lines (ERB/7) because the transgene appeared to integrate into the Y chromosome; all male offspring inherited the transgene but no female transgenic offspring were obtained from this animal (Table 2). All founders and multiple offspring from MMTV/TGFα lines TGF/1 and TGF/2 and from MMTV/c-erbB-2 lines ERB/1 to ERB/3 have been analysed in detail to the second (F_2) generation. To date, we have monitored 29 female MMTV/TGFα transgenics and 34 female MMTV/c-erbB-2 transgenics for the development of mammary lesions that develop before 18 months of age. This analysis is ongoing, and a more complete analysis of the data discussed below will be reported in the future.

Mammary lesions in MMTV/TGFα transgenic rats

MMTV/TGFα female transgenics were fertile and able to nurse their young normally. Virgin mammary epithelium showed no growth abnormalities and did not express the transgene at levels detectable by Northern blotting of poly(A) RNA or by immunocytochemistry. The MMTV promoter is usually activated by the hormones of pregnancy [48]; therefore rats were subjected to repeated rounds of pregnancy and lactation to activate expression of the transgene. The most striking phenotype observed was the development of large, solid, palpable lumps in the mammary glands during pregnancy. These lumps appeared in 41% of transgenic female rats in both transgenic lines after five or more pregnancies. In the most severe cases, lumps developed bilaterally in all the mammary glands. These lumps usually grew so large that the animals became moribund, necessitating culling. The lumps always appeared on day 10 or day 11 of pregnancy and invariably regressed on the day before parturition, suggesting that they were severe hyperplasias rather than neoplasias. The animals were still able to lactate normally and nurse their young in the subsequent lactational period following regression of these lesions. However, the lumps usually reappeared with greater severity during subsequent pregnancies. When these lesions were examined histologically, they were found to consist of solid masses of tissue resembling normal lactating mammary gland (Figs. 2a and 2b). The hyperplastic mammary tissue compressed surrounding normal tissue such

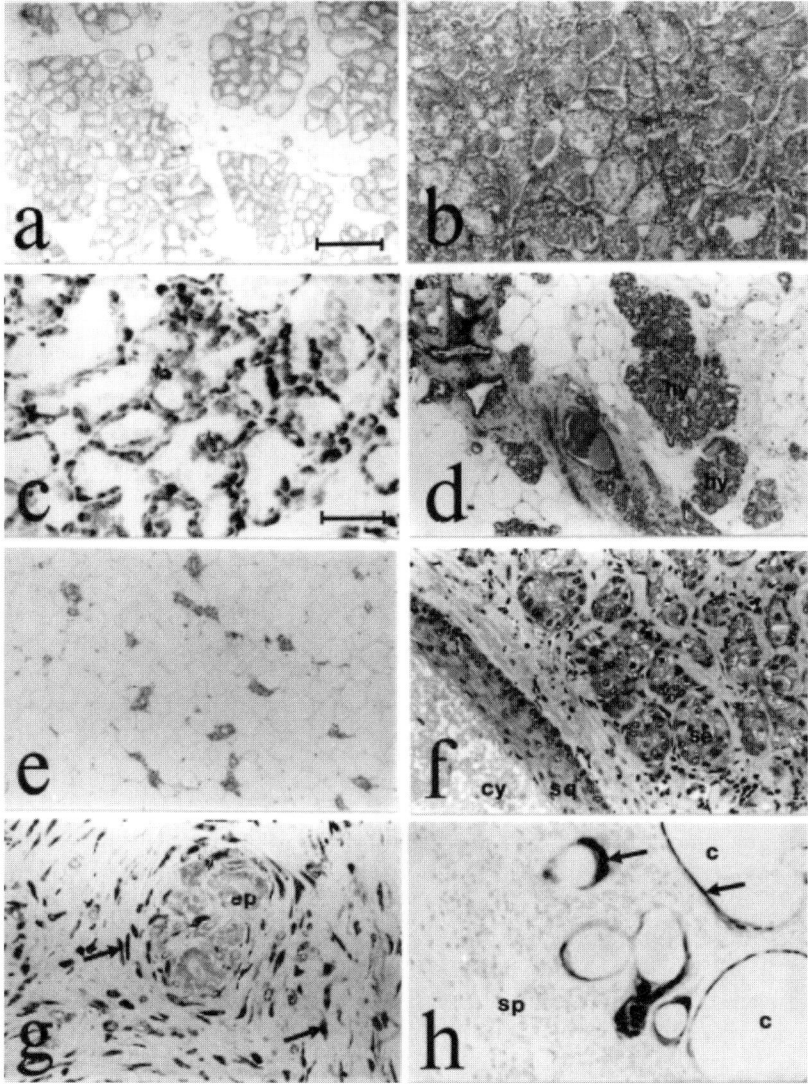

Fig. 2. Histology and immunocytochemistry of mammary lesions and tumours in MMTV/TGFα transgenic rats. (a) Normal mammary gland from a pregnant non-transgenic female rat [stained with haematoxylin and eosin (H&E)]. (b) Severe hyperplasia of the mammary gland at day 16 of pregnancy in a multiparous transgenic rat (H&E). (c) Hyperplastic mammary tissue from a multiparous transgenic rat stained with antiserum to TGFα. The majority of the epithelial cells stain moderately or strongly. (d) Mammary gland from a multiparous female transgenic rat 3 months after weaning of its previous litter. Note the persistence of hyperplastic lactating alveoli (H&E). (e) Normal regressed mammary gland from a non-transgenic female rat of the same strain and reproductive history as the rat in (d). Note the small condensed lobules

as skeletal muscle but did not invade it. The hyperplastic mammary tissue was stained by antiserum to TGFα (Fig. 2c). Whole-mounts of mammary tissues from other pregnant transgenic female animals showed that the mammary tissue was always hyperplastic in comparison with that of non-transgenic litter mates of comparable age and number of pregnancies. In transgenic females the fat pad became completely filled with proliferating mammary epithelium, and individual lobules were impossible to distinguish because they merged together.

The mammary glands of transgenic female animals also failed to regress fully after lactation; dense, focal, hyperplastic lobules with secretions persisted in these animals, even 6 months after their previous lactation (Fig. 2d). These hyperplastic lesions were also stained by anti-TGFα serum. Involuted mammary glands from control litter mates after comparable numbers of pregnancy and lactation cycles were very different, consisting of small condensed ducts and alveoli with no evidence of lactation (Fig. 2e).

Tumours developed stochastically after a long latent period in multiparous females; by 18 months of age, eight out of 29 (28%) of animals had developed tumours. These tumours were variable histologically, and included fibromas, benign papillary tumours with associated severe hyperplasia, ductal carcinoma in situ (DCIS) and carcinomas with squamous metaplasia (Fig. 2f). Transgene expression was variable; in fibromas, the fibroblastic cells that made up the majority of the tumour stained strongly (Fig. 2g), whereas in DCIS and carcinomas, expression of TGFα was either absent or non-uniform (Fig. 2h). However, strong expression of TGFα was always seen in adjacent hyperplastic breast tissue, when present, and in carcinomas where differentiation to squamous elements occurred (Fig. 2h).

Mammary lesions in MMTV/c-erbB-2 transgenic rats

MMTV/c-erbB-2 transgenic females did not develop the severe pregnancy-responsive hyperplasias characteristic of the TGFα transgenics. Indeed, whole-mounted mammary glands of pregnant transgenic females did not reveal any evidence of hyperplasia. Transgene expression was not detectable in virgin females, and it was only just detectable in pregnant animals by immunocytochemistry and by Northern blotting of poly(A)-containing RNA. However,

☞ **Fig. 2 (contd.)** (H&E). (f) Mammary carcinoma with squamous metaplasia (sq) surrounding a cystic space (cy) and sebaceous-gland-like elements in a multiparous transgenic female rat (H&E). (g) Fibroma in the mammary gland of a multiparous female transgenic rat stained with antiserum to TGFα. Note the strong staining of the stromal fibroblastic cells (arrows), whereas the ductal epithelial cells (ep) fail to stain. (h) Mammary carcinoma with squamous metaplasia in a multiparous female transgenic rat stained with antiserum to TGFα. The anaplastic spindle cells (sp) that make up the majority of the tumour fail to stain, but the areas of squamous metaplasia surrounding the cystic spaces (c) stain intensely. Magnification for (a), (b), (d) and (e) ×41; bar = 200 μm; Magnification for (c), (f), (g) and (h) ×161; bar = 50 μm.

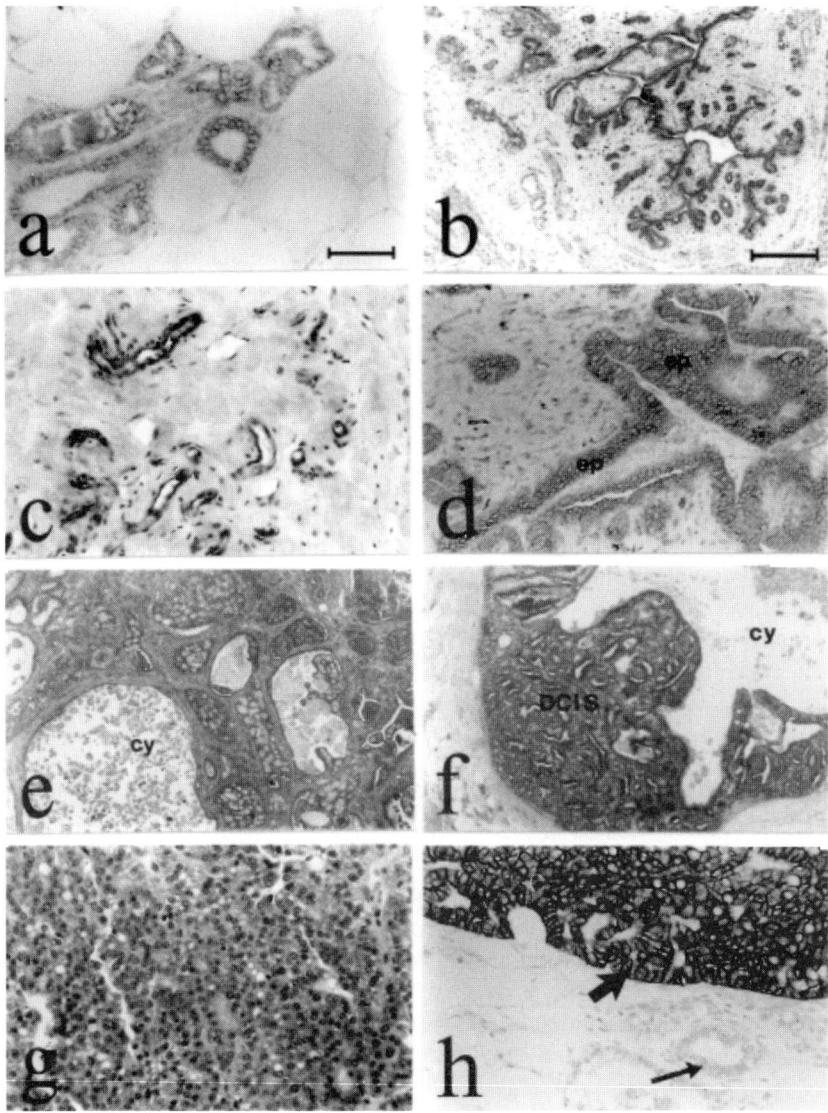

Fig. 3. Histology and immunocytochemistry of mammary lesions and tumours in MMTV/c-erbB-2 transgenic rats. (a) Regressed mammary gland from a multiparous female transgenic animal stained with antiserum to c-*erbB-2*. Note the weak membrane staining of the epithelial cells. (b) Area of fibroadenoma in a multiparous female transgenic rat [stained with haematoxylin and eosin (H&E)]. (c) Area of sclerosing adenosis in a multiparous female transgenic rat (H&E). (d) Fibroadenoma in a multiparous female transgenic rat stained with antiserum to c-*erbB-2*. The epithelial cells (ep) in the lesion stain moderately on their cell membranes. (e) Papillary tumour in a multiparous ☞

whole-mounted mammary glands from females at least 6 weeks after their previous lactation revealed focal areas of mild or moderate adenosis/hyperplasia. These mildly hyperplastic regions stained moderately or weakly on their plasma membranes with antiserum to c-erbB-2 (Fig. 3a), whereas cells in regressed, condensed alveoli in the same mammary gland failed to stain with antiserum to c-erbB-2. Although not as pronounced as in the MMTV/TGFα transgenics, c-erbB-2 expression does appear to be correlated with retention of hyperplastic secretory alveoli.

Analysis of otherwise involuted mammary glands from multiparous transgenic females also revealed a variety of other pathologies. These included collections of thick ducts, which when sectioned appeared to be large cystic expansions, and multiple areas of focally dense tissue. When sectioned, these dense areas were usually found to be small fibroadenomas (Fig. 3b) or other benign lesions, including sclerosing adenosis (Fig. 3c). These benign lesions are likely to be due to transgene expression and not to have arisen spontaneously, for three reasons. First, they were multifocal. Secondly, they were observed very infrequently in mammary glands from control litter mates of comparable age and reproductive history. Out of 20 control females, only one area of mild fibroadenomatous change was found and areas of hyperplasia were not observed. Thirdly, both cystic expansions and fibroadenomas stained with antiserum to c-erbB-2 (Fig. 3d), whereas surrounding normal mammary tissue failed to stain.

As in the MMTV/TGFα transgenics, tumours developed stochastically at low frequency after multiple pregnancies. These tumours included large fibroadenomas and histologically variable tumours with a papillary growth pattern where the papillary epithelium lined cystic spaces in which dense secretions were present (Fig. 3e). Areas of DCIS were also present within these lesions (Fig. 3f), suggesting that a progression occurs from hyperplasia to papillary lesions and then to DCIS. To date, three animals have developed DCIS and only two animals have developed definite carcinomas. Although the carcinomas were well differentiated in comparison with most human breast carcinomas, they were poorly organized in comparison with the benign tumours and contained more malignant-looking cells with large, pleiomorphic nuclei (Fig. 3g). They were classified as definite carcinomas because they failed to stain

☞ **Fig. 3 (contd.)** female transgenic rat. Note the intraductal epithelial proliferation and large cystic spaces (cy) filled with secretory material. (f) Example of an area of DCIS adjacent to a large cystic space (cy) in a multiparous female transgenic rat (H&E). (g) Carcinoma in a multiparous female transgenic rat (H&E). (h) The edge of the carcinoma shown in (g) stained with antiserum to c-erbB-2. Note the strong membrane staining of the carcinoma cells (thick arrow), but the absence of staining in adjacent normal ducts (thin arrow). Magnification for (a), (c), (d), (g) and (h) ×161; bar = 50 μm. Magnification for (b), (e) and (f) ×41; bar = 200 μm.

with antisera to keratin and smooth muscle actin, indicating the absence of myoepithelial cells; moreover, staining with antiserum to laminin revealed that basement membrane was either absent or very fragmented. Although cells in areas of DCIS stained weakly with antiserum to c-erbB-2, cells in carcinomas stained very strongly indeed on their membranes, while adjacent normal mammary ductal epithelium failed to stain (Fig. 3h).

Other non-mammary lesions in transgenic rats

Although the MMTV/TGFα and MMTV/c-erb-B2 transgenes were also variably expressed in several other tissues, including the epithelial cells of the male reproductive tract (Figs. 4a and 4b), salivary glands (Fig. 4c) and areas of the kidneys and spleen, no apparent pathologies were observed in these tissues, with the notable exception of the salivary glands, where hyperplasia sometimes occurred in both MMTV/TGFα and MMTV/c-erbB-2 transgenic rat lines. These results suggest either that these other tissues are not susceptible to TGFα- and c-erbB-2-induced carcinogenesis or that the level of transgene expression is not sufficient to induce a neoplastic phenotype in these tissues.

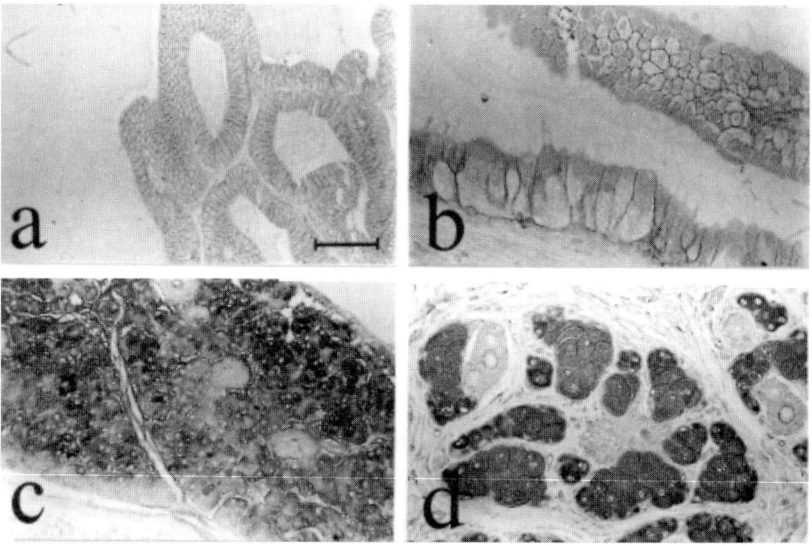

Fig. 4. Immunocytochemistry of non-mammary tissues in transgenic rats. (a) Seminal vesicle from a male ERB/1 transgenic rat stained with antiserum to c-erbB-2. The epithelial cells stain weakly on their cell membranes. (b) Vas deferens from a male ERB/1 transgenic rat stained with antiserum to c-erbB-2. The epithelial cells stain moderately on their cell membranes. (c) Salivary gland from a male ERB/1 transgenic rat stained with antiserum to c-erbB-2. Variable cytoplasmic staining is seen in the cells of the secretory acini. (d) Sebaceous gland hyperplasia in the dermis of the skin of a TGF/1 female transgenic rat stained with antiserum to TGFa. The sebaceous glands stain intensely with this antiserum, whereas other structures fail to stain. Magnification ×161; bar = 50 mm.

The only other striking phenotype of note was areas of hair loss, especially ventrally, in many of the MMTV/TGFα transgenics. Transverse sections through the skin revealed areas of sebaceous gland hyperplasia. These hyperplastic sebaceous glands stained intensely with antiserum to TGFα, whereas the remainder of the dermis failed to stain and appeared to be normal (Fig. 4d). Dense hyperplastic mammary tissue was nearly always found in close proximity to these sebaceous gland hyperplasias, but it did not invade the sebaceous glands and hair follicles of the dermis. Therefore sebaceous gland hyperplasia is most probably responsible for hair loss in these animals.

Model for the role of TGFα and c-erbB-2 overexpression in rat mammary carcinogenesis

The results from our transgenic rat models suggest that overexpression of human cDNAs for TGFα and c-erbB-2 in the rat mammary gland can predispose such animals to tumour development. However, the spectrum of preneoplastic and benign lesions and the pattern of transgene expression in the various lesions suggest that the two genes act at different stages in the pathogenesis of the disease (Fig. 5).

Expression of TGFα appears to cause predominantly hyperplasia. Although a certain degree of mammary hyperplasia is always present in MMTV/TGFα transgenic rats, even during the first pregnancy, the severe, macroscopically identifiable hyperplasias that resemble lactating adenomas only appeared after five or more pregnancies, and then only in approximately half of the animals. This suggests either that a critical threshold level of transgene expression is needed for the severe hyperplasias or that a second, co-operating, genetic event needs to take place for these hyperplasias to develop. In addition to the induction of secretory hyperplasias, the TGFα transgene also appears to prevent involution of the lactating mammary gland by enhancing epithelial cell survival. Hyperplasia and failure of the mammary glands to involute fully are two phenotypes that have been described in certain lines of transgenic mice expressing TGFα in the mammary gland [19–25]. Sebaceous gland hyperplasia has also been observed in one line of MMTV/TGFα transgenic mice [20]. However, the severe, pregnancy-associated, hyperplasias that are characteristic of our transgenic rats have not been described in TGFα transgenic mice, although pregnancy-dependent lesions similar to those seen in the BR6 mouse strain have been described in MMTV/int-2-expressing mice [49]. This may be because these lesions are hormone-dependent, and lends further support to the rat as a model of hormone-responsive mammary tumour development. We are not sure at this stage whether these severe hyperplastic lesions can progress to hormone independence, because their severity has necessitated early culling of the animals; it will be necessary either to resect them partially or to attempt to transplant them into oophorectomized or hypophysectomized recipient rats to prove this progression.

MMTV/TGFα transgenic rats develop tumours at low frequency, but expression of the transgene in the carcinomas is frequently low or absent, suggesting that further, undetermined, genetic events are responsible for the development of these more advanced lesions, and that TGFα expression is

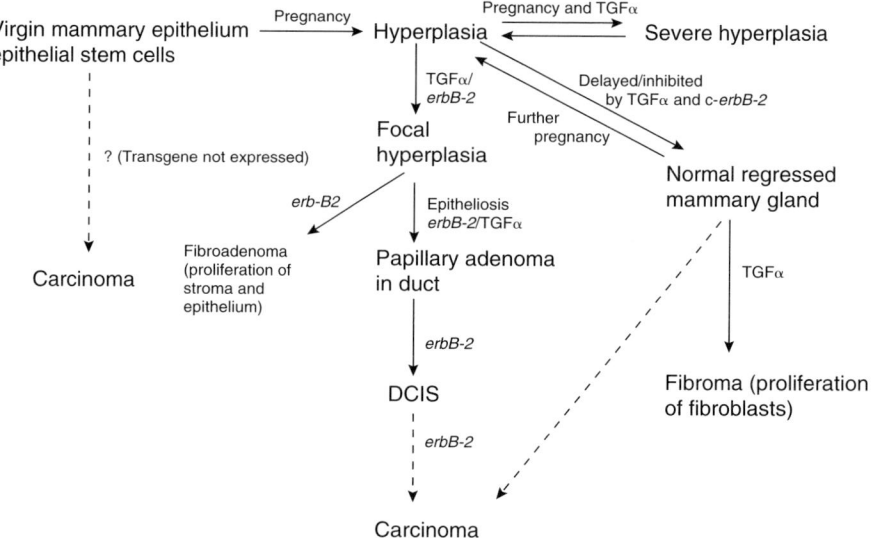

Fig. 5. Model for the role of TGFα and c-erbB-2 overexpression in transgenic rat mammary carcinogenesis. The model of a possible carcinogenic pathway operating in our transgenic rats is based on the expression profile of the transgenes in the various lesions and the gradations between the various different pathologies in individual animals. Transgene expression is activated during pregnancy; expression of TGFα above a certain threshold level or in combination with other oncogenes leads to the development of severe hyperplasia. Expression of either transgene inhibits full regression of the mammary gland after the lactation period, but this is more severe in TGFα-expressing transgenics. Focal expression of either transgene causes focal hyperplasia; this can lead to either fibroadenoma (c-erbB-2) or papillary adenoma forming in ducts (either transgene). Progression to DCIS and carcinoma is accompanied by expression of c-erbB-2, but not TGFα. TGFα can also contribute to the development of fibroma.

unnecessary. However, areas of hyperplasia and papillary lesions adjacent to and continuous with such advanced lesions stain intensely with antiserum to TGFα; this result suggests that the more advanced lesions can develop from these preneoplastic lesions which express the transgene. TGFα clearly can also stimulate proliferation of the stromal fibroblastic cells of the mammary gland; the large fibromas that develop in our MMTV/TGFα transgenic rats strongly express TGFα.

Whereas TGFα overexpression has been detected in both mammary epithelial and fibroblastic cells, c-erbB-2 overexpression has only been detected in epithelial cells in the various lesions that developed in MMTV/c-erbB-2 transgenic rats. The c-erbB-2 gene is expressed in epithelial cells of fibroadenomas, mild hyperplasias and large cystic expansions induced in such animals, but not in fibroblasts. Overexpression of c-erbB-2 appears to play a role in the induction of benign breast diseases and in benign tumours in these animals;

fibroadenomas are particularly commonly found. However, expression of c-*erbB-2* was strongest in the carcinomas that developed in these transgenics. Our MMTV/c-*erbB-2* transgenic rat model most closely resembles the transgenic mouse model of Bouchard et al. [41], in which tumours developed stochastically after a long latent period, although the occurrence of benign lesions was not reported in this model. However, the development of benign lesions such as adenosis, sclerosing adenosis and the preneoplastic lesion DCIS was reported when *neu* was expressed in the reconstituted mouse mammary gland [50].

Taken together, these results suggest a model where TGFα acts at an early stage in breast cancer pathogenesis, predominantly causing hyperplasia and retention of lactating alveoli, and c-*erbB-2* induces certain benign breast lesions and is important in the development of carcinoma (Fig. 5).

Role of mammary differentiation in MMTV-driven transgenics: possible limitations to malignant development

The development of malignant carcinomas is infrequent in our MMTV/c-*erbB-2* transgenic rats. One possible reason for this may lie in the choice of the MMTV promoter for creating the models. The MMTV LTR promoter is known to be activated by hormones during pregnancy and lactation, such as glucocorticoids and prolactin [48]. In our models, we have confirmed that transgene expression is absent in virgin mammary epithelium and is induced during pregnancy. In humans over a whole lifetime, epidemiological evidence has shown that pregnancy protects against the development of breast cancer. This is particularly true of pregnancy early in reproductive life [51,52]. It has been suggested that an early first pregnancy protects the breast by causing some of the stem cell population to differentiate, thus removing these cells from the pool of dividing cells. Fewer cells are therefore available to mutate and form tumours. Late first pregnancy is not as protective, because mutations accumulate over time in the stem cell population and the growth-inducing effects of pregnancy may then encourage expansion of the mutated cell population [52]. Moreover, in the rat, completion of pregnancy and lactation before exposure to carcinogens such as DMBA markedly reduces the susceptibility of the mammary gland to chemical carcinogenesis [6]. Studies of carcinogen-induced rat mammary tumours have shown that malignant mammary carcinomas mainly arise from undifferentiated terminal end buds (TEBs) of the gland. Administration of DMBA to virgin 45–55-day-old rats during the period in which TEBs are decreasing in number due to their differentiation into alveolar buds (ABs) causes affected TEBs to develop large intraductal proliferations of epithelial and intermediate cells instead of differentiating into ABs. These proliferations become progressively larger, and may eventually develop into DCIS and further if transplanted against an immunological barrier [53]. In contrast, those TEBs that have differentiated already into ABs before DMBA administration do not develop DCIS, but remain unmodified, undergo dilation giving rise to hyperplastic lobules or cystic dilations, or exhibit ductular proliferation to form benign tumours such as adenomas or fibroadenomas [6]. The observation that mammary carcinomas probably arise from the undifferentiated stem-cell-containing structures of the gland (TEBs), whereas benign tumours such as adenomas and fibroadenomas arise from structures that were more differentiated at the time of carcinogen administration, suggests that the more differentiated the structure at the time of carcinogenic insult, or indeed oncogene activation, the more benign and organized is the tumour that develops. Similar results have been obtained when the *neu* oncogene is expressed in the reconstituted mouse mammary gland [50]. Moreover, in our transgenic rats, benign intraductal proliferations, intraductal papilloma and DCIS occur together, suggesting progressive steps in a carcinogenic pathway (Fig. 5).

Improvements in the transgenic model

In view of the above, carcinoma development may have been more frequent in our transgenic rats if the animals had remained virgins for a long period of time before their first pregnancy. During this period the additional mutations needed to co-operate with the c-*erbB-2* gene to induce carcinoma development may occur; carcinomas may then develop during the first pregnancy/lactation period, when expression of the c-*erbB-2* transgene is induced. Further studies will be necessary to test this hypothesis. Ideally it would be preferable to obtain a promoter that is active in a mammary stem cell population to target expression of the oncogene to rat mammary epithelial stem cells before differentiation occurs to ABs. However, to our knowledge, such a promoter has not yet been cloned and characterized.

Despite the limitations of the MMTV promoter, the transgenic rat models we have developed have provided some insight into the roles of these genes in the development of rat mammary cancers. In future studies we hope to address the following questions. (i) Can the frequency of carcinoma development be increased by keeping the animals in a virgin state for a long period of time before first pregnancy, or by crossing our outbred transgenic rats with an inbred strain? (ii) Can the TGFα and c-*erbB-2* gene products co-operate in breast cancer development? (iii) Are the transgenic rats more sensitive to chemical carcinogenesis? (iv) Can the TGFα-induced hyperplasias progress to hormone-independent growth and are they are transplantable? It may be possible to achieve a reproducible model of breast carcinoma expressing c-*erbB-2* in our rats by transplantation of one of the infrequent malignant lesions that develop in the transgenic rats. Moreover, it is hoped that we can culture cell lines from the various preneoplastic lesions and transfect them with further candidate oncogenes, antisense constructs to tumour suppressor genes and metastasis-associated genes to gain further insight into the multi-step process of carcinogenesis in the rat mammary gland.

We thank Caroline Harrison for assisting with the microinjection, Dr. Paul Edwards for helpful discussions, Angela Platt-Higgins for assistance with histological sectioning, and colleagues Michael Davies, Paul Jolley and John Hale (Cambridge), Kathy Edwards and Barry Cotterill (Liverpool) for animal care. Special thanks are given to Professor Bruce Ponder for his support in the later stages of this project. This work was funded in part by the Cancer and Polio Research Fund.

References

1. Muller, W.J. (1991) Cancer Metastasis Rev. **10**, 217–227
2. Cardiff, R.D. and Muller, W.J. (1993) Cancer Surv. **16**, 97–113
3. Merlino, G. (1994) Cancer Invest. **12**, 203–213
4. Edwards, P.A.W. (1993) Cancer Surv. **16**, 79–96
5. Young, S. and Hallowes, R.C. (1973) in Pathology of Tumours in Laboratory Animals, vol. 1 (Turusov, V.S., ed.), pp. 31–74, IARC Science Publishers, Lyon, France
6. Russo, J., Gusterson, B.A., Rogers, A.E., Russo, I.H., Wellings, S.R. and van Zweiten, M.J. (1990) Lab. Invest. **62**, 244–278
7. Foulds, L. (1949) Br. J. Cancer **3**, 345–375
8. Sullivan, N., Gatehouse, D. and Tweats, D. (1993) Mutagenesis **8**, 167–174
9. Marquardt, H., Klunkapillar, M.W., Hood, L.E., Twardzik, D.R., DeLarco, J.E., Stephenson, J.R. and Todaro, G.J. (1983) Proc. Natl. Acad. Sci. U.S.A. **80**, 4684–4688
10. Smith, J.A., Barraclough, R., Fernig, D.G. and Rudland, P.S. (1989) J. Cell. Physiol. **141**, 363–370
11. Massague, J. (1983) J. Biol. Chem. **258**, 13614–13620
12. McGready, M.L., Kerby, S., Shankar, V., Ciardiella, F., Salomon, D. and Siedman, M. (1989) Oncogene **4**, 1375–1382
13. Shankar, V., Ciardiella, F., Kim, N., et al. (1989) Mol. Carcinogen. **2**, 1–11
14. Mormanno, N., Ciardiello, F., Brandt, R. and Salomon, D.S. (1994) Breast Cancer Res. Treat. **29**, 11–27
15. Parham, D.M. and Jankowski, J. (1992) J. Clin. Pathol. **45**, 513–516
16. McAndrew, J., Rudland, P.S., Platt-Higgins, A.M. and Smith, J.A. (1994) Histochem. J. **26**, 355–366
17. Lundy, J., Schuss, A., Stanick, D., McCormack, E.S., Kramer, S. and Sorvillo, J.M. (1991) Am. J. Pathol. **138**, 1527–1534
18. Umekita, Y., Enokizono, N., Sagara, Y., Kuriwaki, K., Takasaki, T., Yoshida, A. and Yoshida, S. (1992) Virchows Arch. A. Pathol. Anat. **420**, 345–351
19. Matsui, Y., Halter, S.A., Holt, J.T., Hogan, B.L.M. and Coffey, R.J. (1990) Cell **61**, 1147–1155
20. Halter, S.A., Dempsey, P., Matsui, Y., Stokes, M.K., Graves-Deal, R., Hogan, B.L.M. and Coffey, R.J. (1992) Am. J. Pathol. **140**, 1131–1146
21. Coffey, R.J., Meise, K.S., Matsui, Y., Hogan, B.L.M., Dempsey, P. and Halter, S.A. (1990) Cancer Res. **54**, 1678–1683
22. Sandgren, E.P., Luettke, N.C., Palmiter, R.D., Brinster, R.L. and Lee, D.C. (1990) Cell **61**, 1121–1135
23. Jhappan, C., Stahle, C., Harkins, R.N., Fausto, N., Smith, G.H. and Merlino, G.T. (1990) Cell **61**, 1137–1146
24. Smith, G.H., Sharp, R., Kordan, E.C., Jhappan, C. and Merlino, G.T. (1994) Am. J. Pathol. **147**, 1081–1096
25. Sandgren, E.P., Schroeder, J.A., Qui, T.H., Palmiter, R.D., Brinster, R.L. and Lee, D.C. (1995) Cancer Res. **55**, 3915–3927
26. Coussens, L., Yang-Feng, T.L., Liao, Y.-C., et al. (1985) Science **230**, 1132–1139
27. Yamamoto, T., Ikawa, S., Akiyama, T., et al. (1986) Nature (London) **319**, 230–234
28. Shih, C., Padhy, L.C., Murray, M. and Weinberg, R.A. (1981) Nature (London) **290**, 261–264
29. Bargmann, C.I., Hung, M.C. and Weinberg, R.A. (1986) Cell **45**, 649–657
30. Press, M.F., Cordon-Cardo, C. and Slamon, D.J. (1990) Oncogene **5**, 953–962
31. McCann, A., Johnston, P.A., Dervan, P.A., Gullick, W.J. and Carney, D.N. (1989) Ir. J. Med. Sci. **158**, 137–140
32. Winstanley, J.H.R., Cooke, T., et al. (1991) Br. J. Cancer **63**, 447–450

33.   Slamon, D.J., Clark, G.M., Wang, S.G., Levin, W.J., Ullrich, A. and McGuire, W.L. (1987) Science **235**, 177–182

34.   Lui, E., Thor, A., He, M., Barcos, M., Ljung, B.M. and Benz, C. (1992) Oncogene **7**, 1027–1032

35.   Gusterson, B.A., Machin, L.G., Gullick, W.J., et al. (1988) Int. J. Cancer **42**, 842–845

36.   Van de Vijver, M.J., Peterse, J.L., Moori, W.J., Wiseman, P., Lomons, J., Dalesio, O. and Nusse, R. (1988) N. Engl. J. Med. **319**, 1239–1245

37.   Gullick, W.J. (1990) Int. J. Cancer **5**, 55–61

38.   Muller, W.J., Sinn, E., Pattengale, P.K., Wallace, R. and Leder, P. (1988) Cell **54**, 105–115

39.   Guy, C.T., Webster, M.A., Schaller, M., Parsons, T.J., Cardiff, R.D. and Muller, W.J. (1992) Proc. Natl. Acad. Sci. U.S.A. **89**, 10578–10582

40.   Luccini, F., Sacco, M.G., Hu., N., et al. (1992) Cancer Lett. **64**, 203–209

41.   Bouchard, L., Lamarre, L., Tremblay, P.J. and Jolicoeur, P. (1989) Cell **57**, 931–936

42.   Suda, Y., Aizawa, S., Furuta,Y., et al. (1990) EMBO J. **9**, 181–190

43.   Stocklin, E., Botteri, F. and Groner, B. (1993) J. Cell Biol. **122**, 199–208

44.   Muthuswamy, S.K., Siegel, P.M., Dankort, D.L., Webster, M.A. and Muller, W.J. (1994) Mol. Cell. Biol. **14**, 735–743

45.   Armstrong, D.T. and Opavsky, M.A. (1988) Biol. Reprod. **39**, 511–518

46.   Hogan, B., Constantini, F. and Lacy, E. (1986) in Manipulating the Mouse Embryo: A Laboratory Manual, Cold Spring Harbor Laboratory, Cold Spring Harbor, NY

47.   Warren, J. and Blakemore, S. (1993) Theriogenology **9**, 337

48.   Haraguchi, S., Good, R.A., Engelman, R.W. and Day, N.K. (1992) Int. J. Cancer **52**, 928–933

49.   Stamp, G., Frantl, V., Poulsden, R., Jamieson, S., Smith, R., Peters, G and Dickson, C. (1992) Cell Growth Differ. **3**, 929–938

50.   Bradbury, J.M., Arno, J. and Edwards, P.A.W. (1993) Oncogene **8**, 1551–1558

51.   Pike, M.C., Krailo, M.D., Henderson, B.E., Casagrande, J.T. and Hoel, D.G (1983) Nature (London) **303**, 767–770

52.   Vatten, L.J. and Kvinnsland, S. (1992) Eur. J. Cancer **28A**, 1148–1153

53.   Kim, U. (1979) in Breast Cancer (McGuire, W.L., ed.), vol. 3, pp. 1–36, Plenum Press, New York

Biochem. Soc. Symp. **63**, 185–191
Printed in Great Britain

16

Impact of molecular biology on the clinical management of breast cancer

S.J. Leinster

Department of Surgery, University of Liverpool, Liverpool L69 3GA, U.K.

Abstract

The use of molecular markers is being explored in the prediction of risk of developing breast cancer, in the assessment of prognosis and in the identification of appropriate treatment. Rational selection of treatment for a patient requires an accurate assessment of the prognosis and prediction of the response to a given treatment. Neither of these is possible with current clinicopathological markers. As a result, the current management of breast cancer is empirical, based on the outcome of randomized clinical trials that examine average effects within populations. Clinicopathological factors can be used to separate patients into broad prognostic groups, and treatment decisions are made on this basis. With this approach up to 70% of patients receive adjuvant treatment that is either unnecessary or ineffective. Molecular biological markers have the potential to improve this situation. A wide range of markers have been shown to be predictors of prognosis, but added individually to current prognostic indicators they do not improve the functional accuracy of prognosis or response prediction. There is a need for a molecular prognostic index that combines the results of a number of markers and can be used in conjunction with a clinical index to produce a more useful prognosis. There is also a need for an index that will predict responses to specific treatments. The impact of molecular biology on clinical management is a revolution waiting to happen.

Introduction

In order to undertake rational treatment, a clinician requires three things. The first is rapid, reliable diagnosis; the second is accurate prognosis; and the third is the ability to predict the effectiveness of a given treatment in a particular case. Traditionally, clinicians have depended on clinical and histopathological features of the tumour to give some guidance in these areas, but the data are crude and the information derived from them is imprecise. The great hope of the clinician is that molecular biology may provide some insights that will enable us to refine our practice.

Diagnosis

The diagnosis of a fully fledged carcinoma is relatively straightforward. A combination of clinical examination, imaging and fine-needle aspiration cytology (the triple approach) is almost 100% accurate [1,2]. The major diagnostic headaches are the so-called borderline lesions that may give rise to abnormal cells on cytology and may be difficult to diagnose even on histology. The transition from the normal breast epithelial cell to the cancer cell is assumed to proceed in a stepwise fashion (although there is no absolute evidence to support this belief). The progression runs: normal cell → hyperplasia → atypical hyperplasia → carcinoma *in situ* → invasive carcinoma

Atypical hyperplasia is not malignant, but carries an increased risk for the later development of cancer [3]. Carcinoma *in situ* may remain non-invasive or may progress to frank invasive cancer. At the most basic level, it can be difficult to distinguish atypical hyperplasia from carcinoma *in situ*, but the distinction may radically affect the treatment undertaken. If the patient has atypical hyperplasia she should be monitored closely, but if she has carcinoma *in situ* it may be appropriate to perform a mastectomy. At a more subtle level, it would be useful to be able to identify those cases of atypical hyperplasia or ductal carcinoma *in situ* (DCIS) that were going to progress.

One of the more difficult observations to explain is the overexpression of c-*erbB-2* in DCIS [4]. Only 20% of invasive cancers express c-*erbB-2*, and in these it is associated with a poorer prognosis. In contrast, 50% of DCIS express the receptor. It is not clear whether these cases are the ones that go on to become invasive tumours, although there is an association with large-cell, high nuclear-grade, comedo-type DCIS, which is thought to be the type that is more likely to recur and progress. This type is also more likely to express p53, but there does not appear to be any correlation between the expression of the two markers, and two different cell populations seem to be involved [5,6]. Once again, the significance of p53 expresssion in terms of progression to invasive carcinoma is not clear.

Some cases of atypical ductal hyperplasia show a loss of heterozygosity at some loci, but it is not clear whether there is an association between this and progression to carcinoma.

Prediction of prognosis

The most widely used prognostic index is the Nottingham index [7], which was derived by multivariate analysis of the factors affecting outcome in a large number of patients, and has been well validated with different groups of patients. The independent predictors of prognosis turned out to be tumour size, tumour grade (on the modified Bloom and Richardson grading system) and lymph node status (scored from 1 to 3).

An equation linking these factors has been derived which produces a score (Prognostic Index; P.I.) that can be related to prognosis:

$$P.I. = [0.3 \times \text{size (cm)}] + \text{grade} + \text{lymph node status}$$

A P.I. of <2.4. is associated with a 5-year disease-free survival rate of >90%, whereas a P.I. of >4.5 is associated with a disease-free survival of <60%. The authors of this index suggest that it should be used to select patients for different forms of treatment, particularly adjuvant treatment; however, while it is useful for grouping patients into broad prognostic categories for large-scale population studies, it is not precise enough to use in individual treatment decisions. The obvious inference is that patients with a P.I. of <2.4 would not benefit from adjuvant therapy if that therapy has a significant side-effect profile, because they are going to do well anyway. That ignores the 10% who are going to get recurrence, and what is needed is a method of determining which of the so-called good prognosis group are the ones who are going to experience recurrence.

Because the prognostic categories are so broad and imprecise, treatment is empirical and is based (at best) on the results of large-scale randomized trials that determine average outcomes. The decisions made are statistical rather than scientific. As a result, patients are exposed to treatments that are unnecessary for some and ineffective for others. For example, adjuvant chemotherapy results in a 30% decrease in odds of death [8]. This means that, in a group of patients with a 70% 5-year survival, the addition of adjuvant treatment will result in an 80% 5-year survival. Only 10% of the patients will have received a clear benefit; 20% will have died despite treatment, so for them the treatment was ineffective; 70% would have survived anyway, so for them the treatment was unnecessary.

A large number of molecular markers have been associated with poor prognosis [9]. To the cynical clinical eye it appears that each of the markers of poor prognosis occurs in 20–30% of the tumours and accounts for an approx. 10% difference in survival at 5 years.

The longest established of the molecular markers is the oestrogen receptor (ER). The early publications hailed it as a strong predictor of outcome, with patients whose tumours were ER-positive having a better survival than those whose tumours were ER-negative [10]. This effect was independent of the lymph node status of the patient, and the patient who did not show involvement of the lymph nodes but whose tumours were ER-negative did as badly as those who were node-positive but ER-positive. The effect of ER status is certainly true for the first 5 years, but thereafter the survival curves approach one another, and the difference between ER-positive and ER-negative disappears by 10 years [11].

This loss of predictive power in the long term is also seen with the standard clinicopathological markers such as tumour size, lymph node status and tumour grade [12].

There is conflicting evidence with regard to the prognostic value of a number of other markers. c-*erbB-2* overexpression correlates well with other markers of poor prognosis [13]. It is an accepted marker of poor prognosis in lymph-node-positive patients [14], but the evidence is evenly balanced in node-negative patients [9]. Some of the disparity may be due to differences in methodology and reagents, but some may be due to the low frequency of c-*erbB-2* alteration in the patients and the low number of events (death or recurrence) that occur. From the pragmatic point of view, it means that c-*erbB-2* cannot be used on its own as a prognostic indicator, and it may not contribute much of practical value even when combined with other indicators. Similar considerations hold for other markers.

Other markers are of little practical value because of either the difficulty or the expense of measuring them. Measures of cell proliferation correlate well with prognosis. The thymidine labelling index is particularly effective in lymph-node-negative patients [15], but it requires fresh tissue and autoradiography, which make it impracticable for routine use. The measurement of S-phase fraction and ploidy also correlates well with survival [16], but when included in multivariate analyses with grade, these two factors fail to display independent significance. Grading does not require expensive equipment and is available to a wider range of service laboratories than is measurement of S-phase fraction. It has been claimed that grading is subjective and, therefore, unreliable, but when Elston's modification of Bloom and Richardson's original method is used, high rates of inter-observer reliability can be achieved [17]. It makes more practical sense to continue to use grading for clinical purposes.

Currently, the axillary lymph node status is the best predictor of the later development of metastatic disease, but this can be determined only by axillary surgery, which carries an attendant morbidity. A method of predicting metastatic disease without recourse to surgery would save the patients considerable problems. Abnormalities of the mechanisms that are necessary for metastases may in future allow the patients at risk to be identified. Studies have been reported on Nm23, adhesion molecules, proteases and angiogenesis, but none are sufficiently advanced to be of routine clinical value [9].

Selection of treatment ·

From the earliest use of hormone manipulation in breast cancer, it was noted that not all tumours responded. It became apparent that, in an unselected group of patients with breast cancer, 30% would respond to hormonal manipulation. When that manipulation was major ablative surgery, it was a matter of priority to attempt to identify those who would respond. The detection of the ER allowed some discrimination. Using conventional ligand binding assays, it was found that 50–60% of women with ER-positive tumours responded to hormone treatment, whereas less than 10% of ER-negative patients responded [18]. This level of response still meant that a number of women were receiving treatment that was bound to be ineffective. It also posed the theoretical question as to why a patient with detectable ERs did not respond. The usual explanation is that, although detectable in a binding assay, the receptor is not functional. The search turned to the detection of proteins that are dependent on the presence of a functional ER. The first candidate to enter clinical practice was the progesterone receptor. The response rate for ER-positive, progesterone-receptor-positive tumours is 77%, while for ER-positive, progesterone-receptor-negative tumours it is only 27% [18]. pS2, a protein of unknown function, is also oestrogen-dependent. In one study, 76% of pS2-positive patients responded to hormone therapy compared with 37% of pS2-negative patients [19].

In the U.S.A., it became the standard practice to prescribe hormone therapy for only those women who had ER-positive tumours. In the U.K. a different approach became commonplace with the launching of tamoxifen, which was alleged to be an oestrogen antagonist but achieved 15–20% response rates even in ER-negative tumours. Since the side-effect profile of tamoxifen was so favourable in comparison with chemotherapy (which was the alternative), it was felt that the best way to determine responsiveness to tamoxifen was to give it and see what happened. The clinical importance of ER status was thus reduced. On this basis the NATO trial of adjuvant tamoxifen gave the drug to all comers irrespective of ER status. The results of this trial showed that tamoxifen had some effect in prolonging survival even in those cases that were ER-negative [20].

In the 1960s, oophorectomy was an accepted adjuvant treatment for premenopausal women. Eventually, controlled trials of oophorectomy compared with no adjuvant treatment were carried out, and consistently appeared to show no benefit from oophorectomy. As a result, oophorectomy ceased to be a routine treatment. A meta-analysis carried out by the Early Breast Cancer Trialists Co-operative Group showed that the apparent lack of effect was a result of the small numbers entered into each of the trials. When the results of the trials are combined, adjuvant oophorectomy is found to have an effect roughly equal to that of adjuvant chemotherapy [8]. This led to the setting up of trials directly comparing oophorectomy with chemotherapy. The initial reports from these trials suggest that there is a difference in response depending on the ER status. When the treatment groups are compared as total groups, the effects of chemotherapy and tamoxifen are similar. When the groups are subdivided on the basis of ER status, it is found that the outcome is better for those ER-positive tumours treated with hormone therapy and for those ER-negative tumours treated with chemotherapy [8].

It seems that there needs to be a re-evaluation of the role of ER status in the determination of adjuvant therapy, and rapid assessment of ER status using immunohistochemical methods should now be routinely reported in the histopathology report.

A major requirement for clinicians at present is the ability to predict which patients are going to respond to chemotherapy. Having identified a high-risk group who would potentially benefit from adjuvant therapy, it would be useful to know in which patients it will actually be effective. Those patients where the treatment is unlikely to be effective can be spared the stress of undergoing the treatment. (Some patients will, of course, opt for the treatment even when the chance of benefit is low, as the alternative of no treatment is even more unsettling to contemplate). It would be of particular help if response to treatment could be predicted in those women at a very high risk of recurrence in whom high-dose chemotherapy with marrow rescue might be contemplated.

In some studies, overexpression of c-erbB-2 has been correlated with a poor response to adjuvant chemotherapy [21,22], and in one study there was a dose–response effect in patients with c-erbB-2 overexpression [23]. Thus c-erbB-2 might be one modality that could be used in treatment selection.

Cells that lack wild-type p53 are resistant to chemotherapy and radiotherapy. Cells that possess wild-type p53 undergo death by apoptosis when exposed to these agents [24]. If these findings were verified in clinical studies, they would provide a useful means of selecting patients who were likely to respond to therapy.

Conclusion

At present, the application of molecular biology to clinical practice is in its infancy. The majority of studies have concentrated on a single modality and have examined correlations with other indicators of poor prognosis, or have made retrospective correlations with outcomes. What are needed, as McGuire [25] has pointed out, are multivariate prospective studies to identify those factors that are independently relevant to prognosis. Clinicians would like similar studies to be conducted on diagnosis and treatment.

References

1.   Green, B., Leinster, S.J., Turnbull, L., Smith, P. and Winstanley, J. (1995) Br. J. Surg. **82**, 1509–1511
2.   Layfield, L.J., Glasgow, B.J. and Cramer, H. (1989) Pathol. Annu. **24**, 23–62
3.   Dupont, W.D. and Page, D.L. (1985) N. Engl. J. Med. **312**, 146–151
4.   Barnes, D.M., Bartkova, J., Camplejohn, R.S., Gullick, W.J., Smith, P.J. and Millis, R.R. (1992) Eur. J. Cancer **28**, 644–648
5.   Walker, R.A., Dearing, S.J., Lane, D.P. and Varley, J.M. (1991) J. Pathol. **165**, 203–211
6.   Poller, D.N., Roberts, E.C., Bell, J.A., Elston, C.W. and Blamey, R.W. (1993) Hum. Pathol. **24**, 463–468
7.   Haybittle, J.L., Blamey, R.W., Elston, C.W., et al. (1982) Br. J. Cancer **45**, 361–366
8.   Early Breast Cancer Trialists Collaborative Group (1992) Lancet **339**, 1–15; 71–85
9.   Leong, A.S.-Y. and Lee, A.K.C. (1995) J. Clin. Pathol. Mol. Pathol. **48**, M221–M238
10.   Cooke, T., George, W.D. and Shields, R. (1979) Lancet **i**, 995–997
11.   Winstanley, J., Cooke, T., George, W.D., et al. (1991) Br. J. Cancer **64**, 99–101
12.   Lipponen, P., Aaltomaa, S. and Eskelinen, M. (1992) Int. J. Cancer **19**, 1479–1485
13.   Berger, M.S., Locher, G.W., Saurer, S., Gullick, W.J. and Waterfield, M.D. (1988) Cancer Res. **48**, 1238–1243
14.   Winstanley, J., Cooke, T., Murray, G.D., Platt-Higgins, A. and George, W.D. (1991) Br. J. Cancer **63**, 447–450
15.   Silvestrini, R., Diadone, M.G. and Di Fronzo, G. (1986) Breast Cancer Res. Treat. **7**, 161–169
16.   O'Reilly, S.M. and Richards, M.A. (1992) Eur. J. Cancer **28**, 504–507
17.   Elston, C.W. and Ellis, I.O. (1991) Histopathology **19**, 403–410
18.   Osborne, C.K., Yochmowitz, M.G., Knight, W.A. and McGuire, W.L. (1980) Cancer **46**, 2884–2888

19. Schwartz, L.H., Koerner, F.C. and Edgerton, S.M. (1991) Cancer **46**, 2884–2888
20. Nolvadex Adjuvant Trial Organisation (NATO) (1988) Br. J. Cancer **57**, 608–611
21. Allred, D.C., Clark, G., Tandon, A.K., Molina, R. and Tormey, D.C. (1992) J. Clin. Oncol. **10**, 599–605
22. Gusteson, B.A., Gelber, R.D. and Golhirsch, A. (1992) J. Clin. Oncol. **10**, 1049–1056
23. Muss, H.B., Thor, A.D., Berry, D.A., Kute, T. and Liu, E.T. (1994) N. Engl. J. Med. **330**, 1260–1266
24. Lowe, S.W., Ruley, H.E., Jacks, T. and Housman, D.E. (1993) Cell **74**, 957–967
25. McGuire, W.L. (1990) J. Natl. Cancer Inst. **83**, 154–155

Biochem. Soc. Symp. **63**, 193–198
Printed in Great Britain

17

Type 1 growth factor receptors: current status and future work

W.J. Gullick

ICRF Oncology Unit, Hammersmith Hospital, Du Cane Road, London W12 0NN, U.K.

Abstract

The type 1 family of growth factor receptors consists of the epidermal growth factor receptor (EGFR), and ErbB-2, ErbB-3 and ErbB-4. Six ligands are known to bind directly to EGFR, none (at present) to ErbB-2, and a family of ligands collectively called the neuregulins bind to both ErbB-3 and ErbB-4. It is now apparent that the receptors function in various heterodimeric pairs, depending on their concentrations, the concentrations of particular ligands in the environment and some intrinsic degree of dimer selectivity. Overexpression of EGFR, ErbB-2 and ErbB-3 has been found commonly in solid human tumours. ErbB-4 has not yet been examined. The EGFR is also activated by various mutations in brain tumours and possibly in other tumour types. These changes appear to be one of the causes of malignant transformation. They may also provide information regarding the course of disease and response to current treatments. Finally, they are targets for a variety of new forms of treatment being developed in the laboratory, in preclinical models and in a few cases in clinical trials.

Introduction

Epidermal growth factor (EGF) was first identified in the early 1960s, and its receptor (EGFR) in 1976. Their cDNAs were cloned and sequenced in 1983 and 1984 respectively. A second receptor, related in structure to the EGFR and called variously Neu, HER-2 or ErbB-2, was cloned in 1985, a third called HER-3 or ErbB-3 in 1989 and a fourth, HER-4 or ErbB-4, in 1993. In addition to EGF, five related ligands, each of which bind to the EGFR, have now been identified: transforming growth factor-α, amphiregulin, heparin binding EGF, betacellulin and epiregulin (Fig. 1) [1]. Recently it was shown that betacellulin also binds to and activates ErbB-4 [2]. Finally, proteins originally identified in the rat (termed Neu differentiation factor) and in humans

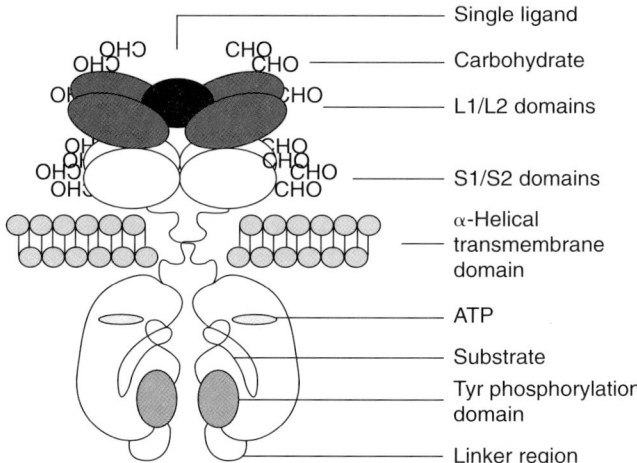

Fig. 1. Model for a type 1 growth factor receptor dimer.

(termed heregulin) have been purified and characterized. These are encoded by a single gene in humans on 8p12–22 which is spliced into at least 12 different protein species, all of which bind to both ErbB-3 and ErbB-4. Neu differentiation factor/heregulins are divided into two classes, α and β, based on the presence of two possible sequences forming the C-terminal half of their EGF-like region. The α class bind to both ErbB-3 and ErbB-4 with about 10-fold lower affinity than the β forms [3].

Thus it is apparent that there are now many more receptor and ligand species making up this family with appreciably more complex interactions than were known even 5 years ago. This brief article attempts to outline the current concepts of how this family of receptors and their ligands interact and to list some outstanding questions in this field, some of which may be answered in the near future.

Present status

Most evidence supports a model in which, in the absence of ligand, type 1 receptors are in equilibrium between monomeric and dimeric forms. It is also proposed that, at concentrations of receptors found in normal cells, the monomeric form predominates. Ligand binding, which stabilizes receptor interactions, promotes a shift towards the dimeric form. Increased expression of receptors in a cell will increase the numbers of both monomers and dimers, but presumably not affect their proportions. This would, it is argued, in some cases mimic the effect of ligand activation, causing increased growth or transformation.

EGF was first shown to promote EGFR homodimerization. Although no ligand is known that binds to ErbB-2 when expressed alone, a mutation identified in rat tumours also stabilizes the homodimeric form of this receptor.

Thus most models originally envisaged homodimers as the principal physio-logically relevant activated state (Fig. 2). Latterly, however, it has become apparent, first for the EGFR and ErbB-2 and then for the EGFR and ErbB-3, that heterodimers can also form. Recent work has shown that all possible per-mutations (10; the factorial of 4) can probably occur (Fig. 2) [4]. Importantly, some evidence shows that heterodimers display a higher affinity for their lig-ands than do homodimers. In principle, therefore, at low ligand concentrations, heterodimers will predominate over homodimers if more than one receptor species is expressed in a cell.

Finally, different receptors interact with their own selection of the array of available second messenger proteins due to the nature of the primary sequences surrounding their autophosphorylation (or transphosphorylation)

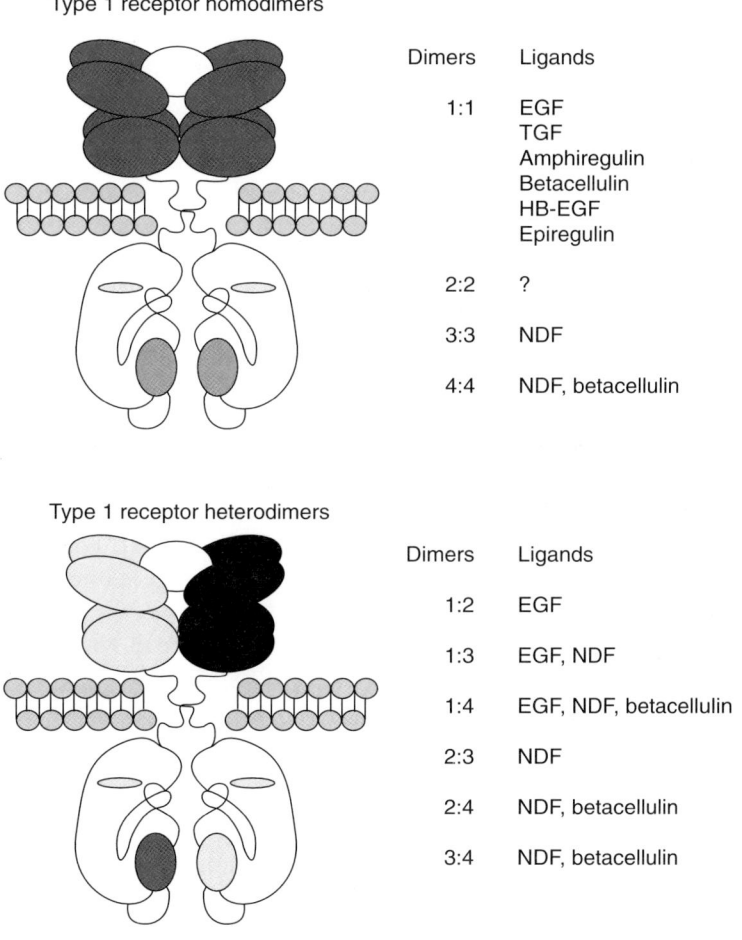

Type 1 receptor homodimers

Dimers	Ligands
1:1	EGF
	TGF
	Amphiregulin
	Betacellulin
	HB-EGF
	Epiregulin
2:2	?
3:3	NDF
4:4	NDF, betacellulin

Type 1 receptor heterodimers

Dimers	Ligands
1:2	EGF
1:3	EGF, NDF
1:4	EGF, NDF, betacellulin
2:3	NDF
2:4	NDF, betacellulin
3:4	NDF, betacellulin

Fig. 2. Type I growth factor receptor homodimers and het-erodimers, and the ligands with which they are currently thought to interact. TGF, transforming growth factor-α; HB-EGF, heparin binding EGF; NDF, Neu differentiation factor.

sites. An example of selective interaction is PtdIns 3-kinase, which binds much more extensively (or avidly) to ErbB-3 than to EGFR or ErbB-2 [5]. The Shc protein, on the other hand, appears to interact more or less equally efficiently with all four receptor types [6]. Over time, the exact receptor choices will need to be determined in detail and may depend upon the cell type examined and its state of differentiation.

Outstanding questions

Surprisingly, after so many years of research, it has not yet been determined how many ligands bind to a type 1 receptor and the mode of association [7]. It has been proposed (and frequently appears in text books) that one ligand binds to each receptor monomer, rather like a cherry on a cupcake, and that this promotes dimerization by allosterically altering the shape of the receptor's extracellular domain, revealing surfaces that now interact physically to stabilize the dimeric form. There is no indication in this model that the ligand interacts with more than one receptor surface.

Other models may, however, be envisaged in which a single ligand binds to one receptor and then this forms a ternary complex with a second receptor. In this case the ligand interacts simultaneously with surfaces of both receptors. This model, despite appreciable thermodynamic advantages, has not been favoured for one principal reason, which is that EGF-like ligands are asymmetrical and are assumed to act as monomers. With the elucidation of the three-dimensional structure of the growth hormone receptor, this objection becomes less powerful, as it is formed of exactly such a ternary complex of two identical receptors and a single asymmetrical ligand [8]. Somewhat more complicated variations of this structure can also be proposed in which two ligands form bridges between the receptor pair (in this case the structure could, of course, be symmetrical). It is also predicted that, at high (perhaps supraphysiological) ligand concentrations, single receptors, each with one ligand bound, would be the predominant and presumably inactive form [8]. Thus the experimental elucidation of which of these models is the correct one by anything other than three-dimensional structural determination is not trivial. It does, however, provoke a final possible twist, which is that, in such a 'bridging' model, different ligands might prefer to form different receptor heterodimers (or even homodimers as, for instance, EGF and betacellulin bind to both EGFR and ErbB-4). This possibility is, however, only theoretical at present.

A second outstanding problem is whether a member of a homodimer is phosphorylated on the same sites as the same molecule present in a receptor heterodimer. As interactions with second messengers via SH2 or PTB (phosphotyrosine binding) domains are apparently dependent on the location of a phosphorylation site, this becomes critical. In fact, the question depends on the assumption that receptor phosphorylation on tyrosine is occurring by transphosphorylation rather that the previously assumed autophosphorylation. Two main experiments support the occurrence of transphosphorylation. Firstly, a 'kinase dead' receptor (generally made by mutating a single lysine residue in the catalytic site) expressed with an active equivalent receptor does become phosphorylated on ligand addition. To digress, this questions the approach of 'dominant negative' receptors, since in some instances this can apparently amplify receptor signalling rather than diminish it, and is certainly reflected in the very different phenotype of Waved 2 (kinase dead) compared with EGFR knockout mice. The second experiment involves receptor transphosphorylation in heterodimers where the low or absent kinase activity of ErbB-3 provides a natural model system.

The answer to this question will come from meticulous examination of phosphorylation at particular sites in homodimers compared with heterodimers. The traditional approach of phosphotryptic peptide mapping as well as new approaches such as the use of site-specific, phosphorylation-dependent, antibodies will probably both prove useful.

As mentioned above, a still intriguing point, although perhaps a nuance to some, is whether ErbB-3 possess any ligand-stimulated tyrosine kinase activity. Without going over old ground, the consensus now is that it has low levels of activity or none. The distinction, however, may be important, as low levels may be quite sufficient to signal under some circumstances. In addition it remains unclear, if ErbB-3 truly has no kinase activity, why in a ErbB-2/ErbB-3 heterodimer there is an apparent increase in tyrosine phosphorylation of ErbB-2. This question should, however, be reasonably easy to answer if the right experimental systems can be designed.

This leads me to my last point in this brief and very speculative article. What are the best experimental systems to determine type 1 receptor interactions and intracellular signalling? Basically, two approaches have been used: cell lines naturally expressing one or more type 1 receptor, and cell lines apparently lacking all expression into which receptors can be introduced using expression vectors. The former system can be manipulated experimentally to reduce expression of an individual receptor type, most originally and effectively by the expression of an antibody fragment made against the extracellular domain of a receptor engineered to prevent from it exiting the endoplasmic reticulum or Golgi apparatus [9]. This approach, although very elegant, suffers from the variable ability of available antibodies to effectively prevent receptor expression on the cell surface. One can therefore never entirely exclude the possibility that a small fraction of these receptors are in a functionally relevant compartment. None the less, interesting results have been obtained this way.

Although superficially more simple, the use of cells lacking type 1 receptor expression has in fact several disadvantages. Firstly, how can one be sure that these receptors are not expressed, even at low levels? In one cell line for instance, Ba/F3 (a pro-B-lymphocyte), it was found using PCR, after the production of a range of lines apparently expressing single receptors and receptor combinations, that the parental line expressed a low level of endogenous ErbB-3 [4]. Secondly, in experiments designed to detect signalling by assays such as growth or survival, the absence of an effect is not informative, as that cell type may lack the necessary second messenger type normally utilized by that receptor.

At this stage, therefore, despite their complexity, 'natural' receptor-expressing cells remain the best model for 'vertical' signalling. If, however, one can be assured to a reasonable degree that a cell lacks type 1 receptor expression (either wholly or of a single member), this system is quite suitable for 'horizontal' interactions, i.e. combinational interactions between receptor monomers. In the long run the ideal model, however, may be cells that normally express type 1 receptors but now cannot do so due to knockout of the receptor gene. These should possess a relevant complement of second messenger proteins and provide a good background for the introduction of mutant receptors, disabled or activated in desired ways.

In summary, therefore, despite 35 years of research, there remain many unanswered and rather fundamental questions regarding the mechanism of action of these receptors. Not least of these is their action in normal and pathological situations in complex tissues, an area of research almost unexplored so far.

References

1.   Prigent, S.A. and Lemoine, N.R. (1992) Prog. Growth Factor Res. **4**, 1–24
2.   Riese, D.J., Bermingham, Y., van Raaij, T.M., Buckley, S., Plowman, G.D. and Stern, D.F. (1996) Oncogene **12**, 345–353
3.   Ben-Baruch, N. and Yarden, Y. (1994) Proc. Soc. Exp. Biol. Med. **206**, 221–227
4.   Riese, D.J., van Raaij, T.M., Plowman, G.D., Andrews, G.C. and Stern, D.F, (1995) Mol. Cell. Biol. **15**, 5770–5776
5.   Prigent, S.A. and Gullick, W.J. (1994) EMBO J. **13**, 2831–2841
6.   Culouscou, J.M., Carlton, G.W. and Aruffo, A. (1995) J. Biol. Chem. **270**, 12857–12863
7.   Gullick, W.J. (1994) Eur. J. Cancer **30A**, 2186
8.   Wells, J.A. (1994) Curr. Biol. **6**, 163–173
9.   Beerli, R.R., Graus-Porta, D., Woods-Cook, K., Chen, X., Yarden, Y. and Hynes, N.E. (1995) Mol. Cell. Biol. **15**, 6496–6505

Biochem. Soc. Symp. **63**, 199–210
Printed in Great Britain

18

Role of epidermal growth factor receptor family members in growth and differentiation of breast carcinoma

Bruce D. Cohen*‡, Clay B. Siegall*, Sarah Bacus†, Linda Foy*,
Janell M. Green*, Ingegerd Hellström*, Karl Erik Hellström*
and H. Perry Fell*

Molecular Immunology Department, Bristol-Myers Squibb, Pharmaceutical
Research Institute, Seattle, WA 98121, and †Advanced Cellular Diagnostics,
Inc., Elmhurst, IL 60126, U.S.A.

Abstract

Members of the epidermal growth factor (EGF) family of tyrosine kinase receptors are involved in the regulation of cell growth and differentiation, and are found to be expressed in many types of cancers. Activation of these receptors can be elicited by multiple ligands, resulting in the formation of a spectrum of heterodimer complexes and a number of biological outcomes. A clear demonstration of biological activation by a single complex has been difficult to address because of the endogenous expression of HERs (human EGF-like receptors) in many cell lines. We have generated a collection of cell lines expressing all HERs alone or in all pairwise combinations in a clone of NIH 3T3 cells (3T3-7d) devoid of detectable EGF receptor family members. Transformation, as measured by growth in soft agar, only occurred in cells expressing two different HER family members. Transformation with activated Neu and the rate of *in vivo* tumour formation were also correlated with the expression of multiple HERs in the same cell. To further our understanding of the role of heterodimer signalling, we demonstrated that, within a breast carcinoma cell line, activation of HER-3 results in cellular differentiation, prolonged activation of extracellular-signal-related kinase 1 (ERK1) activity and an increase in $p21^{CIP1/WAF1}$ nuclear staining. In contrast, activation of HER-4 is mitogenic, induces transient activation of ERK1 activity and decreases the nuclear staining of $p21^{CIP1/WAF1}$. These differences in biochemical

‡To whom correspondence should be addressed.

and biological responses are correlated with the contrasting abilities of HER-3 and HER-4 to be down-regulated from the cell surface. The cell-surface localization of HER-3 does not change in response to ligand, whereas activation of HER-4 results in a loss of cell-surface staining followed by accumulation into a perinuclear compartment.

Introduction

Members of the epidermal growth factor (EGF) family of tyrosine kinase growth factor receptors are expressed in a broad spectrum of tumour types, which classifies them as one of the most frequently implicated cell-surface markers for human cancers. This family consists of four members: EGF receptor (EGFR)/HER-1, Neu/ErbB-2/HER-2, ErbB-3/HER-3 and ErbB-4/HER-4 [1–5]. One or more EGFR family members (hereinafter called HERs, for human EGF-like receptors) have been shown to be overexpressed in tumours of the brain, stomach, bladder, breast, ovary and lung, and in adenocarcinomas [3,6–9]. Much emphasis has been placed on one family member, HER-2, whose expression is up-regulated in 30% of breast and ovarian cancers, is an indicator of a poor prognosis [9–12] and can itself induce tumours in animals when mutated or overexpressed [13–15].

The activation of HER family members can be elicited by multiple EGF-like ligands [16–21], resulting in the formation of both homo- and heterodimeric complexes [22–26]. This provides a very complex system of potential signals leading to diverse biological responses. In many cell lines, EGF stimulation of HER-1 results in a mitogenic response [27]. There is no identified ligand as of yet for HER-2. Examination of the biological responses generated by HER-3 or HER-4 has been difficult due to the fact that each is stimulated by the same ligand, heregulin [24,25,28].

Overexpression of these receptors by gene transfection confers a ligand-dependent transformed phenotype [14,26,29–31]. Unlike the other family members, which require ligand for activation, overexpression of HER-2 alone is sufficient to promote transformation [14,15]. Since all of these receptors can associate with and activate each other, it is difficult to interpret the activities of receptor-transfected cell lines due to the fact that the parent cell line may express low levels of endogenous HERs. This was clearly the case for HER-4 when expressed in NIH 3T3 cells, in which transformation was promoted in response to both heregulin and EGF [26]. To avoid such problems, we have generated a collection of cell lines expressing all HERs alone or in all pairwise combinations in a clone of NIH 3T3 cells (3T3-7d) devoid of detectable EGFR family members. Unlike other studies that analysed a subset of HERs, we set out to investigate the entire repertoire of HER combinations in a cell system that is commonly used for evaluating the transforming activity of proteins. We then furthered our investigation into the biological consequences of heterodimer function into a breast carcinoma cell line. Using receptor-specific ligands we were able to demonstrate that signalling through HER-3 and HER-4 delivers contrasting biochemical and biological signals, when analysed in the context of cells that normally express this class of growth factor receptors.

Results

The 3T3-7d cell line, which is devoid of detectable HER expression, was transfected with expression plasmids encoding each of the HER family members. Cell lines were isolated that expressed the receptors individually or as heterodimers in all possible combinations. The level of receptor expression, as determined by immunoprecipitation and Western analysis, was similar in all cell lines (Fig. 1). The level of receptor activity in response to ligand, as measured by the change in receptor tyrosine phosphorylation, was investigated. Cells were stimulated with EGF or heregulin and the HERs were immunoprecipitated with receptor-specific antibodies followed by immunoblotting with anti-phosphotyrosine antibody (Fig. 2). With respect to the cell lines that expressed only one family member, HER-1 was partially tyrosine phosphorylated in the absence of ligand and was further stimulated by the addition of EGF. Similarly, HER-2 was phosphorylated in the absence of ligand; however, its level of phosphorylation did not change in response to either EGF or heregulin. HER-3, previously shown to be a defective tyrosine kinase [31], demonstrated a weak response to heregulin. HER-4 was partially activated in the absence of ligand, and could be phosphorylated further in response to heregulin. In cells expressing two different receptors, stimulation of either receptor partner by EGF or heregulin resulted in the increased phosphorylation of both receptors, indicative of a heterodimer complex. However, in the context of a HER-1/-3 heterodimer, we were unable to demonstrate a heregulin-dependent increase in HER-1 phosphorylation.

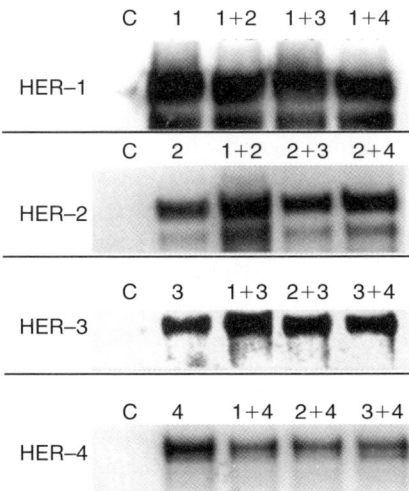

Fig. 1. HER expression levels in transfected 3T3-7d cells. Cell lysates from transfected 3T3-7d cells were immunoprecipitated with specific anti-HER monoclonal antibodies, and the level of receptor expression was determined by immunoblot analysis. C refers to the untransfected parent cell line. The receptors expressed in each cell line are noted above each lane.

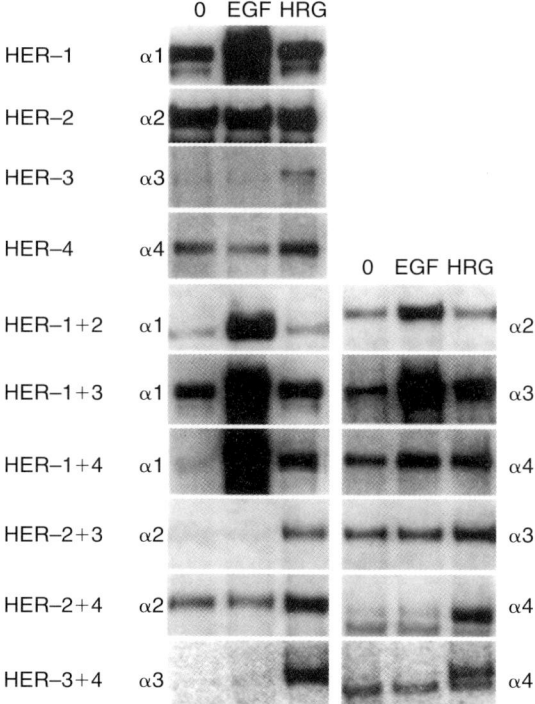

Fig. 2. Levels of HER tyrosine phosphorylation in response to ligand.
HER-transfected cell lines were stimulated with 100 ng/ml EGF or heregulin
(HRG) for 10 min at room temperature. Cells were extracted and receptors
immunoprecipitated with specific monoclonal antibodies. The level of receptor
phosphorylation was determined by immunoblotting using an anti-phosphotyrosine antibody.

In the absence of added ligand, the steady-state level of receptor phosphorylation was affected by the co-expression of other HER family members.
HER-1 phosphorylation was elevated when expressed as a homodimer as well
as when co-expressed with HER-3. However, when co-expressed with HER-2
or HER-4, the level of ligand-independent phosphorylation decreased. HER-2
phosphorylation was elevated when expressed as a homodimer and heterodimer, except when co-expressed with HER-3. HER-3 phosphorylation
was stimulated when co-expressed with HER-1 and HER-2, but not with
HER-4. HER-4 phosphorylation was high as a homodimer and when co-
expressed with HER-1, but low when co-expressed with HER-2 or HER-3.
These data suggest that receptor complexes can form in the absence of ligand,
and that the level of receptor phosphorylation varies from one heterodimer to
another.

To address the transforming activity of the 3T3-7d/HER transfectants,
cells were seeded in soft agar to determine if colony formation occurred in the
presence or absence of ligand stimulation (Fig. 3). All cell lines expressing only
one family member were unable to form colonies, even in the presence of lig-

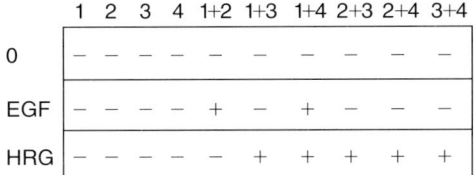

Fig. 3. Transforming activity of HER-transfected 3T3-7d cells in response to ligand. Each cell line, transfected with the HER family members indicated at the top, was mixed with 4 ml of 0.4% agar and added on top of a 6 ml layer of 0.6% agar containing 200 ng/ml EGF or heregulin (HRG). Cells were incubated for 2 weeks, and then analysed.

and. In contrast, all cell lines expressing a combination of HERs were able to form colonies in agar in response to ligand, with the exception of the HER-1+3 cell line. Ligand stimulation of HER-1+3 cells responded positively to heregulin, but not to EGF. This was surprising given the fact that EGF is able to activate both HER-1 and HER-3 tyrosine phosphorylation (Fig. 2).

To further support the hypothesis that heterodimer formation is required for efficient growth in agar, the oncogenic form of Neu (TNeu) was tested for its ability to induce colonies in agar when expressed in the 3T3-7d cell line. TNeu contains a point mutation in the transmembrane domain that induces receptor dimerization, ligand-independent transformation and tumour formation in animals. Cell lines were generated by transfecting a TNeu expression vector into 3T3-7d parent cells or 3T3-7d HER-1-, HER-2-, HER-3- or HER-4-expressing cell lines, and the level of TNeu expression was determined by immunoblot analysis (Fig. 4a). Since the antibody used for the immunoblot cross-reacts with HER-2, we are unable to demonstrate clearly the presence of TNeu expression independent of HER-2 expression. The transforming activity of TNeu was only evident in cells that co-expressed HER-1, HER-3 or HER-4 (Fig. 4b). TNeu- or TNeu/HER-2-expressing cells were unable to form colonies in agar.

The requirement for multiple HER expression in cells to promote a transforming signal was further tested *in vivo* by determining the tumorigenic potential of 3T3-7d HER transfectants in nude mice. 3T3-7d cell lines expressing both HER-1 and HER-2 were highly tumorigenic as compared with those in which either receptor was expressed individually (Fig. 5). Together, these data demonstrate that co-expression of multiple HER family members within a cell is more efficient in generating signals that lead to a transformed phenotype, and imply that heterodimer formation plays an important role in this process.

The transfection of genes into NIH 3T3 cells is a common approach to investigating the transforming potential of a particular protein. Having shown that pairwise expression of HERs is more efficient at transforming 3T3 cells, we were interested in determining whether the activation of different HER complexes generated similar or different biological outcomes in tumour cells known to express these receptors. We focused our attention on HER-3 and HER-4, both of which are activated by heregulin. Stimulation of breast carci-

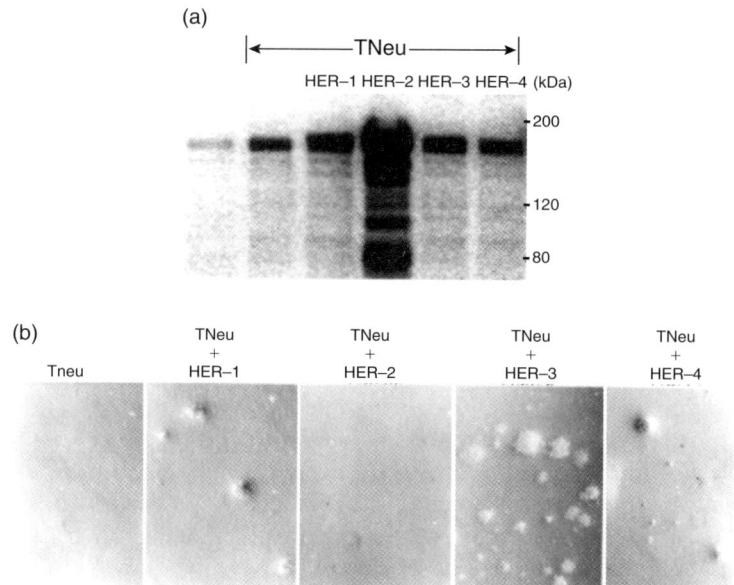

Fig. 4. HER compliments TNeu transforming activity. 3T3-7d parent and derivative cell lines expressing HER-1, HER-2, HER-3 or HER-4 were transfected with a TNeu expression plasmid and a histidinol selection plasmid. Histidinol-resistant colonies were pooled and analysed for TNeu expression by immunoblotting of cell extracts with an anti-HER-2 antibody (a). The transforming activity of these cell lines was analysed by growth in 0.4% agar (b).

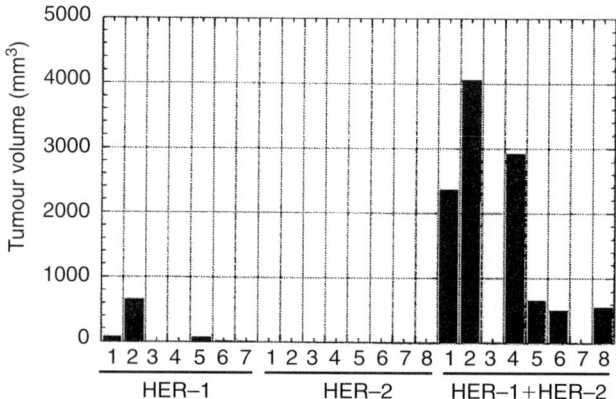

Fig. 5. Enhanced tumour formation by cells expressing multiple HERs. Transfected 3T3-7d cell lines expressing HER-1, HER-2 or HER-1+2 were injected subcutaneously into nude mice (1×10^5 cells), and tumour formation was determined at 4 weeks post-injection.

noma cell lines with heregulin is able to induce cellular differentiation, resulting in decreased cell growth, altered cell morphology and increased synthesis of differentiation markers such as casein [19]. Since heregulin is able to activate both HER-3 and HER-4, it is unclear what each of the receptors is contributing to this biological response. We and others have recently determined that betacellulin, a ligand initially identified for its specificity for HER-1, is also able to bind to and activate HER-4, but not HER-3 [32]. Taking advantage of the contrasting specificities of heregulin and betacellulin, we investigated whether the signals generated by activating HER-3 or HER-4 receptor complexes promoted different biological and biochemical responses. The H3396 breast carcinoma cell line, which expresses HER-2 and HER-3 on its cell surface, was transfected with a HER-4 expression plasmid to generate a cell line that expressed HER-2, HER-3 and HER-4 (H3396/HER-4). H3396/HER-4 cells were stimulated with either betacellulin or heregulin, and changes in cell proliferation as well as the induction of two differentiation markers, p21$^{CIP1/WAF1}$ and extracellular-signal-related kinase 1 (ERK1) [33,34], were measured. Betacellulin, but not heregulin, provided a mitogenic signal that could be inhibited by addition of the HER-4 blocking antibody 10-4 into the growth medium (Fig. 6a). Exposure to betacellulin also decreased the number of nuclei stained for p21$^{CIP1/WAF1}$ (Fig. 6b) and stimulated a transient activation of ERK1 (Fig. 6c). In contrast, heregulin did not stimulate cell growth; it up-regulated the level of p21$^{CIP1/WAF1}$ and promoted a stronger and more prolonged activation of ERK1, which has been shown previously to be associated with cellular dif-

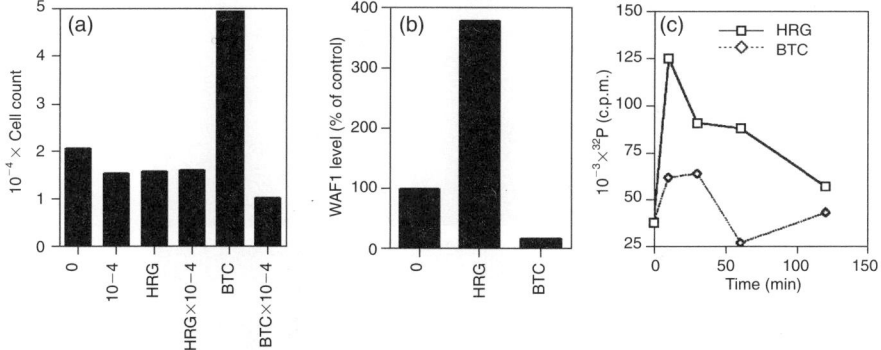

Fig. 6. Activation of HER-3 or HER-4 sends contrasting biological signals. (a) H3396/HER-4-transfected cells were plated at 5000 cells/well in a 24-well dish and grown in the presence of 15 nM (100 ng/ml) heregulin (HRG) or 23 nM (200 ng/ml) betacellulin (BTC) in the presence or absence of the HER-4 blocking antibody 10-4 (10 μg/ml). After 6 days, cells were trypsinized and counted in a cell Coulter counter. (b) H3396/HER-4 cells were treated with heregulin or betacellulin and the level of p21$^{CIP1/WAF1}$ was determined by immunohistochemistry on fixed cell monolayers using an anti-p21$^{CIP1/WAF1}$ antibody and quantified by image analysis. (c) ERK1 activity was determined by immunoprecipitating ERK1 from H3396/HER-4 cells that were stimulated with ligand for increasing amounts of time. ERK1 activity was measured as the incorporation of [γ-^{32}P]ATP into myelin basic protein.

B.D. Cohen et al.

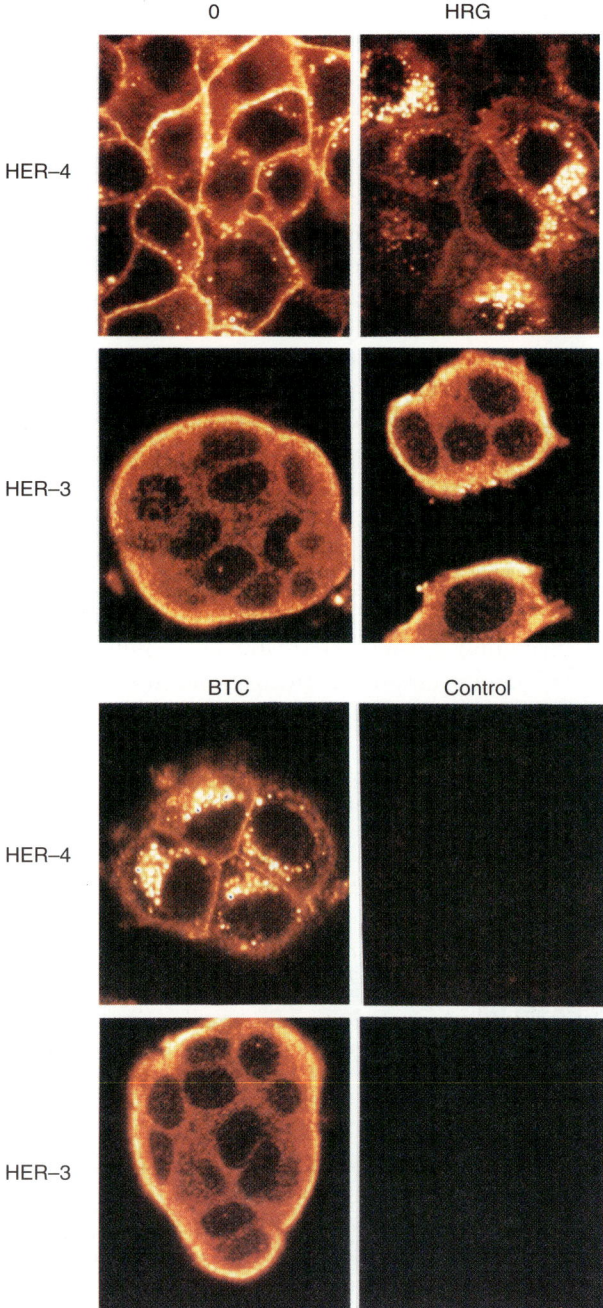

Fig. 7. Cellular redistribution of HER-3 and HER-4 after ligand stimulation. H3396/HER-4 cells were stimulated with heregulin (HRG) or betacellulin (BTC) for 90 min at 37 °C, fixed and stained with monoclonal antibodies specific for either HER-3 or HER-4, followed by FITC-labelled antimouse secondary antibody. Receptor localization was visualized by confocal microscopy.

ferentiation [33,34]. Heregulin-stimulated parental H3396 cells expressing only HER-2 and HER-3 behaved identically in all assays to the heregulin-stimulated H3396/HER-4 transfectant (results not shown). Therefore activation of HER-4 delivers a mitogenic signal, whereas stimulation through HER-3 in the presence or absence of HER-4 induces differentiation.

Previous studies have suggested that the duration of receptor activity may dictate the nature of the biological response [34]. We investigated whether the differential activation of ERK1 was correlated with differences in the expression and subcellular localization of HER-3 and HER-4 in response to ligand. H3396/HER-4 cells were stimulated with betacellulin or heregulin, and the level of HER-4 or HER-3 was analysed by confocal microscopy using receptor-specific monoclonal antibodies (Fig. 7). Cell-surface staining was observed for both receptors in unstimulated cells. Continuous stimulation with betacellulin or heregulin resulted in the loss of HER-4 from the cell surface and its concomitant accumulation within the perinuclear region, suggestive of a lysosomal degradative pathway. In contrast, the subcellular localization of HER-3 did not change in response to ligand stimulation, and it remained at the cell surface without any accumulation into the perinuclear region. The lack of HER-3 down-regulation in response to ligand correlates with a prolonged ERK signal, and suggests that receptor trafficking may play an important role in the duration of signalling and the subsequent biological response evoked by specific HER family members. The biological significance of HER-3 peripheral staining on clusters of cells is unknown.

Conclusions

In analysing the expression profile of HER family members in both normal and tumour tissues, it is often the rule and not the exception that multiple members are expressed within a given cell type. Our data suggest that expression of multiple HERs is required for efficient transformation of cells in response to ligand. None of the receptors when expressed alone could efficiently induce growth in soft agar, even in response to ligand. If the agar plates were maintained for 4 weeks post-plating, small but detectable colonies could be seen in ligand-stimulated HER-1-, HER-3- and HER-4-expressing cells, as well as in HER-2-expressing cells in the absence of ligand. The lack of efficient colony formation was surprising, since we and others have demonstrated previously that expression of one HER member in 3T3 cells confers soft agar growth in response to ligand, and HER-2 overexpression alone was transforming [3,14,15,26,29,30]. The biological differences seen between the parental NIH 3T3 cells and the 3T3-7d cell lines may be due to the low-level expression of EGFR and c-Neu in the parent cell line which may be able to synergize with the transfected gene product. This was clearly evident when HER-4 was transfected into the parent 3T3-7 cell line and was able to form colonies in agar in response to both EGF and heregulin [26]. It is also possible that the level of expression of each receptor is not high enough to elicit a transforming signal. Nevertheless, even at these expression levels, the cells expressing two different HERs are efficiently transformed. This is further supported by the observation that expression of TNeu induced colony formation only in cells that co-expressed HER-1, HER-3 or HER-4. Expression alone or with HER-2 was transformation-negative, even when expression was at high levels (Fig. 4). Similar transfection experiments have demonstrated identical results. Lastly, cells expressing HER-1+2 were able to form aggressive tumours in animals in a short time frame. Cells expressing HER-1 were able to form tumours in animals, albeit slowly, and cells expressing HER-2 were negative for tumour formation. Together, these data demonstrate that the expression of multiple HERs in a cell provides a stronger transforming signal than the expression of only one HER.

Although all of the cell lines expressing multiple HERs were transformed in response to ligand, the cells expressing HER-1 plus HER-3 were only transformed by heregulin and not by EGF. This is in contrast with the cell line expressing HER-1 plus HER-4, which was transformed by the addition of either heregulin or EGF. This was surprising, since EGF can induce both HER-1 and HER-3 tyrosine phosphorylation, as well as activating the phosphorylation of SHC and the p85 subunit of PtdIns 3-kinase (results not shown). A possible explanation is that EGF stimulation of a HER-1+HER-3 complex may induce a growth-inhibitory or differentiating signal. It was shown recently that nerve growth factor stimulation of 3T3 cells expressing TrkA resulted in cell growth arrest and induction of the differentiation marker p21$^{CIP1/WAF1}$ [35]. Further, the epidermoid carcinoma cell line A431, known to overexpress HER-1 at high levels, is growth-inhibited by the addition of EGF [36].

The level of ligand-independent HER tyrosine phosphorylation varied depending upon which other receptor was co-expressed in the same cell. This suggests that receptors can associate with one another and regulate their kinase activity in the absence of ligand. Addition of ligand induced the phosphorylation of homodimers as well as of both receptor chains within a heterodimer complex. We did not see a significant induction of HER-1 phosphorylation by heregulin in cells expressing HER-1+3. This is in contrast with studies examining HER expression in haematopoetic cells [37]. Our lack of a detectable response could be due to an already elevated level of HER-1 phosphorylation, which would make small changes in phosphorylation difficult to detect. This might have been expected, since previous studies have demonstrated that HER-3 is a partially defective kinase [31]. This is clearly evident in the heregulin-stimulated HER-3-expressing cell line (Fig. 2). The implication that HER-3 is an impaired kinase is in contrast with what was found when analysing the HER-2+3 heterodimer. Heregulin stimulation of HER-2+3-expressing cells resulted in an increase in both HER-2 and HER-3 phosphorylation. We and others have seen similar results in other cell lines expressing HER-2 and HER-3. This suggests that HER-3 may not be a defective kinase, but is limited in its specificity for appropriate substrate sites. An alternative hypothesis is that receptor complexes can exist in multimeric configurations and that the activated receptors can phosphorylate adjacent dimer complexes.

Even though the transforming activities of these receptors could be addressed in NIH 3T3 cells, it wasn't until we changed our cell system to a breast carcinoma cell line that we discovered that HER-3 and HER-4 generate different biological signals. Historically, the dual specificity of heregulin for HER-3 and HER-4 made it difficult to study the specific signalling properties inherent to each receptor. The H3396 breast carcinoma cell line expressing HER-2 and HER-3 in conjunction with the H3396/HER-4 transfectant provided a model system for the specific activation of HER-3 or HER-4 within identical cellular backgrounds. We and others have observed that treatment with low doses of heregulin can be mitogenic, whereas high doses induce differentiation [18,19]. This implies that the strength or duration of receptor signalling may play an important role in determining the biological outcome of receptor activation [34]. With regards to both HER-1 [27] and HER-4, ligand stimulation results in a mitogenic response and a transient activation of both the receptor and intracellular targets, culminating in the down-regulation of the receptor at the cell surface. Activation of HER-3 does not result in the loss of the receptor from the cell surface and is correlated with a sustained activation of downstream targets. The lack of HER-3 down-regulation parallels previous studies in which the cytotoxic activity of heregulin toxin fusions, able to bind with high affinity to both HER-3 and HER-4, was dependent upon the expression of HER-4 at the cell surface [38]. A further understanding of the interplay between HER family members and their ligands, the unique signals they produce and their subcellular trafficking could provide significant insights into the role this receptor system plays in tumour progression and development.

References

1.   Ullrich, A. and Schlessinger, J. (1990) Cell **61**, 203–212
2.   Ullrich, A., Coussens, L., Hayflick, J.S., et al. (1984) Nature (London) **309**, 418–425
3.   Kraus, M.H., Issing, W., Miki, T., Popescu, N.C. and Aaronson, S.A. (1989) Proc. Natl. Acad. Sci. U.S.A. **86**, 9193–9197
4.   Plowman, G.D., Whitney, G.S., Neubauer, M.G., Green, J.M., McDonald, V.L., Todaro, G.J. and Shoyab, M. (1990) Proc. Natl. Acad. Sci. U.S.A. **87**, 4905–4909
5.   Plowman, G.D., Culouscou, J.M., Whitney, G.S., Green, J.M., Carlton, G.W., Foy, L., Neubauer, M.G. and Shoyab, M. (1993) Proc. Natl. Acad. Sci. U.S.A. **90**, 1746–1750
6.   Gullick, W.J. (1990) Int. J. Cancer Suppl. **5**, 55–61
7.   Baselga, J. and Mendelsohn, J. (1994) Pharmacol. Ther. **64**, 127–154
8.   Lemoine, N.R., Barnes, D.M., Hollywood, D.P.,et al. (1992) Br. J. Cancer **66**, 1116–1121
9.   Kraus, M.H., Popescu, N.C., Amsbaugh, S.C. and King, C.R. (1987) EMBO J. **6**, 605–610
10. King, C.R., Kraus, M.H. and Aaronson, S.A. (1985) Science **229**, 974–976
11. Slamon, D.J., Clark, G.M., Wong, S.G., Levin, W.J., Ullrich, A. and McGuire, W.L. (1987) Science **235**, 177–182
12. Slamon, D.J., Godolphin, W., Jones, L.A., et al. (1989) Science **244**, 707–712
13. Bargmann, C.I., Hung, M.C. and Weinberg, R.A. (1986) Nature (London) **319**, 226–230
14. Difiore, P.P., Pierce, J.H., Kraus, M.H., Segatto, O., King, C.R. and Aaronson, S.A. (1987) Science **237**, 178–182
15. Hudziak, R.M., Schlessinger, J. and Ullrich, A. (1987) Proc. Natl. Acad. Sci. U.S.A. **84**, 7159–7163
16. Carpenter, G. and Cohen, S. (1979) Annu. Rev. Biochem. **48**, 193–216
17. Plowman, G.D., Green, J.M., McDonald, V.L., Neubauer, M.G., Disteche, C.M., Todaro, G.J. and Shoyab, M. (1990) Mol. Cell. Biol. **10**, 1969–1981
18. Holmes, W.E., Sliwkowski, M.X., Akita, R.W., et al. (1992) Science **256**, 1205–1210

19. Peles, E., Bacus, S.S., Koski, R.A., Lu, H.S., Wen, D.Z., Ogden, S.G., Benlevy, R. and Yarden, Y. (1992) Cell **69**, 205–216

20. Sasada, R., Ono, Y., Taniyama, Y., Shing, Y., Folkman, J. and Igarashi, K. (1993) Biochem. Biophys. Res. Commun. **190**, 1173–1179

21. Shing, Y., Christofori, G., Hanahan, D., Ono, Y., Sasada, R., Igarashi, K. and Folkman, J. (1993) Science **259**, 1604–1607

22. Wada, T., Zian, X. and Greene, M.I. (1990) Cell **61**, 1339–1347

23. Soltoff, S.P., Carraway, K.L., Prigent, S.A., Gullick, W.G. and Cantley, L.C. (1994) Mol. Cell. Biol. **14**, 3550–3558

24. Sliwkowski, M.X., Schaefer, G., Akita, R.W., et al. (1994) J. Biol. Chem. **269**, 14661–14665

25. Plowman, G.D., Green, J.M., Culouscou, J.M., Carlton, G.W., Rothwell, V.M. and Buckley, S. (1993) Nature (London) **366**, 473–475

26. Cohen, B.D., Green, J.M., Foy, L. and Fell, H.P. (1996) J. Biol. Chem. **271**, 4813–4818

27. Carpenter, G. (1987) Annu. Rev. Biochem.. **56**, 881–914

28. Tzahar, E., Levkowitz, G., Karunagaran, D., et al. (1994) J. Biol. Chem. **269**, 25226–25233

29. Difiore, P.P., Pierce, J.H., Fleming, T.P., et al. (1987) Cell **51**, 1063–1070

30. Velu, T.J., Beguinot, L., Vass, W.C., Willingham, M.C., Merlino, G.T., Pastan, I. and Lowy, D.R. (1987) Science **238**, 1408–1410

31. Guy, P.M., Platko, J.V., Cantley, L.C., Cerione, R.A. and Carraway, K.L. (1994) Proc. Natl. Acad. Sci. U.S.A. **91**, 8132–8136

32. Riese, D.J., Bermingham, Y., Vanraaij, T.M., Buckley, S., Plowman, G.D. and Stern, D.F. (1996) Oncogene **12**, 345–353

33. Halevy, O., Novitch, B.G., Spicer, D.S., et al. (1995) Science **267**, 1018–1021

34. Marshall, C.J. (1995) Cell **80**, 179–185

35. Decker, S.J. (1995) J. Biol. Chem. **270**, 30841–30844

36. Macleod, C.L., Luk, A., Castagnola, J., Cronin, M. and Mendelsohn, J. (1986) J. Cell. Physiol. **127**, 175–182

37. Riese, D.J., Vanraaij, T.M., Plowman, G.D., Andrews, G.C. and Stern, D.F. (1995) Mol. Cell. Biol. **15**, 5770–5776

38. Siegall, C.B., Bacus, S.S., Cohen, B.D., et al. (1995) J. Biol. Chem. **270**, 7625–7630

Biochem. Soc. Symp. **63**, 211–221
Printed in Great Britain

19

Somatic mutations that contribute to breast cancer

Robert Callahan

Oncogenetics Section, Laboratory of Tumor Immunology and Biology, National Cancer Institute, Bethesda, MD 20892, U.S.A.

Abstract

Cytogenetic and molecular analyses of primary sporadic human breast carcinomas have documented at least 12 different chromosome arms affected by loss of heterozygosity (LOH). This has been taken as evidence for the presence of putative tumour suppresser genes in the remaining allele within the affected regions. We have previously identified three regions on chromosome 17q that are affected by LOH in primary human breast tumours. A physical map of one of these regions (17q21) has been prepared. The putative target gene appears to be located between the D17S846 and D17S746 loci. We are currently determining whether either of two genes located in this region is the target for LOH. The mouse mammary tumour model system provides an approach for identifying genes which, when activated or inactivated by mouse mammary tumour virus (MMTV) integration, contribute to specific stages of mammary tumorigenesis. Using this approach we have identified two genes, designated *NOTCH4/INT3* and *INT6* respectively. Interruption of *NOTCH4/INT3* by MMTV represents a gain-of-function mutation that has profound consequences for mammary gland development and tumorigenesis. *INT6* was found to be interrupted by an integrated MMTV genome in a mammary hyperplastic outgrowth line and two independent mammary tumours. In each case the transcriptional orientation of the viral genome was opposite to that of *INT6*. The rearranged allele was expressed as a truncated chimaeric RNA species composed of *INT6* coding sequences, intron sequences and MMTV sequences. Since the non-rearranged allele contained no mutations, we conclude that MMTV integration into *INT6* causes a dominant-negative mutation or biologically activates its function. The nucleotide sequence of *INT6* is unrelated to any of the known genes in the GenBank database, but is evolutionarily highly conserved.

Address for correspondence: National Cancer Institute, Building 10, Room 5B50, Bethesda, MD 20892, U.S.A.

Introduction

The aetiology of breast cancer is influenced by a variety of factors, such as menstrual and reproductive history, family history, long-term treatment with oestrogen, diet and previous atypical benign breast disease [1–3]. It seems probable that these factors could provide a selective environment for the clonal outgrowth of mammary epithelial cells that contain somatic mutations. One could imagine that some of these mutations could uncouple normal mammary gland development or could contribute to the development of neoplasia. Alternatively, they could provide atypical non-malignant as well as malignant cells with a selective growth advantage, the means to metastasize to distant organ sites or evasion of host immunosurveillance. Because of the heterogeneity and multiplicity of factors necessary for the development of most epithelial tumours, the current view is that multiple somatic mutations act in concert to produce an invasive carcinoma with the ability to metastasize to distant organ sites.

A preview of the complexity of somatic alterations that occur during human breast tumour progression was provided by earlier cytogenetic analysis of primary human breast tumour cells in culture [4]. The alterations include aneuploidy (either gain or loss of entire chromosomes) and rearrangements affecting chromosomes 1q (translocations), 6q (deletions and translocations), 7p (translocations, pericentric inversions and isochromosomes) and 11q (translocations). More recently, in a study using comparative genome hybridization methodology to map regions of the genome with increased DNA sequence copy number (amplification), 26 chromosomal subregions were found to be affected in primary human breast tumours and breast tumour cell lines [5]. Although genetic analysis of primary breast tumour DNAs has demonstrated amplification of known proto-oncogenes such as *FLG* (8p12), *myc* (8q24), *BEK* (10q24), *FGF3/PRAD1/cyclin D* (11q13), 15q24-q25 (*IGFR-1/FES*) and *erb-B2* (17q12), it seems probable that amplification of other, as yet unknown, genes contributes to malignant progression in breast cancer (reviewed in [6,7]).

Loss of heterozygosity (LOH) in primary human breast tumours

LOH represents another common genetic alteration in primary human breast tumours, and occurs as a consequence of interstitial deletions, chromosome loss or aberrant mitotic recombinational events. It is thought that LOH reveals within the affected region of the genome the presence of a recessive mutation in the remaining allele of a 'tumour suppresser' gene(s) (reviewed in [8,9]). Tumour suppresser genes are believed to be involved in the normal suppression of cellular proliferation during development [9]. Commonly, one normal allele is lost as a result of LOH, while the other allele contains either a small deletion or a point mutation that inactivates the gene product. At the present time, 12 chromosome arms have been found to be frequently affected by LOH in breast tumours, including chromosomes 1p [10], 1q [11], 3p [12], 6q

[13,14], 7q [15], 11p [16,17], 8q (R. Callahan, unpublished work), 13q [18], 16q [19], 17p [20], 17q and 18q [21]. Moreover, it is not uncommon for multiple regions within these chromosome arms to be independently affected by LOH.

A major thrust of research in this area is the identification of the target genes affected by LOH or DNA amplification. However, the apparent complexity of genetic alterations that are found in primary human breast tumours, and the possibility that some of them are a consequence of tumour progression rather than a cause, makes this a daunting challenge. Therefore several different types of approach are being applied to this problem, including surveys of directional cDNA libraries [22,23] and positional cloning [24]. Another approach is based on the mouse model system in which the mouse mammary tumour virus (MMTV) is the biological carcinogen that induces tumour development as a consequence of insertional mutagenesis.

Definition of target genes within regions affected by LOH on chromosome 17q

We have expanded our initial study of chromosome 17q in primary breast tumour DNAs to include 18 polymorphic loci in this region of the genome [23]. At least three distinct regions located at 17q21.1-q21.3 (region 1), 17q22-qter (region 2) and 17q23-q25 (region 3) could be identified that are independently affected by LOH. Based on the current recombination linkage map of chromosome 17q, a proximal region is located within a 22 cM region defined by D17S73 and NME1 (region 1) and thus is similar in location to the region known to contain the *BRCA1* locus associated with familial breast and breast/ovarian cancer. The central region (region 2) is bordered by the D17S86 and D17S21 loci, which are about 28 cM apart. The distal region (region 3) is bordered by the D17S20 and D17S77 loci, which are 11 cM apart.

We have recently focused our efforts on identifying target genes for LOH to 17q21, or region 1 of chromosome 17q [25]. To date there is no evidence that the *BRCA1* gene is mutated in non-hereditary breast tumours [26]. We surveyed this region of chromosome 17 in 130 sporadic breast cancers using 17 polymorphic sequence tagged-site markers that have been physically mapped between the D17S250 and D17S579 loci [27]. The smallest commonly deleted region occurred in the approx. 120 kb interval between the D17S846 and D17S746 loci. This region is centromeric of the *BRCA1* gene and is physically defined by two overlapping P1 phage clones. Our nucleotide sequence analysis of these two P1 phage clone DNAs identified the plackoglobin gene as a potential target gene. This gene had previously been mapped to chromosome 7, but a human/mouse somatic cell hybrid and fluorescence *in situ* hybridization (FISH) analysis confirmed its location on 17q21. Plackoglobin is involved in intercellular communication and is located in desmosomes and adherens junctions (reviewed in [28]). We have defined its genomic organization to facilitate analysis to determine whether it is mutated in genomic DNA from sporadic breast tumours. No mutations were found in 11 breast tumour cell lines or in 11 primary breast tumours containing LOH in this region of chromosome 17q21 using single-strand conformation polymorphism analysis [29] and hybrid mismatch analysis [30,31]. More recently, we have identified a second gene in this region of 17q21 and are determining whether it is mutated in primary sporadic breast tumours.

Future directions

Although efforts to identify the target genes in the regions of chromosome 17 affected by LOH are continuing in our own laboratory as well as other laboratories, the apparent complexity of putative target genes on this chromosome alone was unexpected. Most of the 'alleletyping' studies of primary breast tumour DNAs have examined one or two polymorphic loci per chromosome arm. Moreover, the locations of some of these loci are imprecisely mapped relative to other loci on the particular chromosome arm. It seems probable, therefore, that as high density maps of the other chromosomes (both those that are known to be affected and those that currently appear to be unaffected by LOH) in breast tumour DNAs are developed, additional regions affected by LOH will be uncovered. The increasing availability of highly polymorphic loci that have been either physically mapped or mapped by linkage analysis on all chromosome arms suggests that identification of the target genes for LOH not only is feasible in the near future but should have the highest priority in the effort to solve the puzzle of the genetic pathology of breast cancer. Answers from these studies will provide a sound foundation for determining the linkage between particular mutations and clinical parameters of the disease, as well as whether particular subsets of tumours can be defined by the mutations they contain and the clinical parameters with which they are associated.

Another approach: the mouse model system

Many of the classical inbred strains of *Mus musculus* were intentionally derived from stocks of mice that had a high incidence of mammary tumours (C3H, GR, BR6 and RIII mouse strains), and have been inbred for the past 50–60 years for a high incidence of mammary tumours (reviewed in [32,33]). Mice of each strain congenitally transmit highly infectious MMTV through the milk to their offspring. MMTV is a non-acute transforming retrovirus. An obligate step in the replication of the MMTV virus is the integration of a DNA copy of its proviral genome into the host cellular genome. This event itself is potentially mutagenic for the host cell when it causes the deregulation of the expression of adjacent cellular genes (designated the *INT* loci) in mammary tumours [34]. To identify affected cellular genes, the viral genome has been used as a molecular tag. Using this approach, five *INT* loci (*INT1/Wnt-1*, *INT2/FGF3*, *Wnt-3*, *HST/k-FGF/FGF4* and *FGF8*) have been identified in mammary tumours of high-incidence inbred mouse strains or MMTV-infected transgenic mouse strains [35–39]. The mechanism by which MMTV activates the expression of these *INT* genes is primarily a consequence of the effect of enhancer sequences within the long terminal repeat (LTR) of the integrated

MMTV proviral genome on the transcriptional promoter of the adjacent affected gene.

MMTV has been detected in feral strains of mice (reviewed in [40]). Although mammary tumorigenesis does not play an important role in the zoological history of feral mice in their natural habitat, when brought into a laboratory setting mice do develop mammary tumours [40–42]. A colony, designated CZECH II, was derived from a single breeding pair of *M. musculus musculus* trapped in Czechoslovakia [41]. The CZECH II mice lack endogenous MMTV genomes but do contain an infectious strain of MMTV that is transmitted congenitally through the milk [41,43]. This colony has a 20% incidence of pregnancy-independent mammary adenocarcinomas that are histopathologically similar to those induced by MMTV (C3H). The frequency with which *Wnt-1* was activated by MMTV was similar (24%) to that observed in Balb/cfC3H (30%) or CZECH IIfC3H (30%) mammary tumours, whereas MMTV-induced activation of *FGF3* and *FGF4* was significantly less frequent. Like high-incidence inbred mouse strains, CZECH II mice also develop mammary preneoplastic hyperplastic alveolar nodules (HANs) which we have developed into mammary hyperplastic outgrowth lines (HOGs). A survey of DNA from 31 CZECH II HOGs revealed that 22.6% (7 out of 31) had MMTV-induced rearrangements of *Wnt-1*, but none had rearrangements of either *FGF3* or *FGF4* (E. Kordon and G.H. Smith, personal communication). Since the frequency of MMTV-induced rearrangements of *Wnt-1* is similar in both CZECH II HOGs and mammary tumours, it seems likely that, in the setting of this mouse strain, activation of *Wnt-1* is primarily an early event in tumorigenesis which disrupts regulatory controls of normal mammary gland development leading to lobular hyperplasia. Mammary tumours arising from within these HOGs frequently contain additional MMTV proviral genomes. Based on the results obtained with the MMTV-infected *Wnt-1* transgenic mice, it seems probable that members of the *FGF* gene family will be found to be activated by MMTV in tumours derived from *Wnt-1*-positive HOGs. Moreover, relative to the results of similar studies of C3H HOGs, where rearrangements of *Wnt-1* rarely occur [44], the observations made in CZECH II HOGs serve to highlight the impact of the host genetic background on the frequency and consequences of MMTV activation of a particular *INT* gene in the context of malignant progression.

New *INT* genes in CZECH II HOGs and mammary tumours

Activation of the *INT3* locus was first detected in CZECH II mouse mammary tumours [45]. The locus was defined by the integration of an MMTV proviral genome within a 100 bp region of the cellular genome of 10 independent mammary tumours corresponding to an exon of the target gene. The *INT3* locus is located in the class II region of the major histocompatibility (*MHC*) locus on chromosome 17 [43,46]. In each case the transcriptional orientation of the integrated viral genome was in the same direction as that of the target gene. A 2.3 kb species of RNA was detected in tumours containing a virally induced rearrangement of *INT3*. This RNA species was not detected in tumours where the locus was intact or in the normal mammary gland. Nucleotide sequence analysis of the *NOTCH4/INT3* gene revealed that it is related to the *Drosophila Notch* gene [47]. However, *INT3* is not the murine homologue of *Notch*; rather, it is one of a four-member gene family [48–50]. The *Drosophila Notch* gene encodes a receptor protein that is involved in cell fate determinations during development [48–50]. It is known that the intracellular domain of this protein represents the functional domain responsible for gene activity, whereas the extracellular region serves mainly a regulatory role through interaction with the ligand. Expression of *NOTCH4/INT3*, as well as of *NOTCH1* and *NOTCH2*, RNAs can be detected in mammary glands of virgin, pregnant and lactating mice (R. Callahan, unpublished work). So far *NOTCH1* and *NOTCH2* have not been found to be rearranged by MMTV (R. Callahan, unpublished work). All of the viral integration events within *NOTCH4/INT3* occurred within one of two exons 5′ to the region encoding the transmembrane domain of the encoded protein. This results in the overexpression of the portion of the gene encoding the intracellular domain of the protein. Experiments in which the same region of the *Drosophila Notch* gene are overexpressed demonstrated that this represents a gain-of-function mutation, mimicking the consequences of the interaction between the Notch protein and its ligand [51].

Examination of differentiating normal mammary epithelium for the distribution of the NOTCH4/INT3 protein by immunoperoxidase demonstrated that normal NOTCH4/INT3 expression is strongly associated with the cap cells at the tip of the proliferating end buds of developing ducts [52]. Later during early pregnancy, NOTCH4/INT3 immunoreactivity shifts to the apical cytoplasm of the mammary epithelium of the proliferating alveolar buds, suggesting an intimate association of NOTCH4/INT3 with growth and development of the secretory mammary epithelium. This conclusion was strengthened in the fully lactating gland, where immunoreactive NOTCH4/INT3 is relocated to a basal position in the secretory epithelium of functional lobules and disappears from the cytoplasm of the mammary ductal epithelium. The shift in immunoreactive NOTCH4/INT3 from a luminal to a basal position in the secretory mammary epithelium at lactational maturity probably reflects a dynamic change in the functional role of NOTCH4/INT3, induced either intrinsically or by an accompanying alteration in the three-dimensional pattern of NOTCH4/INT3-specific ligand localization.

To begin to understand the biological consequences of activated NOTCH4/INT3 for mammary gland development and tumorigenesis, transgenic mouse strains were developed that express activated NOTCH4/INT3 at different times during mammary gland development. In female MMTV-LTR/*NOTCH4/INT3* transgenic mice, expression of the intracellular region of NOTCH4/INT3 in the mammary gland blocks normal ductal branching morphogenesis in post-pubertal females [52,53]. The mammary ductal epithelium penetrates the mammary fat pad only minimally. During the first pregnancy the mammary fat pad fills with ductal epithelium, but there is little lobular-alveolar development and within 4 to 6 months all females develop mammary tumours. To determine whether the lobular developmental defect was associated with early events correlating with the early expression of the transgene, or was a consequence of transgene expression during lobular development, we developed transgenic mice expressing the intracellular region of NOTCH4/INT3 under the transcriptional control of the whey acid protein (WAP) gene promoter, which is specifically active in differentiating secretory mammary epithelium. There are several striking differences between the WAP/*NOTCH4/INT3* and the MMTV/*NOTCH4/INT3* transgenic model systems with respect to mammary gland growth and development. A full and completely branched mammary ductal system develops in virgin WAP/*NOTCH4/INT3* females, and in these mice the ductal epithelium forms the appropriate intercellular connections necessary for proper ductal morphology. Neither of these events are accomplished in the virgin FVB transgenic mouse mammary gland [52]. This suggests that WAP/*NOTCH4/INT3* is not expressed in the non-secretory ductal epithelial progenitor cells. In the first pregnancy there is limited lobular development of the mammary gland in WAP/*NOTCH4/INT3* mice, and dysplastic lesions appear throughout the gland. These lesions do not regress after weaning, but progress to frank carcinoma upon successive pregnancies. We conclude that the effect of expression of truncated NOTCH4/INT3 on mammary gland development and tumorigenesis is exquisitely dependent on the timing of its expression relative to mammary gland development. WAP/*NOTCH4/INT3* and MMTV-LTR NOTCH4/INT3 transgenic lines will therefore be appropriate models for distinguishing, at a molecular level, the effects of *NOTCH4/INT3* on different epithelial cell subsets in the differentiating mammary gland.

A second common insertion site, designated *INT6*, for MMTV has been detected in a CZECH HOG and two independent CZECH mammary tumours [54]. The *INT6* gene is expressed in all adult tissues that have been tested, including the mammary gland, and as early as day 8 of embryonic development. The *INT6* gene encodes a 55 kDa protein with three potential translation start sites (at 27 bp, 174 bp and 189 bp of the mouse sequence). Each of these polypeptides can be detected in the products of *in vitro* translation of *INT6* RNA in the rabbit reticulocyte system. INT6 is a cytoplasmic protein which is unrelated to any of the known gene products in the GenBank database. We have found that purified bacterially expressed INT6 can be phosphorylated by protein kinase C. Cell fractionation studies and immunofluorescence studies have demonstrated that INT6 is primarily localized to the cytoplasm. Moreover, in immunofluorescence studies of mouse embryos, INT6 was localized to the Golgi apparatus.

As with *NOTCH4/INT3*, the MMTV proviral genome integrates within *INT6*. However, in each of these cases the virus integrates within an intron of the *INT6* gene in the opposite transcriptional orientation. This results in the expression of a truncated chimaeric *INT6* transcript from the rearranged allele. The chimaeric transcript is composed of *INT6* exon and intron, and MMTV LTR sequences. *INT6* transcription terminates at a cryptic termination signal within the MMTV LTR in the minus-strand orientation. In the *INT6*-positive HOG and tumours, the unaffected allele was determined by nucleotide sequence analysis to be normal. This suggests either that the truncated gene product of the rearranged allele is biologically activated or that MMTV induces a dominant-negative mutation of *INT6*. The fact that MMTV rearrangement of *INT6* was initially detected in a CZECH II HOG is consistent with it being an early event in mammary tumorigenesis, and suggests that examination of tumours derived from this HOG will lead to the identification of an MMTV-induced mutation which complements *INT6* in mammary tumour progression.

The *INT6* gene has been highly conserved throughout evolution [54]. The amino acid sequences of the mouse and human *INT6* gene products are identical (S. Miyazaki, A. Imatani, L. Ballard, A. Marchetti, F. Buttitta, H. Alberton, H. Nevanlinna, D. Gallahan and R. Callahan, unpublished work), and related sequences have been detected in *Drosophila*, *Candida elegans* and *Saccharomyces cerevisiae*. The human *INT6* gene is located on chromosome 8q22 (S. Miyazaki, A. Imatani, L. Ballard, A. Marchetti, F. Buttitta, H. Alberton, H. Nevanlinna, D. Gallahan and R. Callahan, unpublished work). We have found a polymorphic microsatellite sequence in the seventh intron and have used it to survey primary human breast tumour DNAs for evidence of LOH. LOH was found in 11 out of 40 (25%) tumour DNAs from informative (heterozygous) patients. We are currently determining whether the remaining *INT6* allele is altered by somatic mutations in these primary human breast carcinoma DNAs. In a separate panel of tumours, composed of 36 malignant breast tumours and two preneoplastic lesions (high-grade dysplasia), there were 14 cases (37%) where *INT6* RNA expression, as determined by Northern blot analysis, was significantly reduced or not detectable (A. Marchetti, F. Buttitta and R. Callahan, unpublished work). Of these 14 cases, eight were invasive ductal carcinomas (IDCs), two were comedocarcinomas (IDCs with a prevalent intraductal component), two were lobular and two were preneoplastic lesions.

Similarly, in 14 of 47 non-small cell lung carcinomas there was loss of *INT6* RNA expression (A. Marchetti, F. Buttitta and R. Callahan, unpublished work). Loss of *INT6* RNA expression has a highly significant association ($P = 0.003$) with the non-small cell lung carcinoma histological subtype of lung carcinomas. These results are consistent with the conclusion that loss of *INT6* expression is an early event in human breast cancer and may be a contributing factor in other neoplasias.

Implications for human breast cancer research

One of the major problems in identifying and addressing the impact of somatic mutations on the evolution of breast carcinogenesis is a fundamental lack of information on the identity of the signalling pathways that regulate the growth and development of the mammary gland. It seems likely that the target cells that are susceptible to carcinogenic mutations are those that have been incompletely committed to a particular fate of differentiation, i.e. stem cells [55–58]. However, again the number of molecular tags that identify these cells is limited. The MMTV/mouse model system has provided a productive and experimentally amenable approach, relative to other strategies, to identifying genes and signalling pathways which, when altered by mutation, contribute to the deregulation of normal mammary gland development, leading to mammary tumorigenesis. It seems likely that further analysis of MMTV-induced HOGs, HOG-derived tumours and subsequent distant metastases will lead to the identification of additional MMTV-induced genetic alterations which, taken together, define pathways of mutations that drive malignant progression to its end-point, metastasis.

The mouse model system does, however, have some potentially important limitations, relative to human breast cancer, which should be recognized. For instance, there are endocrinological, hormonal and obvious lifestyle differences between the two biological systems. In addition, within the scientific community there has also been another perceived limitation, namely that the histopathological descriptions of mouse mammary tumours do not correspond to the most frequent forms of human breast tumours, i.e. IDCs. However, in this regard it seems relevant that Wellings [59] found that many of the human mammary lesions observed are localized to the terminal ductal lobular unit. Of these, atypical lobular type A lesions are morphologically similar to the mouse mammary HAN lesions. At the present time the question of whether the genetics of mouse mammary tumorigenesis are directly relevant to human breast cancer remains largely unanswered. *Wnt-1* and *Wnt-3* appear not be frequently rearranged or amplified in IDCs of the breast, but other forms of breast cancer have not been extensively studied [60,61]. Similarly, *FGF3* and *FGF4* are frequently co-amplified in IDCs of the breast; however, whether they are expressed as a consequence is controversial (reviewed in [62]). The human homologues of the other *INT* genes have not, as yet, been tested for genetic alterations in human breast tumours.

In the short term, the MMTV/mouse model system provides an opportunity to identify the genes (or gene families) encoding signalling pathways that are involved in normal mammary gland development. It seems likely that some of these mutations induced by MMTV or the genes involved in the particular signalling pathways will be relevant to human breast cancer. Since the *INT6* type of viral insertion can be functionally similar to LOH, it seems reasonable that the identification of genes affected by this type of virally induced mutation could be prime candidates for mutation in human breast tumours.

References

1. Gompel, G. and van Kerkem, C. (1983) in The Breast, vol. 1, pp. 245–255, Wiley Medical, New York
2. Harris, J.R., Hellman, S., Canellos, G.P. and Fisher, B. (1982) in Cancer of the Breast, pp. 1119–1178, J.B. Lippincott, Philadelphia
3. Lynch, H.T., Albano, W.A., Danes, B.S., et al. (1984) Cancer **53**, 612–622
4. Trent, J.M. (1985) Breast Cancer Res. Treat. **5**, 221–229
5. Kallioniemi, A., Kallioniemi, O.P., Piper, J., et al. (1994) Proc. Natl. Acad. Sci. U.S.A. **91**, 2156–2160
6. Callahan, R. and Salomon, D.S. (1993) Cancer Surv. **18**, 35–56
7. Callahan, R. (1996) Breast Cancer Res. Treat. **39**, 33–34
8. Hollingsworth, R.E. and Lee, W.-H. (1991) J. Natl. Cancer Inst. **83**, 91–96
9. Knudson, A.G. (1989) Br. J. Cancer **59**, 661–666

10. Bieche, I., Champene, M.H., Merlo, G., Larsen, C.J., Callahan, R. and Lidereau, R. (1990) Hum. Genet. **85**, 101–105

11. Merlo, G.R., Siddiqui, J., Cropp, C.S., Liscia, D.S., Lidereau, R., Callahan, R. and Kufe, D.W. (1989) Cancer Res. **49**, 6966–6971

12. Ali, I.U., Meissner, S., Lidereau, R. and Callahan, R. (1989) J. Natl. Cancer Inst. **81**, 1815–1820

13. Devilee, P., van Vliet, M., van Sloun, P. and Kuipers Dijkshoorn, N. (1991) Oncogene **6**, 1705–1711

14. Orphanos, V., McGown, G., Hey, Y., Boyle, J.M. and Santibanez-Koref, M. (1995) Br. J. Cancer **71**, 290–293

15. Bieche, I., Champene, M.H., Matifas, F., Hacene, K., Callahan, R. and Lidereau, R. (1992) Lancet **339**, 139–143

16. Ali, I.U., Lidereau, R., Theillet, C. and Callahan, R. (1987) Science **238**, 185–188

17. Theillet, C., Lidereau, R., Escot, C., et al. (1986) Cancer Res. **46**, 4776–4781

18. Varley, J., Armour, J., Swallow, J.E., et al. (1989) Oncogene **4**, 725–729

19. Devilee, P., Vandenbroek, M., Kuipersdijkshoorn, N., Kolluri, R., Khan, P.M., Pearson, P.L. and Cornelisse, C.J. (1989) Genomics **5**, 554–560

20. Merlo, G., Venesio, T., Bernards, A., et al. (1992) Am. J. Pathol. **140**, 215–223

21. Cropp, C., Lidereau, R., Campbell, G., Champene, M.-H. and Callahan, R. (1990) Proc. Natl. Acad. Sci. U.S.A. **87**, 7737–7741

22. Morrison, B.W. and Leder, P. (1994) Oncogene **9**, 3417–3426

23. Adams, S.M., Helps, N.R., Sharp, M.G.F., et al. (1992) Hum. Mol. Genet. **1**, 91–96

24. Miki, Y., Swensen, J., Shattuckeidens, D., et al. (1994) Science **250**, 66–71

25. Cropp, C.S., Nevanlinna, H.A., Pyrhonen, S., et al. (1994) Cancer Res. **54**, 2548–2551

26. Futreal, P.A., Liu, Q.Y., Shattuckeidens, D., et al. (1994) Science **266**, 120–122

27. Albertsen, H., Plaetke, R., Ballard, L., et al. (1994) Am. J. Hum. Genet. **54**, 516–525

28. Cowin, P. (1994) Proc. Natl. Acad. Sci. U.S.A. **91**, 10759–10761

29. Orita, M., Iwahana, H., Kanazawa, H., Hayashi, K. and Sekiya, T. (1989) Proc. Natl. Acad. Sci. U.S.A. **86**, 2766–2770

30. Myers, R.M., Larin, Z. and Maniatis, T. (1985) Science **230**, 1242–1246

31. Winter, E., Yamamoto, F., Almohuera, C. and Perucho, M. (1985) Proc. Natl. Acad. Sci. U.S.A. **82**, 7575–7579

32. Weiss, R., Teich, N., Varmus, H. and Coffin, J. (1982) in Molecular Biology of Tumor Viruses (Weiss, R., Teich, N., Varmus, H. and Coffin, J., eds.), pp. 16–18, Cold Spring Harbor Laboratory Press, Cold Spring Harbor, NY

33. Marchetti, A., Robbins, J., Campbell, G., Buttitta, F., Squartini, F., Bistocchi, M. and Callahan, R. (1991) J. Virol. **65**, 4550–4554

34. Varmus, H.E. (1982) Cancer Surv. **1**, 309–320

35. Dickson, C., Smith, R., Brookes, S. and Peters, G. (1984) Cell **37**, 529–536

36. Nusse, R. and Varmus, H.E. (1982) Cell **31**, 99–109

37. Peters, G., Brookes, S., Smith, R., Placzek, M. and Dickson, C. (1989) Proc. Natl. Acad. Sci. U.S.A. **86**, 5678–5682

38. MacArthur, C.A., Shankar, D.B. and Shackleford, G.M. (1995) J. Virol. **69**, 2501–2507

39. Roelink, H., Wagenaar, E., Silva, S.L. and Nusse, R. (1990) Proc. Natl. Acad. Sci. U.S.A. **87**, 4519–4523

40. Gallahan, D., Escot, C., Hogg, E. and Callahan, R. (1986) Curr. Top. Microbiol. Immunol. **127**, 354–361

41. Callahan, R., Drohan, W., Gallahan, D., D'Hoostelaere, L. and Potter, M. (1982) Proc. Natl. Acad. Sci. U.S.A. **79**, 4113–4117

42. Escot, C., Hogg, E. and Callahan, R. (1986) J. Virol. **58**, 619–625

43. Gallahan, D., Kozak, C. and Callahan, R. (1987) J. Virol. **61**, 218–220

44. Schwartz, M., Smith, G. and Medina, D. (1992) Int. J. Cancer **51**, 805–811

45. Gallahan, D. and Callahan, R. (1987) J. Virol. **61**, 66–74
46. Siracusa, L.D., Rosner, M.H., Vigano, M.A., Gilbert, D.J., Staudt, L.M., Copeland, N.G. and Jenkins, N.A. (1991) Genomics **10**, 313–326
47. Robbins, J., Blondel, B.J., Gallahan, D. and Callahan, R. (1992) J. Virol. **66**, 2594–2599
48. Lardelli, M., Dahlstrand, J. and Lendahl, U. (1994) Mech. Dev. **46**, 123–136
49. Weinmaster, G., Roberts, V.J. and Lemke, G. (1991) Development, **113**, 199–205
50. Weinmaster, G., Roberts, V.J. and Lemke, G. (1992) Development **116**, 931–941
51. Struhl, G., Fitzgerald, K. and Greenwald, I. (1993) Cell **74**, 331–345
52. Smith, G.H., Gallahan, D., Diella, F., Jhappan, C., Merlino, G. and Callahan, R. (1995) Cell Growth Differ. **6**, 563–577
53. Jhappan, C., Gallahan, D., Stahle, C., Chu, E., Smith, G.H., Merlino, G. and Callahan, R. (1992) Genes Dev. **6**, 345–355
54. Marchetti, A., Buttitta, F., Miyazaki, S., Gallahan, D., Smith, G.H. and Callahan, R. (1995) J. Virol. **69**, 1932–1938
55. Kordon, E.C., McKnight, R.A., Jhappan, C., Hennighausen, L., Merlino, G. and Smith, G.H. (1995) Dev. Biol. **168**, 47–61
56. Medina, D. and Smith, G.H. (1990) Protoplasm **159**, 77–84
57. Smith, G. and Medina, D. (1988) J. Cell Sci. **89**, 173–183
58. Smith, G.H., Gallahan, D., Zwiebel, J.A., Freeman, S.M., Bassin, R.H. and Callahan, R. (1991) J. Virol. **65**, 6365–6370
59. Wellings, S.R. (1980) Pathol. Res. Pract. **166**, 515–535
60. Roelink, H., Wang, J., Black, D.M., Solomon, E. and Nusse, R. (1993) Genomics **17**, 790–792
61. Vande Vijver, M.J., Peterson, J., Mooi, W., et al. (1989) in Molecular Diagnostics of Human Cancer (Furth, M. and Greaves, M., eds.), pp. 385–391, Cold Spring Harbor Laboratoy Press, Cold Spring Harbor, NY
62. Callahan, R., Cropp, C., Merlo, G.R., et al. (1993) Clin. Chim. Acta **217**, 63–73

Biochem. Soc. Symp. **63**, 223–230
Printed in Great Britain

20

Inherited predisposition to breast cancer

B.A.J. Ponder

CRC Human Cancer Genetics Group, Addenbrooke's Hospital, Box 238, Level 3 Lab Block, Hills Rd., Cambridge CB2 2QQ, U.K.

Abstract

Breast and ovarian cancers sometimes occur in families. Linkage studies in these families have led to the mapping and then cloning of two predisposing genes, *BRCA1* and *BRCA2*. Together these genes probably account for rather less than 5% of all breast and ovarian cancers. In the medium term, understanding the function of the proteins encoded by these genes should lead to a better understanding of how the cancers develop, and the design of new approaches to treatment and prevention. Of more immediate concern is the possibility of genetic testing for cancer susceptibility in families. In multiple-case families, where the *BRCA1* or *BRCA2* mutation is likely to be present and there are clear clinical decisions to be taken, genetic testing is not controversial. The costs and benefits of wider testing are much less clear.

Introduction

Breast cancer, like other common cancers, shows a tendency to cluster in families [1]. The mother, sister or daughter of a woman who has breast cancer has an increased risk, which is quite strongly related to the age at diagnosis of the initial case, ranging from about 5-fold for the relatives of a young woman diagnosed aged 39 to 2-fold for one diagnosed aged 70. This familial clustering might, in principle, result from either environmental or inherited factors. There is clear evidence from the existence of multiple-case families, such as those shown in Fig. 1, that strong inherited factors play a role in at least some families, and this has been confirmed by the recent identification of mutations in specific genes in these families [2,3]. It is less clear what the proportion of the total familial risk is accounted for by these genes, and the extent to which commoner but weaker genes and environmental factors may be involved. We also do not know how possible genetic and environmental predisposing influences may interact.

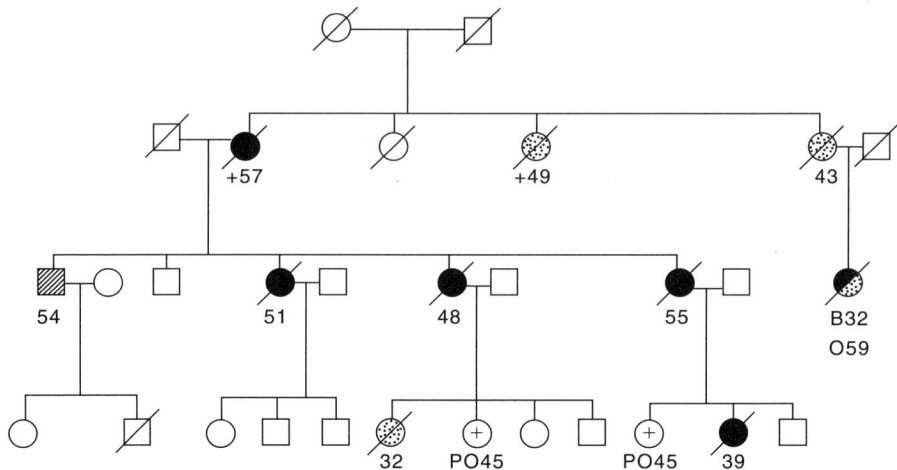

Fig. 1. Family with breast/ovarian cancer syndrome due to mutation in the *BRCA1* gene on chromosome 17q. Key: stippled circles (and semi-circle), breast cancer; solid circles (and semi-circle), ovarian cancer; hatched box, colorectal cancer; PO45, prophylactic oophorectomy at age 45; numbers indicate ages at which cancer was diagnosed or at death (B, breast cancer; O, ovarian cancer).

Highly penetrant predisposing genes

Two genes have been identified by linkage and positional cloning based on families such as those in Fig. 1.

BRCA1

BRCA1 (for <u>Br</u>east <u>C</u>ancer <u>1</u>) was cloned in 1994 [2]. It maps to chromosome 17q21, and encodes a protein of 1863 amino acids. The consistent involvement of the wild-type chromosome in allele losses of 17q21 in familial tumours [4], and the nature of *BRCA1* mutations, which are predicted to inactivate the gene, both suggest that *BRCA1* acts as a tumour suppressor. If *BRCA1* conforms to the retinoblastoma model of a tumour suppressor, one would expect to find somatic mutations of *BRCA1* in sporadic tumours. Curiously, despite the high frequency of allele losses in the *BRCA1* region in sporadic breast cancers, no somatic mutations of *BRCA1* in breast cancer have been found [5]. There are data that suggest reduced levels of *BRCA1* expression in the tumour cells of sporadic breast cancers [6], and so it remains uncertain whether the involvement of *BRCA1* is confined to familial tumours or whether the gene is silenced in sporadic tumours by some mechanism other than coding mutations.

At the time of writing, it is 2 years since *BRCA1* was identified, but there are still few indications as to its function. The predicted BRCA1 protein contains a ring-finger motif at the 5′ end, and a possible 'acidic blob' motif at the 3′ end, which suggested that it might be a transcription factor [2]. Other motifs include putative nuclear localization signals in exon 11, a possible coiled-coil domain in the middle of the molecule, a region of possibly significant identity to the granin family of secreted proteins [7] and a region at the 3' end which appears to have activity as a transcriptional activator [8]. Conservation between human and mouse BRCA1 proteins is not particularly good: the average amino acid identity and similarity are 60% and 70% respectively [9]; but there appear to be several small stretches of consistent identity within the proteins, none of which, however, contain recognizable functional motifs. Apart from the ring finger, the localizations of the known mis-sense mutations do not provide any clues either.

Localization within the cell might provide indications of function, but this has been highly controversial [8,10–12]. Different results have been reported with different antibodies, and with different fixation methods using the same antibody. The main competing hypotheses have been nuclear localization, consistent with a role for BRCA1 as a transcriptional activator or in DNA repair or cell cycle regulation; and cytoplasmic localization, specifically in the trans-Golgi and the cell membrane, and secretion into the extracellular fluid. The latter results, coupled with possible sequence identity, led to the proposal that BRCA1 is a member of the granin family. Members of this family are secreted and proteolytically cleaved outside the cell to release active peptides – a mode of action which, if confirmed, would suggest approaches to restoring BRCA1 function in therapy. At the time of writing, the localization controversy remains unresolved. Evidence is, however, accumulating that suggests a role for BRCA1 in cell-cycle control. Expression (and phosphorylation) of BRCA1 is reported to vary during the cell cycle [13]. Sequence similarities between the predicted BRCA1 protein and a p53 binding protein and the rad-9 protein of yeast, involved in DNA repair, have been proposed [14]. Mice homozygous for a *BRCA1* mutation in exon 5, which would be predicted to abolish protein function, die at around 6 days of gestation, apparently as a result of a failure to complete the burst of cell proliferation necessary at that stage of embryogenesis [15]. Interestingly, however, mice that are homozygous for a mutation in exon 11 (albeit on a different genetic background) survive until embryonic day 11.5 [16]. In addition, one case has been reported of a 32-year-old woman with breast cancer but no evident developmental abnormality who is homozygous for an exon 11 truncating mutation [17].

Roughly 85% of the mutations so far reported in *BRCA1* are predicted to result in a truncated protein; 10% are mis-sense mutations. The mutations are widely scattered across the gene, and a high proportion of mutations have been described only once [18]. This has important implications for genetic testing, as it implies that an extensive search may be needed to detect the mutation in each new family. No mutation hot spots have been identified, but there are founder effects, most notably the 185 del AG mutation which is present in approx. 1% of the Ashkenazi Jewish population [19], and which (together with a similar founder mutation in the *BRCA2* gene) [20] may account for some 15–25% of young-onset breast and ovarian cancer in this population.

An individual who has inherited a *BRCA1* mutation in a multiple-case breast or breast and ovarian cancer family has a high risk of developing one of these cancers. The risk of breast cancer in such families is estimated to be 85% by age 80 [21]; the risk of ovarian cancer appears to vary between families (see below), and has been estimated overall to be about 40%. The risk of male breast cancer is probably not increased, but there may be a somewhat higher risk of cancers of the prostate, colon and rectum. Evidence for effects on the risks of cancer at other sites may emerge as more data become available. The evidence that ovarian cancer risk varies between families came first from a statistical analysis of the occurrence of ovarian cancer in families which showed evidence of linkage to *BRCA1* in studies by the International Breast/Ovarian Cancer Linkage Consortium [21]. Rather than a spectrum of involvement, the data fitted best to a model in which families fell into two groups: a majority with a high risk of breast cancer but only a slightly increased risk of ovarian cancer, and a minority with a high risk of both cancers. Support for this has come from a direct mutational analysis of 28 multiple-case families, which showed a significantly higher ratio of ovarian to breast cancers in families with a truncating mutation 5' to exon 13 of *BRCA1* compared with those where the mutation is 3' to this point [22]. If these observations can be confirmed, they imply either a difference between breast and ovarian epithelium in 3' splicing of the gene or that the truncated proteins encoded by the mutant alleles are stable and have residual positive or negative activity.

BRCA2

Soon after *BRCA1* was mapped by linkage, it became clear that a substantial fraction of families were unlinked, and presumably due to predisposition at a different locus. This was mapped to chromosome 13q12, and the gene *BRCA2* was identified by positional cloning [3]. *BRCA2* is larger than *BRCA1*, encoding a predicted protein of 3418 amino acids. Because it has been identified only recently, rather little is known about it. It appears to resemble *BRCA1* in that it has features of a tumour suppressor gene but, as in *BRCA1*, somatic mutations in sporadic cancers are very uncommon. Mutations are scattered throughout the gene and the majority are predicted to result in a truncated protein. Ovarian cancer risk is strongly associated with truncating mutations in exon 11 [23]. Founder mutations have been identified in the Ashkenazi population (6178 del T) [20] and in Iceland (997 del TT) [24]. The predicted protein has no structural features that give a clue to function, except possible granin identity at the 3' end. A series of structural repeats suggesting globular domains is present in exon 11 [25] and is conserved, at least in part, in the mouse homologue, but the function of these is unclear. No subcellular localization data are yet available.

The pattern of cancers in *BRCA2* mutation carriers is similar to that for *BRCA1*, but with intriguing differences. Both *BRCA1* and *BRCA2* mutations confer a high risk of female breast cancer; the risk of ovarian cancer is lower with *BRCA2* mutations, but *BRCA2* is also associated with an increased risk of male breast cancer. The Icelandic founder mutation 997 del TT has been shown to be responsible for 40% of all male breast cancer in Iceland in the past 30 years [24]; generally the lifetime risk of male breast cancer in a *BRCA2* carrier is probably about 5–10% (based on limited data). *BRCA2* mutations probably confer an increased risk of cancers of the prostate and larynx, and possibly of colorectal and pancreatic cancer and uveal melanoma. Extensive data are needed to define such associations, and this listing is only provisional.

Other highly penetrant predisposing genes

Estimates based on the linkage data from the large set of families in the International Breast/Ovarian Cancer Linkage Consortium suggested that, between them, *BRCA1* and *BRCA2* account for almost all large ($\geqslant 4$ affected members) families with young-onset breast cancer and ovarian cancer, and possibly 80% or so of large families with 'site-specific' breast cancer [26]. Data from direct mutation analyses of families are just becoming available, and are subject to some uncertainty about the proportion of mutations that might be missed by the various techniques used for mutation detection; but the impression is that there may be a substantial minority – perhaps 30% – of 'site-specific' breast cancer families that are due to neither *BRCA1* nor *BRCA2*, and are presumably due to at least one other strong predisposing gene '*BRCA3*'. Assembly of families for a *BRCA3* linkage search is in progress.

Large multiple-case families are quite uncommon. The contribution of *BRCA1* and *BRCA2* to families with two or three relatives affected is much less certain. Estimates based on gene frequencies (see below), and on penetrance derived from larger families, suggest that, of breast cancer sibling pairs both aged under 40 at diagnosis, perhaps 30% may be due to *BRCA1* and 20% to *BRCA2*; for pairs both over 50 at diagnosis, these figures may fall to as little as 2% and 1%. Of the remaining sib pairs, a proportion (which becomes larger, the older the age at diagnosis) will be due to chance, but others may be due to a variety of commoner but less highly predisposing genes of which little is so far known (see below). It will be important to define as accurately as possible, by direct mutational analysis on population-based sample sets, the proportions of these smaller families that are due to *BRCA1* or *BRCA2*. This will help to define the extent of the excess familial risk which is unaccounted for, and indicate the likely yield of searches for other predisposing genes.

Contribution of *BRCA1* and *BRCA2* to breast cancer in the population

Estimates from epidemiological and linkage data suggest that about 1 in 800 individuals carries a strong predisposing *BRCA1* mutation. The prevalence of *BRCA2* mutations is probably a little lower. Assuming that these mutations have a similar penetrance in the population as a whole as they do in multiple-case families (which may not be exactly true), this leads to estimates that *BRCA1* and *BRCA2* each account for about 2% of total breast cancer incidence, and about 10% of cases below the age of 35 years. The very small amount of data from mutation testing in unselected cases so far available is consistent with this. This refers to rare, highly predisposing mutations only. It is possible, in principle, that one or more of the common polymorphisms in *BRCA1* or *BRCA2* which affect amino acids could be associated with small increases in individual risk. Because the polymorphisms are common, these could translate into quite large effects at the level of the population. However, there is currently no evidence for this.

Search for common but weaker predisposing genes

Strongly predisposing genes such as *BRCA1* and *BRCA2* commonly give rise to multiple-case families. In such families, the predisposing genes can be sought empirically by genetic linkage. Weaker predisposing genes – for example, conferring a 15% risk of breast cancer by age 60, which is 5 times the population rate – will only occasionally give rise to small family clusters, and hardly ever to large families. Different strategies must, therefore, be used to find such genes.

It is possible to use linkage-based strategies in small families, but the likelihood of heterogeneity between families (some will be due simply to coincidence, others to different genes) means that the 'noise' in the system will be high. Depending on the strength of the gene to be sought and its overall contribution, analysis of, for example, several hundred pairs of siblings may be required.

An alternative is a case-control approach: the 'association study'. Generally, a candidate gene must first be selected. The frequency of a polymorphism in this gene is then compared between matched series of cancer cases and controls. A significant difference implies that a particular allele of the candidate gene – either the allele defined by the polymorphism itself, or another variant in tight linkage disequilibrium with it – is associated with a higher or lower cancer risk. If the polymorphism used is simply a marker for the functionally significant variant in disequilibrium with it, the method requires that the functional variant has arisen only once or a few times in the population to be studied, otherwise the association with a given marker allele will be too weak. This method can be extended to whole populations as a type of genome-wide linkage search with empirical markers, using the population as an extended family, but only if the population is descended from a small group of founder individuals, so that there is likely to be strong association between given genetic markers and a founding genetic variant which predisposes to the disease.

Using these types of approaches, a number of genes have been tentatively identified that may contribute to breast cancer risk. Of these, the best known is the oncogene Ha-*ras* [27]. The repeat number of a variable number tandem repeat adjacent to the gene defines a set of alleles. Alleles with the lowest repeat number are significantly commoner in individuals with breast cancer (and a variety of other cancers) than in controls, with the odds ratio for breast cancer being 2.29. Because the frequency of the high-risk alleles in the population is about 6% (0.06; compared with about 0.0033 for *BRCA1*), the attributable risk – that is, the proportion of all breast cancer accounted for by these alleles – is about 9%, compared with 2% for *BRCA1*. Other candidate genes, variation in which might affect susceptibility to breast cancer, include members of the cytochrome *P*-450 family, genes involved in oestrogen synthesis and metabolism, and DNA repair genes. Data consistent with an important contribution to breast cancer susceptibility of inherited variation in G2 DNA repair capacity have been published by several groups [28], but the precise nature of the genetic variation is still to be identified.

Future prospects

Elucidation of the function of the *BRCA1* and *BRCA2* genes and the effects of disordered function is now a very active area of research. The results are likely to be of considerable biological interest, but their application to the majority of breast cancers remains unclear while the contribution of *BRCA1* and *BRCA2* to sporadic cases is unknown. The identification of the genes means that predictive genetic testing is now possible in breast cancer families. Because of the size of the genes and the scattered mutations, testing is quite laborious, and it carries with it a number of complex psychological and social issues which are still to be fully explored. For these reasons, although commercial pressures for testing may come to the fore, testing will most appropriately be carried out initially under research conditions, and will be confined mostly to the larger families where the prior probability that there is a *BRCA1* or *BRCA2* mutation is high.

In the longer term, identification of common less strongly predisposing genes will open up several possibilities. Defining the interaction of these genes, and of external factors such as oral contraceptive use, with each other and with genes such as *BRCA1* and *BRCA2* will lead to more precise estimates of risk for individuals. Knowledge of the genes will lead to the definition of sizeable minority groups in the population who should be targeted for, or maybe excluded from, screening or prevention. If the mechanisms of predisposition are known and are open to manipulation, this may provide a rational basis for developing new approaches to prevention.

B.A.J.P. is a Gibb Fellow of the Cancer Research Campaign [CRC].

References

1. Ottman, R., Pike, M.C., King, M.-C., Casagrande, J.T. and Henderson, B.E. (1986) Am. J. Epidemiol. **123**, 15–21
2. Miki, Y., Swenson, J., Shattuck-Eidens, D., et al. (1994) Science **266**, 66–71
3. Wooster, R., Bignell, G., Lancaster, J., et al. (1995) Nature (London) **378**, 789–792
4. Smith, S.A., Easton, D.F., Evans, D.G.R. and Ponder, B.A.J. (1992) Nature Genet. **2**, 128–131
5. Weaverfeldhaus, W., Ding, W., Gholami, Z., et al. (1994) Science **266**, 120–122
6. Thompson, M.E., Jensen, R.A., Obermiller, P.S., Page, D.L. and Holt, J.T. (1995) Nature Genet. **9**, 444–450
7. Jensen, R.A., Thompson, M.E., Jetton, T.L., et al. (1996) Nature Genet. **12**, 303–308
8. Chapman, M.S. and Verma, I.M. (1996) Nature (London) **382**, 678–679
9. Abel, K.J., Xu, J.Z., Yin, G.Y., Lyons, R.H., Meisler, M.H. and Weber, B.L. (1995) Hum. Mol. Genet. **4**, 2265–2273
10. Chen, Y.M., Chen, P.L., Riley, D.J., Lee, W.H., Allred, D.C. and Osborne, C.K. (1996) Science **272**, 125–126

11. Jensen, R.A., Thompson, M.E., Jetton, T.L., et al. (1996) Nature Genet. **13**, 269–272
12. Scully, R., Ganesan, S., Brown, M., et al. (1996) Science **272**, 123–125
13. Chen, Y., Farmer, A.A., Chen, C.-F., Jones, D.C., Chen, P.-L. and Lee W.-H. (1996) Cancer Res. **56**, 3168–3172
14. Koonin, E.V., Altschul, S.F. and Bork, P. (1996) Nature Genet. **13**, 266–267
15. Hakem, R., Luis de la Pompa, J., Sirard, C., et al. (1996) Cell **85**, 1009–1023
16. Gowen, L.C., Johnson, B.L., Latour, A.M., Sulik, K.K. and Koller, B.H. (1996) Nature Genet. **12**, 191–194
17. Boyd, M., Harris, F., McFarlane, R., Davidson, H.R. and Black, D.M. (1995) Nature (London) **375**, 541–542
18. Friend, S., Borresen, A.L., Brody, L., et al. (1995) Nature Genet. **11**, 238–239
19. Struewing, J.P., Abeliovich, D., Peretz, T., Avishai, N., Kaback, M.M., Collins, F.S. and Brody, L.C. (1995) Nature Genet. **11**, 198–200
20. Neuhausen, S., Gilewski, T., Norton, L., et al. (1996) Nature Genet. **13**, 126–128
21. Easton, D.F., Ford, D., Bishop, D.T. and the Breast Cancer Linkage Consortium (1995) Am. J. Hum. Genet. **56**, 265–271
22. Gayther, S.A., Mazoyer, S., Warren, W., et al. (1995) Nature Genet. **11**, 428–438
23. Gayther, S.A., Mangion, J., Russell, P., Barfoot, R., Ponder, B.A.J., Stratton, M. and Easton, D. (1997) Nature Genet. **15**, 103–105
24. Thorlacius, S., Olafsdottir, G., Tryggvadottir, L., et al. (1996) Nature Genet. **13**, 117–128
25. Bork, P., Blomberg, N. and Nilges, M. (1996) Nature Genet. **13**, 22–23
26. Ford, D., Easton, D.F. and Peto, J. (1995) Am. J. Hum. Genet. **57**, 1457–1462
27. Krontiris, T.G., Devlin, B., Karp, D.D., Robert, N.J. and Risch, N. (1993) N. Engl. J. Med. **329**, 517–523
28. Scott, D., Spreadborough, A., Levine, E. and Roberts, S.A. (1994) Lancet **344**, 1444

Biochem. Soc. Symp. **63**, 231–243
Printed in Great Britain

21

Breast cancer metastasis-associated genes: role in tumour progression to the metastatic state

Garth L. Nicolson

Institute for Molecular Medicine, 1761 Kaiser Ave., Irvine, CA 92614, U.S.A.

Abstract

Breast cancer patients usually do not die of their primary cancers; they die of metastatic disease. Thus understanding the progression of breast cancer to the metastatic state and the changes that take place in highly malignant breast cells are important goals that could eventually result in new therapeutic approaches to highly progressive breast disease. Changes in the expression of certain genes or alterations in gene structures and encoded products can result in benign tumour cells progressing to the metastatic state. Experimentally, this has been performed by transferring dominantly acting oncogenes into susceptible cells and then testing the malignant properties of these cells in suitable animal models, but such rapid qualitative changes occur *in vivo* only rarely, and the natural progression of mammary cells to the metastatic state is thought to occur through a slow stepwise process that can take several years. Some of the slow stepwise changes in mammary cancer progression can be reversible and need not involve dominantly acting oncogenes or tumour supresor genes, consistent with clinical observations. An important element of the natural progression of mammary tumours to malignancy may be their ability to circumvent microenvironmental controls that regulate growth and cellular diversity, a process that appears to involve mainly quantitative changes in gene expression, resulting in loss of normal cellular regulation. One of the important mechanisms of cellular regulation in epithelial tissues, such as those found in the breast, is mediated by intercellular junctional communication. Alterations in gene expression can result in loss of gap-junctional communication, concomitant with cellular diversification and progression. It is thought that the highly malignant cancer cells that have slowly evolved *in vivo* with only a few qualitative changes in gene structure have undergone extensive cycles of diversification and the accumulation of several quantitative changes in the expression of various genes that encode products related to malignancy. We have identified some of the genes that are related to progression and metastasis in breast cancer. For example, one of these genes, a novel gene called *mta1* (in rodents) or *MTA1* (in humans) appears to be involved in mammary cell motility and growth regulation. Thus highly malignant cellular phenotypes can arise rapidly due to specific qualitative changes in critical controlling genes, or more slowly via less critical qualitative genetic changes coupled with other cellular changes, such as loss of intercellular communication, and changes in gene expression, such as in the *MTA1* gene, resulting in cellular diversification and ultimately tumour progression to the metastatic state.

Introduction

The progression of tumours from benign to malignant and eventually to the metastatic state is one of the most important but least understood aspects of cancer. Tumour progression from one state to another is thought to occur slowly due to the accumulation of rare qualitative genetic changes (Fig. 1) [1], but these genetic changes may initiate other important events that eventually lead to further progression [2]. The progression of breast cells to the malignant phenotype is mainly typified by quantitative changes in gene expression (oncogenes, suppressor genes, differentiation genes and genes associated with growth, invasion, survival and metastasis) and by some qualitative (DNA sequence) alterations, such as gene amplifications, mutations, deletions, translocations and other changes that are usually associated with earlier states of oncogenesis [1–3]. In addition, the host tissue microenvironment is also important in tumour progression, providing tumours with soluble and insoluble mediators that can modulate tumour cell properties and responses to host-cell, extracellular matrix and electrical signals [4–6]. An important aspect of the

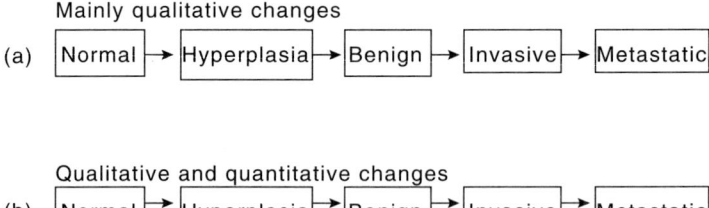

Fig. I. Generalized schemes of tumour progression. In (a), tumour progression is thought to be non-reversible and occurs in a stepwise fashion due to qualitative changes in the DNA coding sequence [15]. In (b), tumour progression is thought to be at least partially reversible and due to qualitative changes in the DNA coding sequence, particularly in the early stages of progression, and to quantitative changes in gene expression, particularly in the later stages of progression or malignancy [9].

tumour microenvironment, especially in epithelial tumours, is the ionic and metabolic co-ordination of cells via junctional communication [5]. Extracellular and cellular signals constitute both positive and negative regulators that usually control the normal aspects of epithelial tissue differentiation, proliferation and death [6,7]. As tumours progress, they are thought to become less responsive to host microenvironments and cellular controls, and they eventually gain autonomy from such regulation [8].

An important general property of malignant tumours is their ability to undergo cellular diversification into heterogeneous phenotypes [9]. Cellular heterogeneity found in malignant tumour cell populations is usually more pronounced than that found in the cells of counterpart benign or normal tissues [2,9,10]. In normal tissues intercellular, cellular and matrix interactions combine to stabilize cellular phenotypes into more narrow states of diversity than is seen in isolated single cells or tumour cells derived from the same tissue. Indeed, once removed from their normal interactions, normal or untransformed cells show increased diversity in their cellular properties [11]. Such diversity may be due to adoptive changes that affect each cell individually and result in individual quantitative differences in gene expression. In malignant cell populations, diversification occurs irrespective of (or at least less dependent of) the host microenvironment, producing heterogeneous cellular phenotypes that are less regulated by normal host cell and other interactions [2,9,11].

As tumour cells diversify in vivo, they also undergo host selection [1]. This can occur because of differences in responses to host mediators or inhibitors, or by active processes such as immune or non-immune host responses [12]. The result of this can be multiple cycles of diversification and subsequent host selection of tumour cells, until dominant malignant cell subpopulations emerge that display highly autonomous phenotypes (Fig. 2) [2,9]. Tumour progression, particularly at the later stages in highly malignant cell populations, probably results in waves of cellular diversification and then restriction of diversity (clonal dominance) [13], until malignant cell subpopulations that have the correct properties to be self-sufficient and highly malignant become dominant (Fig. 2).

Malignant-cell characteristics are not restricted to cancer cells. In normal tissues some highly motile, invasive, normal cells, usually embryonic, are capable of autonomous survival and growth in different tissues (such as neural crest cells and primary gonocytes, among others), and have the capacity for invasion and dissemination as single cells to colonize distant sites [14]. In normal adult tissues, moreover, there is evidence that injury can initiate the events necessary for converting sessile, quiescent cells into motile, invasive cells capable of autonomous cellular division, e.g. during angiogenesis or the development of a new vascular system to feed the injured tissue while it is being repaired [14].

The quantitative changes in gene expression that occur during malignant progression are potentially reversible, and this may explain the inherent instability and potential reversibility of highly malignant states [3,9]. This has been carefully documented in various animal tumours; that is, it has been found that highly metastatic cells can quickly revert to a non-metastatic state and vice versa. However, there are also qualitative (essentially irreversible) changes in

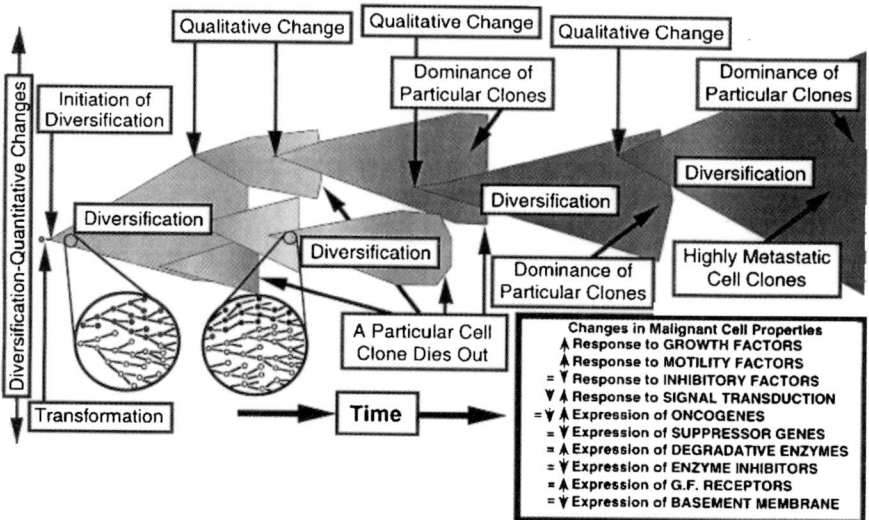

Fig. 2. Example of how qualitative alterations in gene sequence and quantitative changes in gene expression could be related to tumour cell diversification and progression. In this scheme, a single cell is transformed and proliferates, and the progeny undergo diversification due to quantitative changes in gene expression. As the tumour cells diversify, particular cell clones begin to dominate the cell population due to growth advantages and host selection. At some point in time, in one cell clone a qualitative change in a gene occurs that gives this clone an advantage over other clones in the population, and it proliferates and diversifies until clonal dominance again occurs. After several cycles of qualitative genetic changes, proliferation and extensive quantitative changes in gene expression that drive diversification, a tumour cell subpopulation has progressed to a highly malignant state. Abbreviation: G.F., growth factor.

DNA sequences during the progression of cancer cells that may fix certain changes in the genome, preventing reversion [2,15]. Such qualitative events occur rarely and differently among cells in a tumour and among different tumours of the same histological classification [8]. If such qualitative genetic changes are critical to tumour progression and clonal dominance, then it is likely that the most successful cells in a tumour will overgrow the other cells, and eventually almost all of the tumour cells within the tumour should display similar qualitative change(s). The most common examples of such qualitative changes are the genetic changes seen in certain oncogenes and suppressor genes. For example, in colorectal cancers the accumulation of multiple, different qualitative genetic changes in oncogenes and suppressor genes typifies cancer progression [15], but the range of genetic alterations found in each state suggests that other changes (among them quantitative differences in gene expression) may also be important, especially in the most advanced malignant states (metastatic state) [9].

Oncogenes, suppressor genes and tumour progression

Oncogenes encode proteins that function abnormally, inappropriately or at improper concentrations, resulting in the circumvention of the normal cellular controls that regulate cell division and the cell's state of differentiation [2,16]. Although qualitative changes (often gene point mutations) in oncogenes have been found in transformed cells, a more common feature of spontaneously transformed cells is a change in oncogene expression due to chromosome translocations, gene amplifications and other changes. Such single events by themselves are unlikely to be the cause of neoplastic transformation, because further cellular changes are usually necessary [16]. This has been demonstrated in transgenic mice that are homozygous for activated oncogenes and carry the activated oncogene in each and every cell. Although the activated oncogenes are present in every cell, only very few cells are eventually transformed and develop into tumours [17].

Oncogene amplification has been proposed as an important mechanism for driving tumour progression [18]. Although amplification of oncogenes has been seen frequently in various cancers, it is not universal [19]. Oncogene amplification may be symptomatic of other, unrecognized, genetic changes, and the amplification of oncogenes (and other genes) could contribute to progression without being the sole determinant of progression [2,9]. Since the expression of oncogenes can differ between primary tumours and their metastases [19], oncogene expression has also been proposed to be important in the progression of tumour cells to the metastatic state. However, examination of a variety of primary and secondary tumours revealed that oncogenes can be overexpressed, underexpressed or equally expressed in metastases compared with primary tumours [2,19,20]. Thus the qualitative changes seen in oncogenes or the quantitative changes in their expression may contribute to progression, but they are unlikely to be the universal determinants of progression [2,9].

Tumour metastases can show genetic alterations in or overexpression of oncogenes in comparison with the primary tumours from which they were derived, but the data are not convincing in support of a causative role for oncogenes in the progression of tumours to the metastatic state. In examining these data, however, metastases were usually compared with advanced primary tumours that may have already undergone all of the changes necessary to become metastatic [19]. Progression to the metastatic phenotype appears to occur in different tumours by successive cellular changes and evolution via different parallel pathways, only some of which are caused by changes in oncogenes or their expression [2]. Experimentally, the insertion of dominantly acting oncogenes into the genome of a suitable recipient cell can result in acquisition of the metastatic phenotype [20–22]. Unfortunately, such experiments have usually been conducted using aneuploid, unstable, easily spontaneously transformable animal cells as recipients, such as the mouse fibroblast cell lines [20]. In some untransformed cells, conversion into the metastatic state only occurred when two different dominantly acting or activated oncogenes were inserted, an event rarely seen in spontaneous tumours of the same type. These

rapid qualitative changes are unlike the slow, sequential changes that characterize spontaneous transformation and tumour progression to the metastatic state
in vivo [2,15,16].

Some normal cells or even benign tumour cells are highly resistant to
oncogene-mediated conversion into the metastatic phenotype. Within the same
cell type there appears to be heterogeneity in the ability of dominantly acting
activated oncogenes to cause metastatic conversion of individual cells [23,24].
Moreover, in some systems the gene transfer techniques themselves may be as
important as the transferred gene in causing metastatic conversion. For example, the calcium phosphate transfection procedure can modify the tumorigenic
and metastatic properties of benign cells and alter the expression of certain
genes [24,25]. Often multiple gene copies are transferred, and the effects of
their accompanying strong promoter/enhancer elements are not considered. It
is usually assumed that oncogene constructs are incorporated randomly into
the genome, but just the opposite appears to be the case. In addition, consistent
non-random cytogenetic changes may occur concomitant with gene transfer
[26]. Thus it is difficult to conclude from experimental studies that the insertion
of an oncogene is the only event required for conversion into the metastatic
state. Additional changes are probably necessary, and these are likely to include
quantitative changes in gene expression that are reversible in Nature and
unlikely to be the same in every cell. When Gingras et al. [27] examined the
expression of certain proteases and extracellular matrix components in onco-
gene-transfected human fibroblasts, they found that these gene products were
expressed at variable concentrations in different transfected cell subpopulations
but were, in general, expressed in relation to the metastatic properties of the
cells.

Oncogene-mediated conversion of a cell into the metastatic state may be
dependent on the resulting concentration of an oncogene-encoded product.
Support for this has been obtained mostly in fibroblastic cell systems
[20,22,28]. However, others have concluded from their experimental results
that there is no obvious correlation between the level of expression of an oncogene-encoded product and metastatic conversion [24,29]. Thus, in addition to
oncogene insertion and expression, other changes are probably necessary.
Some of these changes may involve other oncogenes, suppressor genes, chromosomal structural alterations and, eventually, cellular diversification [2,9].

In addition to the effects of oncogenes on malignant progression and
diversification, suppressor genes can affect progression and malignancy and
may provide a balance to oncogenes [30]. Cell fusion experiments originally
predicted the existence of metastasis suppressor genes [31,32]. By examining
differences in gene expression in non-metastatic and metastatic cells, several
candidate metastasis suppressor genes have been identified [33,34]. For example, Steeg et al. [35] identified the *nm23* candidate metastasis suppressor gene,
low expression of which was associated with lymph node metastasis of breast
cancers [36]. The predicted Nm23 protein sequence was subsequently found to
be essentially identical to that of the protein encoded by the *Drosophila* developmental gene *awd* [37], which has a high degree of identity with nucleotide
diphosphate kinase [38], suggesting a role for the *nm23* gene product in micro-

tubule assembly/disassembly or in signal transduction and regulation of G-proteins. Thus altered *nm23* structure or expression could result in aberrant signal transduction, gene expression and possibly progression. Other metastasis suppressor genes are those that encode natural protease inhibitors that block invasion or substances that inhibit tumour cell motility. Examples are the tissue inhibitors of metalloproteinases (TIMPs) and plasminogen activator inhibitors. Transfection of antisense TIMP inhibits TIMP-1 expression and enhances the malignant properties of mouse 3T3 cells, and administration of recombinant TIMP-1 inhibits the invasion and lung colonization of mouse melanoma cells [39].

The *MTA1* gene and breast cancer progression to malignancy

The precise roles of most of the products of differentially expressed genes in maintenance of the malignant state are not yet known. Differentially expressed gene products may enhance a malignant cell's metastatic properties by increasing the amounts of degradative enzymes or decreasing the amounts of their inhibitors; by increasing cell adhesion components; by increasing growth factor receptors or modifying their signals; by increasing cell survival and inhibiting apoptosis; or by altering cell–cell communication components, cell motility components or components that allow a malignant cell to escape host surveillance mechanisms. An example of the last possibility was obtained from the examination of differentially expressed genes in mouse lymphoma cell variants, which revealed overexpression of the mitochondrial gene *ND5* [40]. This gene encodes the NADH dehydrogenase in complex I of the electron transport chain, and its overexpression may allow highly metastatic cells to escape macrophage-released cytostatic factors that act at the level of mitochondrial complex I and inhibit cell respiration [40]. Many of the differentially expressed gene products associated with mammary tumour metastasis or non-metastasis, however, have unknown functions. For example, highly metastatic mouse cells appear to overexpress the *mts1* gene, which has high sequence identity with calcium-binding proteins but is of unknown function [41]. This gene has been found to be identical with the *S100A4* gene that encodes a S-100-related, calcium binding, cytoskeleton binding protein. Transfection of the *S100A4* gene into benign mammary cells resulted in these cell acquiring the metastatic phenotype [42].

We have identified another overexpressed novel gene, *mta1*, that is associated with mammary tumour metastasis. This gene appears to function in signal transduction, but its exact role in maintenance of the malignant phenotype is unknown [43,44]. We have now identified and cloned the human *MTA1* gene, also a novel gene that appears to be involved in human breast epithelial cell motility and growth regulation. We set out to investigate the role of the *MTA1* gene by blocking its expression. This was done by making an antisense oligonucleotide to the precise sequence at the transcription start site in the gene. The antisense oligonucleotide, but not a sense oligonucleotide, blocked expression of the gene and inhibited human breast cancer cell motility and pro-

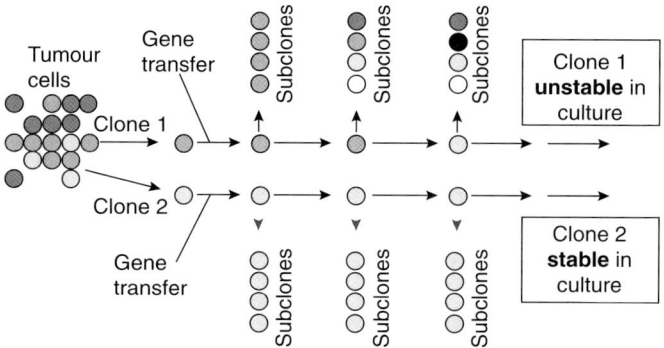

Fig. 3. Schematic representation of an experiment to determine cellular stability and phenotypic diversification. In the upper pathway, a cell population is transfected with a specific gene, the population is cloned and at various times subclones are obtained and tested for malignant and other properties. In the lower pathway, the cell population is transfected with a control gene used in the transfection for antibiotic resistance. The cells transfected with the control gene are subcloned at various times and also examined for malignant and other properties.

liferation. Thus this gene may function in allowing the highly malignant breast cancer cells to move and grow in unusual sites, such as the bone and brain, which are common sites for breast cancer metastasis.

Junctional communication, tumour cell diversification and metastasis

It appears likely that highly malignant cells exhibit rapid rates of phenotypic change due to quantitative differences in gene expression, resulting in a range of different immunological, biochemical, enzymological, structural and other cellular phenotypes [2,9]. That cellular diversification and heterogeneity can be stimulated by oncogene transfer has been demonstrated by transfecting relatively stable benign cell clones with dominantly acting oncogenes, or in some cases with a control gene construct, and observing the diversification of subclones derived from single transfected cells (Fig. 3) [24,45]. For example, we found that stable, benign mammary epithelial cell clones that acquired an oncogene construct diversified rapidly, concomitant with the cells acquiring the metastatic phenotype (Fig. 4a). In addition to increased diversity in metastatic properties, the transfected cells also showed increased diversity in the expression of a metastasis-associated cell-surface mucin-like glycoprotein that may be involved in cell adhesion [45]. In contrast, most of the cell clones that received the control gene construct were relatively more stable, and their subclones were for the most part non-metastatic (Fig. 4b). These results suggest that rapid cellular diversification is an important property of highly malignant cells. *In vivo* a qualitative event, such as sequence alteration of a dominantly acting oncogene, would be expected to occur at a low rate, but the results do demonstrate possible relationships between qualitative gene changes, cellular

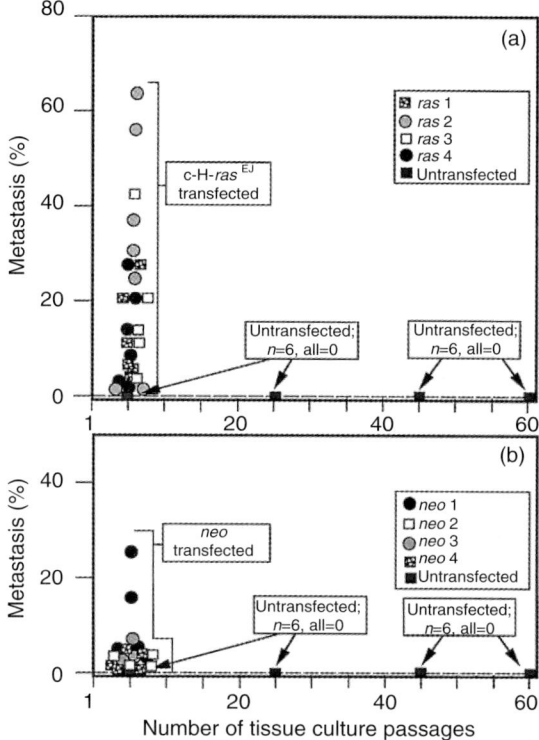

Fig. 4. Initiation of phenotypic diversification in the metastatic properties of a cell clone by transfection of an oncogene (c-H-ras^{EJ}) or control neo constructs. The recipient is a stable, benign rat mammary cell (MTC.4). This cell clone shows no tendency to diversify and progress to the malignant phenotype within 60 tissue culture passages, as shown by the metastatic properties of at least six independent subclones derived at passages 5, 25, 45 and 60. After transfection, however, individual transfected cells (shown by different symbols) undergo rapid diversification into subclones with diverse phenotypes within five tissue culture passages, the minimum time in culture required to expand the cells for examination. In this system the c-H-ras^{EJ}-transfected MTC.4 cells (a) diversify at a more rapid rate than the control neo-transfected cells (b). Diversification was measured by injection of untransfected or transfected subclones into the mammary fat pads of syngeneic F344 rats (nine animals for each subclone), and spontaneous metastases were determined after 45 days. The data are the means from nine animals for each subclone (data from Nicolson et al. [45]).

phenotypic diversification and malignancy, and this suggests that stimulation of cellular diversification could be an important step in tumour progression.

There are several potential ways in which environmental signals could regulate cellular diversity. An important example is the dynamic regulation of electrical, ionic and metabolic coupling between epithelial cells mediated by gap junctions (Fig. 5) [5,7]. This form of cellular communication plays an important role in cell proliferation and differentiation, physiological responses

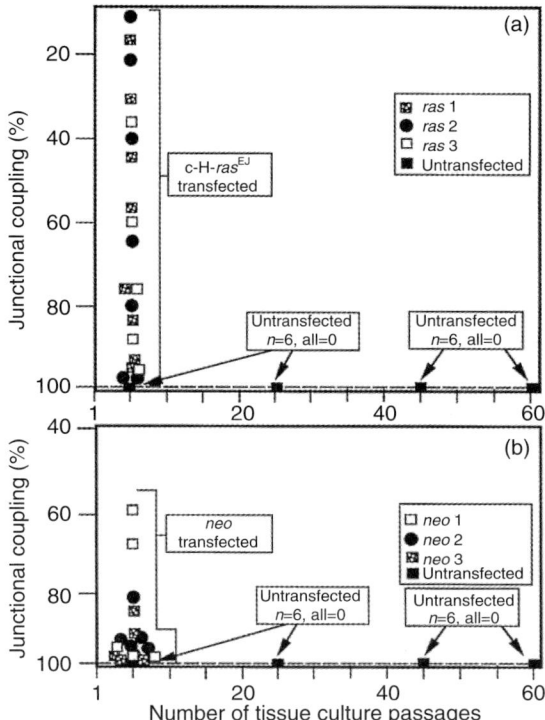

**Fig. 5. Initiation of phenotypic diversification in gap-junctional com-
munication of a cell clone by transfection of c-H-ras^{EJ} or control neo
constructs.** The recipient cells were as in Fig. 4. Junctional communication
was determined by the scrape-loading dye transfer technique. After transfection, individual transfected cells (shown by different symbols) undergo rapid
diversification into subclones with diverse phenotypes within five tissue culture
passages, the minimum time in culture required to expand the cells for examination. In this system the c-H-ras^{EJ}-transfected MTC.4 cells (a) diversify in their
junctional communication properties at a more rapid rate than the control neo-
transfected cells (b) (data from Nicolson et al. [24]).

and carcinogenesis [5,7,46]. Overexpression of oncogenes can disrupt gap-
junctional communication [5,47], and overexpression of tumour suppressor
genes is associated with an increase in gap-junctional communication [5,48].
When we examined the ability of a dominantly acting oncogene to cause diversification in the junctional communication properties of transfected benign
mammary cells, we found that, similar to their metastatic properties, their gap-
junctional communication was inhibited and more diverse among subclones
that were obtained from single-cell clones at various times during subculture
(Fig. 5a). As noted above, most of the cell clones that received the control gene
construct remained relatively more stable and their subclones were for the most
part junctionally coupled and non-metastatic; however, we found more diversity in the control subclones in terms of their junctional communication than in
their metastatic properties (compare Fig. 5b with Fig. 4b), perhaps because the

metastatic state is determined by quantitative levels of several gene products, and many of these would have to be quantitatively altered in expression to induce the metastatic state.

Conclusions on tumour progression and diversification

The cellular and extracellular mechanisms that control tumour as well as normal cellular stability and diversity have not been the subject of many studies, and thus it is difficult to ascribe precise molecular mechanisms for this process. Volpe [3] has proposed that genes exist that control cellular stability, and these may be altered during tumour progression, resulting in extensive tumour cell diversity, evolution and acquisition of malignant and metastatic states. These 'stability genes' could be those involved in karyokinesis and the repair, recombination and replication of DNA. Epigenetic factors, such as those that control tissue and stromal organization, could also control cellular diversity [2,11]. Transformation of cells (or even removal of cells from their usual microenvironments), as proposed by Rubin [11], could also result in the loss of 'hierarchical (tissue-specific) control'. In this elaboration of 'progressive state selection', cells are in a constant dynamic flux due to changes in their microenvironments.

Normal tissues, as well as tumours, experience cellular variations in the concentrations of nutrients, oxygen, growth and differentiation factors and inhibitors, hormones, enzymes, ions and other regulatory factors. Normal cells may be more stable than tumour cells in the face of changes in such components in their microenvironment. However, under certain microenvironmental conditions even malignant cells can be made to undergo 'stabilization' to essentially normal cell states. For example, on inserting certain teratocarcinoma cells into normal blastocysts, the microenvironment of the blastocysts can regulate and decrease the malignancy of the implanted teratocarcinoma cells. Not all malignant cells, however, develop into normal adult cells upon implantation into the blastocyst microenvironment [49], suggesting that neoplastic cells are heterogeneous in these properties and that some can progress beyond a point where they can be regulated by microenvironmental factors. This may be analogous to the changes in growth properties seen during tumour progression. As malignant cells progress, they can reach states where they are no longer regulated by paracrine growth factors and inhibitors, and thus can grow in a variety of microenvironments that would usually not be permissive for growth [50].

The generation of tumour cell diversity is unlikely to be an event that is associated solely with transformation or malignancy. Normal cells also undergo diversification during development, and even in adult organisms some cellular diversification systems remain active [7]. For example, in mammals the diversification of lymphocytes in response to specific antigens results in a highly heterogeneous population of mature B lymphocytes. In this case hypermutable and stable regions of the immunoglobulin gene families are rearranged rapidly into new genes that encode unique immunoglobulin molecules [51]. Many, if not all, of the gene products important in malignancy and metastasis are probably normal gene products that may be inappropriately expressed in malignant cells, and although the identities of these genes and their encoded products are for the most part unknown, it is likely that they will be found to play an important role in normal homoeostasis or differentiation as well as in malignancy [2,37].

References

1. Nowell, P.C. (1976) Science **194**, 23–28
2. Nicolson, G.L. (1987) Cancer Res. **47**, 1473–1487
3. Volpe, J.P.G. (1988) Cancer Genet. Cytogenet. **34**, 125–134
4. Miller, F.R. and Heppner, G.H. (1990) Cancer Metastasis Rev. **9**, 21–34
5. Trosko, J.E., Madhukar, B.V. and Chang, C.C. (1993) Life Sci. **53**, 1–19
6. Christ, G.J., Brink, P.R. and Ramanan, S.V. (1994) Biophys. J. **67**, 1335–1344
7. Iverson, O.H. (1965) in Progress in Biocybernetics (Wiener, N. and Schade, J.P., eds.), pp. 76–110, Elsevier, Amersterdam
8. Foulds, L. (1975) Neoplastic Development, Academic Press, New York
9. Nicolson, G.L. (1991) Bioessays **13**, 337–342
10. Heppner, G.H. (1984) Cancer Res. **44**, 2259–2265
11. Rubin, H. (1990) Cancer Metastasis Rev. **9**, 1–20
12. Frost, P. and Chernajovsky, Y. (1990) Cancer Metastasis Rev. **9**, 93–98
13. Kerbel, R.A., Waghorne, C. and Korczak, B. (1988) Cancer Surv. **7**, 597–629
14. Armstrong, P.B. (1984) in Invasion: Experimental and Clinical Implications, pp. 126–167, Oxford University Press, Oxford
15. Fearon, E.R. and Vogelstein, B. (1990) Cell **61**, 759–767
16. Klein, G. and Klein, E. (1986) Cancer Res. **46**, 3211–3224
17. Hanahan, D. (1989) Science **246**, 1265–1275
18. Gitelman, I,. Dexter, D.F. and Roder, J.C. (1987) Cancer Res. **47**, 3851–3855
19. Yokota, J., Tsunetsugu-Yokota, Y., Battifora, H. and Cline, M.J. (1986) Science **231**, 261–265
20. Chambers, A.F. and Tuck, A.B. (1988) Anticancer Res. **8**, 861–872
21. Muschel, R. and Liotta, L.A. (1988) Carcinogenesis **9**, 705–710
22. Greenberg, A.H., Egan, S.E. and Wright, J.A. (1989) Invasion Metastasis **9**, 360–378
23. Tuck, A.B., Wilson, S.M. and Chambers, A.F. (1990) Clin. Exp. Metastasis **8**, 417–431
24. Nicolson, G.L., Gallick, G.E., Dulski, K.M., Spohn, W.H., Lembo, T. and Tainsky, M.A. (1990) Oncogene **5**, 747–753
25. Kerbel, R.S,. Waghorne, C. and Man, M.S. (1987) Proc. Natl. Acad. Sci. U.S.A. **84**, 1263–1267
26. Muschel, R.J. and McKenna, W.G. (1989) Anticancer Res. **9**, 1395–1406
27. Gingras, M.C., Jarolim, L. and Finch, J. (1990) Cancer Res. **50**, 4061–4066
28. Egan, S.E., McClarty, G.A. and Wright, J.A. (1987) Mol. Cell. Biol. **7**, 830–837
29. Kyprianou, N. and Isaacs, J.T. (1990) Cancer Res. **50**, 1449–1454
30. Liotta, L.A., Steeg, P.S. and Stetler-Stevenson, W.G. (1991) Cell **64**, 327–336
31. Sidebottom, E. and Clark, S.R. (1983) Br. J. Cancer **47**, 399–406
32. Ramshaw, I.A., Carlsen, S. and Wang, H.C. (1983) Int. J. Cancer **32**, 471–478
33. Sobel, M.E. (1990) J. Natl. Cancer Inst. **82**, 267–275
34. Dear, T.N., McDonald, D.A. and Kefford, R.F. (1989) Cancer Res. **49**, 5323–5328
35. Steeg, P.S., Bevilacqua, G., Kopper, L., et al. (1988) J. Natl. Cancer Inst. **80**, 200–204
36. Bevilacqua, G., Sobel, M.E., Liotta, L.A. and Steeg, P.A. (1989) Cancer Res. **49**, 5185–5190
37. Rosengard, A.M., Krutzsch, H.C., Shearn, A., et al. (1989) Nature (London) **342**, 177–180
38. Kimura, N., Shimada, N., Nomura, K. and Watanabe, K. (1990) J. Biol. Chem. **265**, 15744–15749

39. Khokha, R., Waterhouse, P., Yagel, S., and Denhardt, D. (1989) Science **243**, 947–950

40. LaBiche, R.A., Mitsuzi, Y., Gallick, G.E. and Nicolson, G.L. (1988) J. Cell. Biochem. **36**, 393–403

41. Ebralidze, A.K., Tulchinsky E.M., Grigorian, M.S., Afanasyeva, A., Senin, V., Revazova, E. and Lukanidin, E. (1989) Genes Dev. **3**, 1086–1093

42. Davies, B.R., Davies, M.P.A., Gibbs, F.E.M., Barraclough, R. and Rudland, P.S. (1993) Oncogene **8**, 999–1008

43. Toh, Y., Pencil, S.D. and Nicolson, G.L. (1994) J. Biol. Chem. **269**, 22958–22963

44. Toh, Y., Pencil, S.D. and Nicolson, G.L. (1994) Gene **159**, 99–104

45. Nicolson, G.L., Gallick, G.E., Spohn, W.H., Lembo, T. and Tainsky, M.A. (1992) Oncogene **7**, 1127–1135

46. Lowenstein, W.R. (1979) Biochim. Biophys. Acta **560**, 1–65

47. Dotto, G.P., El-Fouly, M.H., Nelson, C., et al. (1989) Oncogene **4**, 637–641

48. Lee, S.W., Tomasetto, C. and Sager, R. (1991) Proc. Natl. Acad. Sci. U.S.A. **88**, 2825–2829

49. Pierce, G.B., Lewis, S.H., Millter, G.J., et al. (1979) Proc. Natl. Acad. Sci. U.S.A. **76**, 6649–6655

50. Nicolson, G.L. (1993) Exp. Cell Res. **204**, 171–180

51. Tonegawa, S. (1983) Nature (London) **302**, 575–581

Biochem. Soc. Symp. **63**, 245–259
Printed in Great Britain

22

Adhesion molecules in breast cancer: role of α2β1 integrin

Deborah Alford*, Paula Pitha-Rowe†
and Joyce Taylor-Papadimitriou*‡

*Laboratory of Epithelial Cell Biology, Imperial Cancer Research Fund, 44 Lincoln's Inn Fields, London WC2A 3PX, U.K., and †Oncology Centre and Department of Molecular Biology and Genetics, The Johns Hopkins University School of Medicine, Baltimore, MD 21231, U.S.A.

Abstract

An early event in the development of breast carcinomas is the loss of normal tissue architecture. In benign lesions and *in situ* tumours both luminal and myoepithelial cells are present, but in most invasive cancers the malignant cell has the phenotype of the luminal cell, and proliferates without contacting the myoepithelial cells or the basement membrane. The reduction in cell contacts is clearly crucial for the initiation of metastatic growth, and is accompanied by a loss of expression or function of cell adhesion molecules. Immunohistochemical studies using tissue and tumour sections indicate that a decrease in the level of expression of the α2β1 integrin is observed in many breast cancers. A specific and crucial role for this molecule in the maintenance of normal morphological differentiation has also been demonstrated in *in vitro* studies. The evidence from these studies suggests that, in mammary epithelial cells, oncogenes may be upstream regulators of the expression of the α2β1 integrin and of other specific molecules important for epithelial differentiation. These findings implicate oncogenes in the initial events relating to the disruption of tissue architecture that is seen in invasive breast cancer.

Introduction

The changes in oncogenes that have been reported to occur in breast cancers are, in general, changes in levels of expression of proto-oncogenes involved in signalling pathways and the cell cycle [e.g. c-*myc*, epidermal growth factor receptor (EGFR), c-*erbB-2*, *bcl-2*, H-*ras*, cyclin D1], and expression may or

‡To whom correspondence should be addressed.

may not be associated with gene amplification; mutations in these genes are seldom seen [1,2]. While mutations in the tumour suppresser gene p53 are relatively common, the tumours that develop in p53 null mice are not mammary tumours, but lymphomas, suggesting that the loss of p53 function may not be a dominant initiating event in the development of mammary carcinomas [3]. Moreover, changes in the *BRCA1* gene associated with familial breast cancer are not found in the sporadic disease [4]. Thus the available data on changes in the genes associated with cell proliferation and the cell cycle suggest that amplification or overexpression is the common change, with mutational changes being less common.

While the search for genetic changes in breast cancer is clearly important, the identification of the changes in phenotype resulting from these changes is also necessary (Table 1). In examining changes in phenotype, emphasis has been placed on effects on parameters related to cell proliferation. In this context it is important to remember that the hallmark of the developing adenocarcinoma cell is not so much that it is proliferating, but that it is doing so without retaining the normal structure of the gland. Indeed, the classification of tumours as benign, *in situ* or invasive still depends on the identification of specific alterations in tissue architecture. This loss of tissue architecture, which occurs in carcinomas, reflects the loss of a differentiated function of the normal epithelial cell, i.e. the ability to form an ordered three-dimensional structure. Fig. 1 illustrates the difference between the ordered growth of normal mammary epithelial cells seen during pregnancy and lactation compared with the loss of glandular structure seen in the proliferation associated with an infiltrating ductal carcinoma (Fig. 1C) and a metastasis developing from it (Fig. 1D). An important question then to ask is: what are the features of the cancer cell that allow it to negate or ignore the signals that result in morphologically ordered growth, and what are these signals to which the normal cell responds? To answer this question, an analysis of the normal process of morphogenesis and the identification of molecules that play a crucial role in this process are

Table 1. Development of carcinomas.

Changes	Loss or gain of function
Genetic changes	Loss: mutation or deletion
	Gain: mutation or amplification;
	change in a gene affecting expression of a normal gene
Phenotypic changes	Signalling pathways
	Cell-cycle-related components
	Apoptosis-related factors
	Specific parameters related to cell phenotype
	(differentiation)
Malignancy	Loss of normal tissue architecture
	Subsequent invasion
	Proliferation out of context

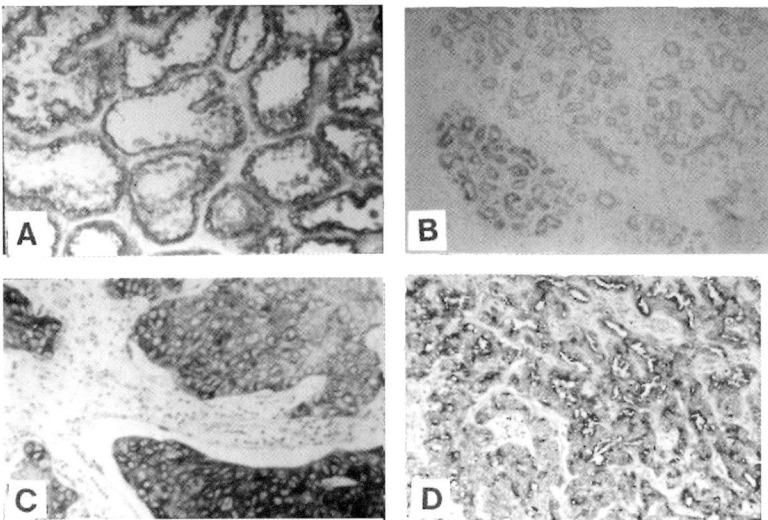

Fig. 1. Loss of tissue architecture in breast cancer. Histological sections are shown of (A) lactating breast, (B) resting breast, (C) a primary infiltrating ductal carcinoma and (D) a breast cancer metastasis to a lymph node. The sections were stained with an antibody to an epithelial mucin which shows apical localization in the normal gland. In the cancers epithelial polarity is lost, and staining is all around the cell and can be intracellular. Magnifications: (A) × 100; (B) × 50; (C) × 200; (D) × 100.

required, in order to recognize any relevant changes that occur at the molecular level in breast cancers. It is clear that cell–cell and cell–matrix interactions are pivotal in maintaining tissue architecture, so changes in the levels or functions of the molecules involved in such interactions need to be investigated. These interactions are particularly important in epithelial cells, which are normally strongly attached to each other and to the basement membrane, forming an impermeable barrier at the luminal surface.

In order to analyse the molecular basis for the loss of morphogenetic potential in breast cancer, an *in vitro* experimental system is required. Moreover, if comparisons are to be made between normal and malignant cells, it is crucial to define the phenotype of the malignant cell in terms of the normal cell lineage, and to work with normal cells that show a phenotype corresponding to that of the malignant cell. Since 90% of primary breast cancers show the phenotype of the keratin 19 positive luminal cell [5], we have chosen to analyse the molecular mechanisms underlying normal morphogenesis using this cell type. Luminal cells can be cultured from milk, but have a short life span *in vitro*. A cell line, MTSV1-7, was therefore developed by immortalizing luminal epithelial cells cultured from human milk [6], and this cell line and a subline, HB2, developed from it [7] have been used in some of the studies described here. By analysing morphogenesis in a collagen matrix *in vitro*, we have found the α2β1 integrin and its interaction with the extracellular matrix to be of crucial importance. Since this is the major integrin expressed by the luminal mammary epithelial cell, and since it is frequently lost or expressed at lower levels in breast cancers, it is likely that changes in integrin expression or function relate to the loss of morphogenetic potential of human breast cancer cells.

Phenotype of the breast cancer cell

The cells lining the ducts and alveoli of the normal breast fall into two major categories: the basal or myoepithelial cells, which are firmly attached to the basement membrane by hemidesmosomes and by specific adhesion molecules; and the luminal epithelial cells, which sit on the basal cells, form junctions with them and each other and line the lumen. Although the contact with the basement membrane is less extensive than with the basal cells, projections from the luminal cells extend down to and interact with the basement membrane [8]. The two cell types can be distinguished by the profile of intermediate filaments that they express, with all luminal cells expressing the simple epithelial keratins 7, 8 and 18 and the basal cells expressing keratins 5 and 14 and vimentin [9]. Subgroups can also be identified, and of particular importance is the subgroup of luminal cells that expresses keratin 19 [10], since this profile of keratins is expressed by most primary and metastatic breast cancers [5]. Other molecules that distinguish the two epithelial cell types are growth factor receptors, with EGFRs being more dominantly expressed in the basal cells, and oestrogen receptors, which are expressed by only a fraction of luminal cells and not by basal cells [11,12]. The common leucocyte antigen (CALLA) and basement membrane components are also expressed by the basal cells [13,14] and an epithelial mucin, MUC1, is expressed at the apical surface of luminal cells [15].

From the earliest changes seen in the development of abnormal lesions, it is clear that the luminal cells appear to proliferate and form multilayers instead of the single layer evident in the normal gland. However, in benign lesions, particularly in fibroadenomas, myoepithelial cells and basement membranes are evident. Moreover, it is clear from immunohistochemical studies that, in most breast cancers, the invasive breast cancer cell has a phenotype of the keratin 19+ expressing luminal epithelial cell. This phenotype is shown by the cancer cells in *in situ* tumours, where the malignant cells are contained by a layer of apparently normal myoepithelial cells sitting on a basement membrane, and is also maintained in many metastatic lesions and in cell lines derived from them [5]. Expression of one or more basal markers (EGFR, keratin 14, vimentin) can occur in a small proportion of breast cancers, and their expression is generally associated with a poor prognosis [16].

Although the phenotype of the breast cancer cell suggests that, in most cases, it develops from the luminal lineage, the lack of information on the kinetic relationship between different phenotypes in the normal gland does not allow unequivocal identification of the luminal cell as the initial target cell, which may have been a stem cell retaining the ability to develop into a differentiated luminal cell. However, for comparative studies between normal and malignant cells that might identify changes in phenotype associated with malignancy, the normal luminal epithelial cell must be the cell of choice.

Adhesion molecules in the mammary gland

Cell–cell and cell–matrix interactions play a particularly important role in maintaining the architecture and polarity of epithelial tissues. Of the cell–cell junctions, the tight junctions, desmosomes and adherens junctions are characteristic of epithelial cells and act to maintain polarity, resulting in an impermeable protective cell barrier which is held in place by these junctions and by those made between the cells and the basement membrane. The epithelial junctions are complex, each involving several proteins. Studies in the mammary gland have focused on a component of the adherens junction, E-cadherin, and the intracellular molecules (catenins) that associate with it, and on the integrin family of molecules, which are involved in cell–matrix and cell–cell interactions. While E-cadherin clearly plays a central role in maintaining the polarity of the normal epithelial cells, and the decrease in level or function seen in breast cancers is undoubtedly relevant to malignant progression, here we will focus our discussion on the α2β1 integrin.

Integrins

Integrins are transmembrane glycoproteins that are important in the adhesion of cells to extracellular matrix components, and may also play a role in cell–cell adhesion [17,18]. Integrins are expressed in all cell types examined to date, and consist of α and β heterodimers, of which 15 α subunits and eight β subunits have been identified and cloned. Individual β subunits can heterodimerize with different α subunits and vice versa (although the latter case is less frequent), forming a large number of different integrin family members. Further diversity is achieved by the fact that individual integrins can often bind more than one extracellular matrix ligand, and individual ligands may be recognized by more than one integrin. The ligands that an integrin can bind will also vary between cell types, making it important to consider integrin function within the context of cell phenotype [19].

Three members of the integrin family are found to be abundantly expressed in the resting and lactating mammary gland, namely α2β1, α3β1 and α6β4 [7]. Being a component of hemidesmosomes [20], the α6β4 complex is found to be localized exclusively where the cells contact the basement membrane. In contrast, the α2β1 integrin is found evenly distributed along the basolateral cell surface in both cell layers, as well as in regions of cell–basement-membrane contact. Monoclonal antibodies to the α3β1 integrin show strong staining of the basolateral surface of myoepithelial cells (with stronger staining in the cell–basement-membrane contacts) and weaker staining of the basolateral surfaces of luminal cells [7].

It can be seen from these expression patterns that the integrins are in the correct position to be involved in cell–cell and cell–matrix adhesions in the mammary gland *in vivo*; the disruption of such interactions, due to either a decrease in expression or function, or a change in organized position, could be involved in malignant progression. It is also clear that, although the α2β1 integrin is expressed strongly in both luminal and myoepithelial layers, a higher level of integrin expression tends to be found in the myoepithelial rather than the luminal cells. Since the α2β1 integrin is the major integrin expressed by the luminal epithelial cells, we will focus our discussion on the role of the α2β1 integrin in mammary morphogenesis, and on the molecular mechanisms underlying changes in the expression or function of this integrin in breast cancers.

Changes in integrins in breast cancers

Immunohistochemical studies using tumour sections indicate that, in general, integrin levels are reduced in many breast cancers, and also that integrins are expressed in a more disorganized way. In interpreting the results, however, it is important to remember that the majority of breast cancers are derived from luminal epithelial cells and that, with the exception of α2β1, integrin expression in these cells is normally quite low compared with that in the myoepithelial cells.

Levels of the α2β1 integrin have been found to be reduced in breast carcinomas [21], and several studies show that increased loss of expression correlates with increasing tumour grade [22–24]. However, it is very important to consider the phenotype of cells in the tumour when interpreting these results. Berdichevsky and colleagues [25] subdivided breast tumours for analysis into those with a completely luminal phenotype (group L) and those with basal elements (group B), and found that, while most of the high-grade ductal carcinomas in group L showed a reduced expression of α2β1 integrin, the same category of tumours in group B expressed high levels [25]. These results show that, while reduced α2β1 integrin expression is frequent in undifferentiated tumours with the luminal phenotype, integrin expression can also be regarded as a marker for basal elements in a tumour.

Morphogenesis of mammary epithelial cells *in vitro*

A major advantage of working with cells in culture is that they can be experimentally manipulated in a variety of ways. *In vitro* studies using non-tumorigenic cell lines derived from luminal epithelial cells point to a crucial role for the α2β1 integrin in normal morphogenesis.

For the formation of three-dimensional structures, the presence of an extracellular matrix is essential. While Matrigel may be more physiological, since all the components of the basement membrane are represented, collagen type I provides a single ligand for the integrins, and therefore the integrin–ligand interactions are less complex and more readily analysed. Moreover, when the breast cancer cell invades *in vivo*, it invades a collagen-containing matrix, making this a relevant system. The actual type of structure formed by normal mammary epithelial cells in collagen *in vitro* depends on the profile of intermediate filaments expressed [26,27], and the specific process of branching morphogenesis can be induced by fibroblast-derived factors, including hepatocyte growth factor (HGF) [7]. On the other hand, cells from breast cancers, cultured either in primary culture or as cell lines, cannot form these organized structures [25,28].

Reflecting the situation *in vivo*, the loss of morphogenetic ability *in vitro* appears to be an early event, and cell lines derived from primary cancers that do not exhibit the changes in growth properties generally associated with overt malignancy (anchorage-independent growth or growth in the nude mouse) also exhibit this loss of morphogenetic potential *in vitro* [28]. The *in vitro* system therefore is an appropriate model for analysing the role of adhesion molecules in normal morphogenesis, and for investigating how the changes in levels or function of these molecules that occur in malignancy affect morphogenetic potential.

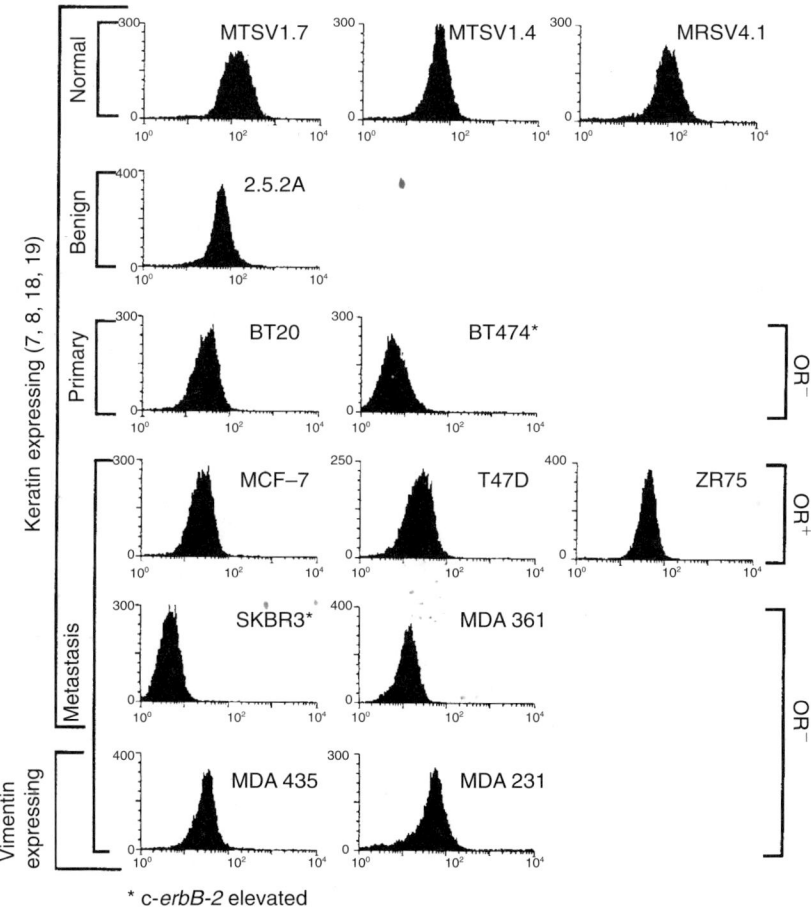

* c-*erbB-2* elevated

Fig. 2. Comparison of expression of the α2 integrin subunit by non-tumorigenic breast cell lines and breast cancer cell lines. Expression of the α2 integrin subunit was determined by FACS analysis using a monoclonal antibody (HAS4) to the α2 integrin subunit. x axis, fluorescent intensity; y axis, number of cells. OR, oestrogen receptor. Reproduced, with permission, from [25].

Importance of the α2β1 integrin in morphogenesis

As indicated above, the α2β1 integrin is the major integrin expressed by luminal epithelial cells. This integrin is well expressed by non-tumorigenic breast cell lines developed from human milk [6,7], while many breast cancer cell lines express a reduced level, suggesting a correlation with the loss of morphogenetic ability (Fig. 2). Like the loss of morphogenetic potential *in vitro*, the decrease in α2β1 integrin expression appears to be an early event, and is seen in cell lines developed from primary breast cancers that are non-tumorigenic in nude mice. However, cell lines expressing vimentin (MDA 435 and MDA 231), like the tumours expressing basal markers *in vivo*, can express high levels of the α2β1 integrin. Notably, this expression does not confer the ability to create organized structures in gels when other epithelial specific molecules such as E-cadherin are missing, emphasizing the importance of cell phenotype in the context of a molecular function.

Direct evidence for a crucial role for the α2β1 integrin in morphogenesis can be obtained by modifying either integrin expression or integrin function. Inhibition of expression of the α2β1 integrin by antisense oligonucleotides has been shown to inhibit morphogenetic potential [29], and increasing expression of the α2β1 integrin by transfection of the α2 integrin cDNA improves the morphogenetic potential of a mouse mammary epithelial cell line [30]. We have used antibodies to the α2 and β1 integrin subunits to examine the effects of modulating α2β1 integrin function on the morphogenesis of a human mammary epithelial cell line, HB2, in collagen gels, paying particular attention to the branching of structures induced by fibroblast-derived factors. These results are discussed below.

Effect on morphogenesis of antibodies regulating function of the α2β1 integrin

The interaction of an antibody with either of the integrin subunits may modify the interaction of the integrin with the extracellular matrix, by increasing or decreasing the strength of the interaction depending on the epitope recognized. Fig. 3 shows diagramatically the domains of the α2 and β1 subunits in which epitopes reactive with antibodies have been located. The antibodies reactive with the α2 integrin that block the interaction with the collagen matrix map to the I domain [31]. Strikingly, antibodies reactive with the β1 integrin that either block or enhance binding to collagen map to the same domain, which lies between two putative ligand binding sites [32].

The importance of the α2β1-integrin–collagen interaction is emphasized by the fact that high concentrations of antibodies that block this interaction inhibit the growth of the non-tumorigenic HB2 cells [7] or MCF-10 cells [33] in collagen gels. Whatever signal(s) is/are generated by the interaction does not, however, seem to be required for the growth of breast cancer cell lines in collagen, which continue to proliferate in the presence of high concentrations of blocking antibodies [33].

Analysis of the effects of lower concentrations of antibodies on the branching morphogenesis of HB2 cells induced by HGF has led to a very interesting observation. In the presence of HGF, antibodies to either the α2 or β1

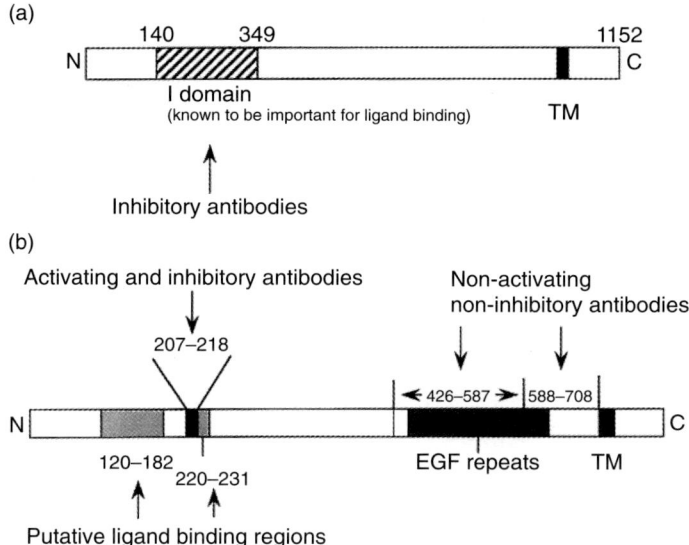

Fig. 3. Diagram of the α2 (a) and β1 (b) integrin subunits illustrating important domains containing antibody-reactive epitopes. TM, trans-membrane domain. Numbers indicate residue numbers within the protein.

subunits that inhibit binding to collagen induce a marked separation of the cells that normally form compact branching structures. This effect on cell–cell inter-actions, illustrated in Fig. 4, is an indirect effect which depends on inhibition of the cell–matrix interaction. This is shown by the fact that the same anti-α2 anti-bodies have no effect on the branching structures formed in fibrin gels (in the presence of HGF), where the matrix interaction is not mediated by the α2β1 integrin. Thus complete impairment of the interaction of the α2β1 integrin with the collagen matrix can lead to apoptosis of normal epithelial cells, while a decrease in the strength of the interaction in the presence of a motility factor such as HGF leads to cell–cell separation, an event that may be important in the initial stages of invasion.

The level of expression and the affinity of the α2β1 integrin for the colla-gen matrix is important not only in allowing the development of three-dimensional structures but also in influencing their form. When HB2 cells are embedded in collagen, the levels of expression of all of the integrins expressed by these cells (α2β1, α3β1, α6β4) are reduced. This response probably reflects the need for motility in generating form. In line with this, we have found that an 'activating' antibody to the β1 integrin (TS2/16), which has been shown to increase the affinity of the integrin for ligand [34], can inhibit branching mor-phogenesis induced by HGF (Fig. 4).

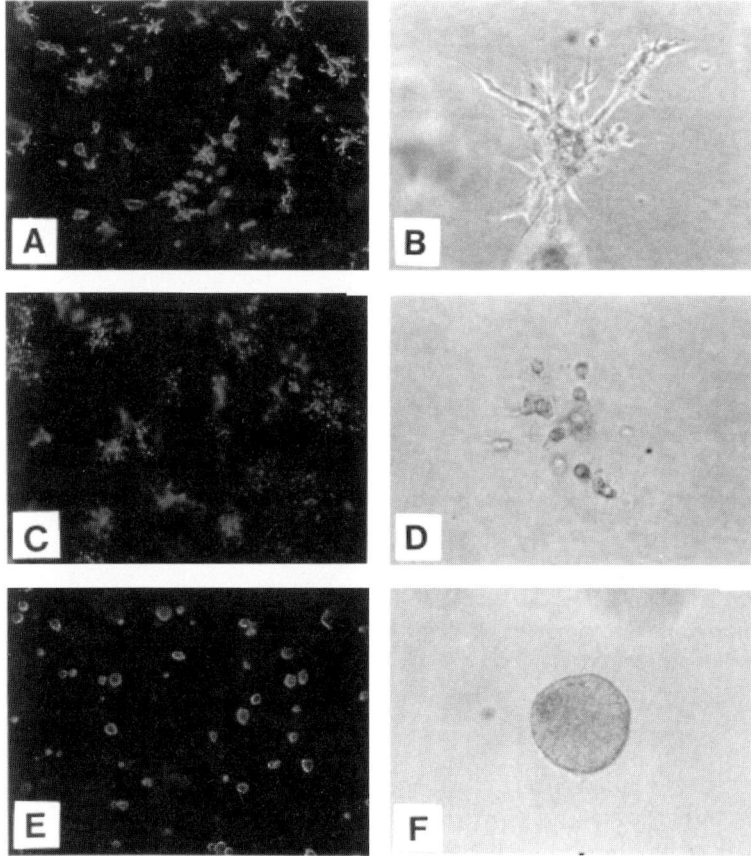

Fig. 4. Effects of antibodies to integrin subunits on the formation of three-dimensional structures in collagen gels. Cells were pretreated with medium (A and B), with antibody P1E6 to the α2 subunit, which blocks the collagen interaction (C and D), or with antibody TS2/16 to the β1 integrin subunit, which increases binding to collagen (E and F). All samples were cultured in collagen gels in medium containing 10 ng/ml HGF. Magnification × 80.

Regulation of expression of adhesion molecules: effects of oncogenes

If changes in the α2β1 integrin are important in the loss of tissue morphology and in the evolution of the breast cancer cell, then it is important to know which factors act to induce the loss of function or down-regulation of expression of this molecule. Oncogenes are obvious candidates, particularly in view of the observation that transformation of epithelial cells with oncogenes *in vitro* often leads to their conversion into an undifferentiated fibroblastic/mesenchymal phenotype. Many of these *in vitro* studies have been carried out using mammary epithelial cells, and it has been shown that expression of c-*erbB-2* [35,36], *bcl-2* [27], activated *ras* oncogenes [37] and c-*fos* [38] can all lead to epithelial–mesenchymal conversion of mammary epithelial cells and loss of adhesive function. However, the level of expression of the α2β1 integrin has only been examined in human mammary epithelial cells (MTSV1-7 or HB2 cells) overexpressing the c-*erbB-2* or *bcl-2* genes. In both cases, a high level of expression of the transfected gene in MTSV1-7 cells was associated with a dramatic decrease in the level of expression of the α2 integrin subunit. In the case of the c-*erbB-2* transfection there was a clear correlation between the level of expression of the proto-oncogene, the decrease in expression of the α2β1 integrin (and of E-cadherin) and morphogenesis [36]. The relationship between the level of expression of the *bcl-2* gene, α2 integrin expression and morphogenesis was more complex. Very high levels of expression of the gene, which reduced dramatically the expression of the α2β1 integrin and epithelial specific markers, did indeed inhibit the formation of compact, organized three-dimensional structures. However, both the detailed phenotype of the target cell (MTSV1-7 or HB2) and the level of expression of the α2β1 subunit influenced the effect on morphogenesis, and in some cases branching occurred in the absence of a stimulatory factor. Branching is in part a reflection of a motility response, but the *bcl-2*-expressing cells did not produce a factor showing such a function. It is, however, possible that, in collagen, selective release of a protease occurred in response to the cell–collagen interaction [27].

Down-regulation of the activity of the α2 integrin promoter by oncogene signalling

Since the decrease in expression of the α2 subunit was seen at the RNA level, changes in the functioning of the α2 promoter [39] may be expected, and have recently been demonstrated [40]. Changes in the transcription of another adhesion molecule, E-cadherin, have been shown to become irreversible after only 24–48 h of expression of the c-*fos* proto-oncogene [38], and both methylation and mutation are implicated in silencing this gene in breast cancers showing reduced expression [41,42]. While such irreversible changes may also be implicated in the reduced expression of the α2 integrin subunit in c-*erbB-2*- or *bcl-2*-expressing mammary epithelial cells, *in vitro* transfection experiments show that the profile of factors affecting transcription from the α2 promoter may be altered by c-*erbB-2*. Thus expression of a reporter gene driven by the α2 promoter in T47D or HB2 cells is dramatically reduced when co-transfected with a plasmid expressing c-*erbB-2* [40]. Signalling from c-*erbB-2* can occur via Grb2/Sos, feeding into the Ras signalling pathway [36,43,44], and also via the Src kinase pathway [45]. Significantly, co-transfection of a *ras*-expressing plasmid into normal or malignant mammary epithelial cells together with the α2 promoter reporter gene construct also resulted in down-regulation of expression of the reporter gene. Moreover, co-transfection of a dominant-negative *ras* mutant abrogated the inhibitory effect of c-*erbB-2* on the transcriptional activity of the α2 integrin promoter [40].

Activated *ras* has also been shown to induce epithelial–mesenchymal conversion by affecting E-cadherin function [37]. In this case the level of expression of the E-cadherin molecule was unchanged, but normal interactions between E-cadherin, β-catenin and the cytoskeleton were disrupted, resulting in loss of E-cadherin function. The modification of the function of integrins has not been well documented. However, the fact that many tumour cells expressing the α2β1 integrin are unable to undergo normal morphogenesis, and apparently do not require integrin-generated signals for survival in collagen gels, suggests that the function of the integrin is altered in these cells.

The available data suggest that several proto-oncogenes or oncogenes, which have different functions and act at different steps in signalling pathways (from surface receptors such as c-erbB-2 to transcription factors such as c-fos), converge by affecting the expression or function of adhesion molecules, just as they converge in stimulating cell growth. The α2β1 integrin is the major integrin expressed at the basolateral surface of the luminal epithelial cells from which breast cancers develop, and undoubtedly this receptor plays a central role in maintaining the integrity of the epithelial layer through attachments to the basement membrane and adjacent cells. It is highly likely that a reduction in the level or function of the integrin (and other adhesion molecules such as E-cadherin) is required for the loosening of cell–matrix and cell–cell contacts that is necessary for cell division and morphogenesis. If so, the down-regulation of expression of the α2 integrin subunit in response to growth factor signalling may represent a normal but reversible event in dividing cells undergoing morphogenesis. In breast cancer, the ras pathway can be constitutively activated [46,47], and the down-regulation of the function or expression of the integrin could become irreversible, possibly involving other mechanisms such as methylation. This in turn would lead or contribute to the disruption of tissue architecture seen in primary breast cancers.

Finally, it is important to note that the α2β1–ligand interaction is crucial for the survival of normal mammary epithelial cells, while breast cancer cells can survive when this interaction is abrogated [7,33]. Clearly, not only can the level of the α2β1 integrin be changed in breast cancers, but the signals generated by the integrin–ligand interaction, which are normally required for survival, either are not generated or are ignored by the breast cancer cell. How oncogenes or proto-oncogenes such as c-erbB-2 might affect integrin signalling is therefore another aspect of malignant progression that needs addressing.

Relevance to the evolution of the breast cancer cell

In this chapter we have focused on trying to understand, at the molecular level, what must be one of the early events in the evolution of the breast cancer cell, namely loss of the ability to grow with the ordered morphology exhibited by normal mammary epithelial cells. This change apparently involves losing some functions, such as the ability to adhere to other cells and to the extracellular matrix, and acquiring others, such as the ability to proliferate or avoid apoptosis when not adherent. Available studies point to a crucial role for the α2β1 integrin in the maintenance of normal tissue architecture and suggest that changes in the level of expression or function of these molecules, which may be regulated by oncogenes, are associated with early events in the development of primary breast cancers.

The process of invasion and metastasis must also involve other changes related to protease activities and to the expression of factors allowing independent growth in a distant site. Moreover, it is probable that, when metastases arise, increases in the amounts of adhesion molecules are seen. These could relate to binding to endothelial cells, or to the matrix, or cells in the final metastatic site. It is therefore relevant to ask whether the changes in expression and/or function of adhesion molecules are reversible and whether their expression will, in fact, be required at a later stage for survival. Certainly many breast cancer cell lines that have been developed from late metastases (pleural effusions) still exhibit an epithelial phenotype with reduced, but not complete loss of, expression of the adhesion molecules discussed here. Possibly some capacity for reforming a group after initial separation may be conducive to colonizing a new environment. It is therefore crucial to put any phenotypic changes in the context of the stage of development of the tumour.

Another point that requires clarification in the context of an epithelial–mesenchymal conversion is not only what triggers the changes in the cell adhesion molecules but also whether expression of one of these molecules can affect expression of the other, or control the epithelial phenotype in a more general way. The use of oncogenes, which down-regulate the expression or function of the α2β1 integrin and the epithelial-specific molecules that appear to be so crucial to epithelial cell polarity, should allow an analysis of the interdependence of the expression of the different genes, and the functions of the proteins, and of the events leading to the down-regulation of function or expression. Human mammary epithelial cell lines showing normal morphogenesis *in vitro* are appropriate recipients for these oncogenes, and if such genes are expressed from an inducible promoter, or can be regulated in some other way, the sequence of events leading to the loss of morphogenetic potential (and their reversibility) can be analysed. The changes in expression of the α2β1 integrin occur early in the development of breast cancers. An understanding of the mechanisms involved not only will contribute to our understanding of the factors involved in the regulation of their expression and function but also could lead to the development of strategies for intervention at an early stage of malignant progression.

References

1. Callahan, R. and Salomon, D.S. (1993) Cancer Surv. **18**, 35–56
2. Fantl, V., Smith, R., Brookes, S., Dickson, C. and Peters, G. (1993) Cancer Surv. **18**, 77–94
3. Eeles, R.A., Bartkova, J., Lane, D.P. and Bartek, J. (1993) Cancer Surv. **18**, 57–75
4. Miki, Y., Swensen, J. and Shattuck-Eidens, D. (1994) Science **266**, 66–71
5. Bartek, J., Taylor-Papadimitriou, J., Miller, N. and Millis, R. (1985) Int. J. Cancer **36**, 299–306
6. Bartek, J., Bartkova, J., Kyprianou, N., et al. (1991) Proc. Natl. Acad. Sci. U.S.A. **88**, 3520–3524
7. Berdichevsky, F., Alford, D., D'Souza, B. and Taylor-Papadimitriou, J. (1994) J. Cell Sci. **107**, 3557–3568
8. Taylor-Papadimitriou, J. and Lane, E.B. (1987) in The Mammary Gland (Neville, M.C. and Daniel, C.W., eds.), pp. 181–215, Plenum, New York

9.   Taylor-Papadimitriou, J., Wetzels, R. and Ramaekers, F. (1991) in Genes, Oncogenes and
       Hormones: Advances in Cellular and Molecular Biology of Breast Cancer (Dickson, R.B.
       and Lippman, M.E., eds.), pp. 355–378, Kluwer Academic Publishers, Boston

10.   Bartek, J., Durban, E.M., Hallowes, R.C. and Taylor-Papadimitriou, J. (1985) J. Cell Sci. **75**,
       17–33

11.   Petersen, O.W., Hoyer, P.E. and Van Deurs, B. (1987) Cancer Res. **47**, 5748–5751

12.   Taylor-Papadimitriou, J. (1992) in European School of Oncology: Endocrine Therapy of
       Breast Cancer V (Goldhirsch, A., ed.), pp. 3–13, Springer-Verlag, Berlin and Heidelberg

13.   Gusterson, B.A., Monaghan, P., Mahendran, R., Ellis, J. and O'Hare, M.J. (1986) J. Natl.
       Cancer Inst. **77**, 343–349

14.   Wetzels, R.H.W., Holland, R., van Haelst, U.J.G.M., Lane, E.B., Leigh, I.M. and
       Ramaekers, F.C.S. (1990) Am. J. Pathol. **134**, 571–579

15.   Girling, A., Bartkova, J., Burchell, J., Gendler, S., Gillett, C. and Taylor-Papadimitriou, J.
       (1989) Int. J. Cancer **43**, 1072–1076

16.   Domagala, W., Lascota, J., Bartkowiak J., Weber, K. and Osbourn, M. (1990) Am. J. Pathol.
       136, 219–227

17.   Symington, B.E., Takada,Y. and Carter, W.G. (1993) J. Cell Biol. **120**, 523–535

18.   Sriramarao, P., Steffner, P. and Gehlsen, K.R. (1993) J. Biol. Chem. **268**, 22036–22041

19.   Hynes, R.O. (1992) Cell **69**, 11–25

20.   Sonnenberg, A., Calafat, J., Janssen, H., et al. (1991) J. Cell Biol. **113**, 907–917

21.   Jones, J.L., Critchley, D.R. and Walker, R.A. (1992) J. Pathol. **167**, 399–406

22.   Zutter, M.M., Mazoujian, G. and Santoro, S.A. (1990) Am. J. Pathol. **137**, 863–870

23.   Zutter, M.M., Krigman, H.R. and Santoro, S.A. (1993) Am. J. Pathol. **142**, 1439–1448

24.   Pignatelli, M., Hanby, A.M. and Stamp, G.W. (1991) J. Pathol. **165**, 25–32

25.   Berdichevsky, F., Wetzels, R., Shearer, M., Martignone, S., Ramaekers, F.C.S. and Taylor-
       Papadimitriou, J. (1994) Mol. Cell. Differ. **2**, 255–274

26.   Berdichevsky, F. and Taylor-Papadimitriou, J. (1991) Exp. Cell Res. **194**, 267–274

27.   Lu, P.J., Lu, Q.L., Rughetti, A. and Taylor-Papadimitriou, J. (1995) J. Cell Biol. **129**,
       1363–1378

28.   Shearer, M., Bartkova, J., Bartek, J., Berdichevsky, F., Barnes, D., Millis, R. and Taylor-
       Papadimitriou, J. (1992) Int. J. Cancer **51**, 602–612

29.   Keely, P.J., Fong, A.M., Zutter, M.M. and Santoro, S.A. (1995) J. Cell Sci. **108**, 595–607

30.   Zutter, M.M., Santoro, S.A., Staatz, W.D. and Tsung, Y.L. (1995) Proc. Natl. Acad. Sci.
       U.S.A. **92**, 7411–7415

31.   Kamata, T., Puzon, W. and Takada, Y. (1994) J. Biol. Chem. **269**, 9659–9663

32.   Takada, Y. and Puzon, W. (1993) J. Biol. Chem. **268**, 17597–17601

33.   Howlett, A.R., Bailey, N., Damsky, C., Petersen, O.W. and Bissell, M.J. (1995) J. Cell Sci.
       108, 1945–1957

34.   Arroyo, A.G., Garcia-Pardo, A. and Sanchez-Madrid, F. (1993) J. Biol. Chem. **268**,
       9863–9868

35.   D'Souza, B., Berdichevsky, F., Kyprianou, N. and Taylor-Papadimitriou, J. (1993)
       Oncogene **8**, 1797–1806

36.   D'Souza, B. and Taylor-Papadimitriou, J. (1994) Proc. Natl. Acad. Sci. U.S.A. **91**,
       7202–7206

37.   Kinch, M.S., Clark, G.J., Der, C.J. and Burridge, K. (1995) J. Cell Biol. **130**, 461–471

38.   Reichmann, E., Schwarz, H., Deiner, E.M., Leitner, I., Eilers, M., Berger, J., Busslinger, M.
       and Beug, H. (1992) Cell **71**, 1103–1116

39.   Zutter, M.M., Santoro, S.A., Painter, A.S., Tsung, Y.L. and Gafford, A. (1994) J. Biol.
       Chem. **269**, 463–469

40.   Ye, J., Xu, R.H., Taylor-Papadimitriou, J. and Pitha, P.M. (1996) Mol. Cell Biol. **16**,
       6178–6189

41.   Graff, J.R., Herman, J.G., Lapidus, R.G., et al. (1995) Cancer Res. **55**, 5195–5199

42. Berx, G., Cleton-Jansen, A.-M., Nollet, F., de Leeuw, W.J.F., van de Vijver, M.J., Cornelisse, C. and van Roy, F. (1995) EMBO J. **14**, 6107–6115
43. Janes, P.W., Daly, R.J., deFazio, A. and Sutherland, R.L. (1994) Oncogene **9**, 3601–3608
44. Xie, Y., Pendergast, A.-M. and Hung, M.-C. (1995) J. Biol. Chem. **270**, 30717–30724
45. Muthuswamy, S.K. and Muller, W.J. (1995) Oncogene **11**, 1801–1810
46. Spandidos, D.A. and Agnantis, N.J. (1984) Anticancer Res. **4**, 269–285
47. Clair, T., Miller, W.R. and Cho-Chung, Y.S. (1987) Cancer Res. **47**, 5290–5295

Biochem. Soc. Symp. **63**, 261–271
Printed in Great Britain

23

Nm23 and tumour metastasis: basic and translational advances

José M.P. Freije*, Nicholas J. MacDonald and Patricia S. Steeg

Women's Cancers Section, Laboratory of Pathology, National Cancer Institute, Building 10, Rm. 2A33, Bethesda, MD 20892, U.S.A.

Abstract

The *nm23* genes were discovered on the basis of their reduced expression by highly metastatic cell lines. This trend was confirmed in cohorts of several types of human carcinomas and melanomas. Several transfection studies have demonstrated the suppressive effect of *nm23* overexpression on the metastatic aggressiveness of melanoma and breast carcinoma cells *in vivo*. These transfection experiments have also demonstrated an effect of *nm23* overexpression on cellular functions involved in the metastatic phenotype, such as cell motility, and point to a regulatory role for Nm23 proteins in cellular signalling pathways. Nm23 homologues from various species are also involved in normal tissue development and differentiation. Transfection of *nm23-H1* into breast cancer cells provided a functional demonstration of the involvement of this gene in the differentiation of mammary epithelial cells. However, the molecular mechanism of these biological effects remains unknown. Several biochemical activities have been reported for Nm23, including NDP kinase activity, serine autophosphorylation and protein-histidine kinase activity. To define the possible significance of these biochemical activities, we carried out site-directed mutagenesis of the relevant codons of *nm23-H1* cDNA and studied the effects upon transfection into MDA-MB-435 human breast carcinoma cells. We have also used Nm23 expression as a molecular marker to identify novel compounds that are active against the most aggressive tumour cells. This approach revealed that none of the standard agents currently in clinical use is preferentially active against the most aggressive tumour cells, and allowed us to identify new compounds that are preferentially inhibitory towards low-Nm23-expressing breast carcinoma and melanoma cell lines. This analysis also revealed a significant correlation between Nm23 levels and sensitivity of the tumour cells to alkylating agents. A functional implication of Nm23 proteins in this phenomenon was

*To whom correspondence should be addressed.

demonstrated after transfection of *nm23* cDNAs into melanoma and breast and ovarian carcinoma cells.

Introduction

The presence of metastases, and the complications from treating them, are major contributors to cancer mortality. In order to develop new strategies to limit metastatic spread, we must first understand the cell biological, biochemical and genetic controls over this process. Unfortunately, metastasis research spanning the past 20 years has taught us that tumour cells can accomplish this process by many alternative routes. Here we describe our basic and translational research into one gene that exerts metastasis suppressive activity in several model systems, *nm23*.

The first cDNA belonging to the *nm23* family was identified after differential colony hybridization between two related murine K-1735 melanoma cell lines with different metastatic potentials *in vivo* [1]. Expression of *nm23-1*, at the mRNA [1] and protein [2] levels, was quantitatively greater in five highly metastatic K-1735 cell lines than in two low-metastatic K-1735 lines derived from the same tumour. Besides the K-1735 murine melanoma cell lines, reduced *nm23* RNA levels have been correlated with high tumour metastatic potential in several *in vitro* cell systems, including chemically induced rat mammary carcinomas [1], mouse mammary tumour virus (MMTV)-induced tumours [3], *ras* or *ras* + adenovirus 2 *E1a*-transfected rat embryo fibroblasts [4,5] and B16 murine melanomas [6]. In other model systems, however, this correlation has not been observed (reviewed in [7]), confirming the known heterogeneity of the tumour metastatic process.

Members of the family of *nm23* genes have been cloned from many species. In humans, three members of this gene family have been identified: *nm23-H1* [2], *nm23-H2* [8] and *DR-nm23* [9]. For most species, two members are currently known, including the murine *M1* and *M2* isoforms [1,10], and rat *NDPKb* and *NDPKa* [11,12]. Other closely related genes are *Drosophila awd* [13,14] *Myxococcus ndk* [15], *Escherichia coli ndk* [16] and *Dictyostelium gip17* and *guk 7.2* [17,18].

Human tumour cohort studies

We have asked whether decreases in *nm23* expression are correlated with high tumour metastatic potential in human tumours. In these experiments, tumour sections were assayed for Nm23 expression, typically by immunohistochemistry, a scale of positive–negative ratings developed, and the data correlated with parameters of human metastatic potential, such as disease-free or overall survival, presence of metastases, and/or other histopathological criteria. These data are reviewed in detail elsewhere [7].

Decreases in *nm23* RNA or protein levels have been correlated with histological or clinical parameters of high metastatic potential in cohorts of human breast [19–25], gastric [26], cervical [27,28], ovarian [29,30] and hepatocellular

[31–33] carcinomas, as well as melanomas [31,34]. These data do not establish Nm23 as an independent prognostic factor. However, they do suggest the hypothesis, testable in transfection experiments, that restoration of Nm23 expression may exert a suppressive effect on tumour metastatic potential.

The opposite trend was detected in neuroblastoma [35,36] and pancreatic carcinoma [37], while in other cases no correlation was detected (reviewed in [7]). For neuroblastoma, gene amplification [36] and *nm23* mutations [36,38] were detected. While the functional significance of these mutations is now under study using transfection of site-directed mutant constructs [39], these data suggest that Nm23 can be deregulated by mechanisms other than reduced expression. The data also suggest that Nm23 may be irrelevant to several other types of human cancer progression.

Transfection experiments

The evidence for a functional involvement of *nm23* genes in the regulation of tumour metastasis was provided by its transfection into highly metastatic cell lines, and subsequent analysis of the metastatic potential of overexpressing transfectants when injected into experimental animals. Five studies have now reported that transfection of *nm23* cDNAs into cell lines of melanoma or breast carcinoma origins resulted in significant decreases in metastatic potential (discussed below). Not all *nm23* cDNAs exerted equivalent metastatic suppressive capacities, suggesting specificity in the biochemical mechanism of action.

When the murine *nm23-M1* cDNA was transfected into K-1735 TK melanoma cells, the transfectants showed a clear decrease (58–96%) in the number of experimental pulmonary metastases after injection into the tail vein of immunodeficient mice [40]. In spontaneous metastasis assays, where control and *nm23-1* transfectants were injected subcutaneously, primary tumour size was unaffected by *nm23-1* expression, but the incidence of spontaneous metastases was reduced.

The transfection of human *nm23-H1* cDNA into the human MDA-MB 435 breast carcinoma cell line gave similar effects. Overexpressing cells produced 65–90% less pulmonary or draining lymph node metastases than control transfectants when injected in the mammary fat pad of nude mice in spontaneous metastasis experiments [41]. Primary tumour size was again unaffected.

A 93% decrease in experimental metastasis has been reported after transfection of murine *nm23-M1* into murine B16 F10 melanoma cells [42]. In this experiment, the median survival time of mice injected with *nm23*-transfected tumour cells was significantly higher than that of animals injected with control transfected cells (223 days compared with 31 days).

Baba et al. [43] reported that a 78–86% reduction in experimental metastatic potential resulted from transfection of *nm23-M1* or *nm23-M2* into murine B16 FE7 melanoma cells. Interestingly, transfection of human *nm23* cDNAs into the same tumour cell line failed to alter tumour metastatic potential, suggesting species specificity in the protein(s) with which Nm23 functionally interacts.

It has also been reported that transfection of rat *NDPKa* (the homologue of the murine *M2* and human *H2* genes) into rat MTLn3 mammary carcinoma cells resulted in a 44–52% reduction in spontaneous metastatic potential [44].

Nm23 effects on cell biology

The transfection of *nm23* cDNAs into metastatic tumour cells not only provides a functional demonstration of the effect of these genes in metastasis suppression, but also constitutes the most powerful tool with which to investigate the mechanisms by which these effects take place. Characterization of *nm23*-transfected cell lines has revealed an effect on cellular function in several components of the metastatic phenotype, including chemotaxis [45], invasiveness through Matrigel-coated filters [42] and soft agar colonization in response to transforming growth factor-β [40,41] (reviewed in [46]). However, no effect was observed on the proliferation of the transfected cells under standard tissue culture conditions, which is in good agreement with the lack of effect on the primary tumour size upon injection into immunodeficient mice [40,41,43]. This points to a role in the regulation of specific signal transduction pathways. Inhibition of the response to diverse cytokines, including insulin-like growth factor, transforming growth factor-β, platelet-derived growth factor and serum, has been reported, suggesting an action on some point of the intracellular signalling network downstream of the point of convergence of all these different receptors. The fact that all the above cellular responses involve interactions with extracellular matrix components or three-dimensional cultures is particularly suggestive that pathways where integrin and growth factor signalling meet may be relevant.

Venturelli et al. [9] described the isolation of a third human *nm23* gene, called *DR-nm23*, which was identified by differential colony hybridization of a chronic myelogenous leukaemia–blast cell (CML-BC) cDNA library with RNA from myelogenous and lymphoblastic leukaemia cells. Overexpression of this gene in the myeloid precursor 32Dc13 cell line inhibits differentiation in response to colony-stimulating factor and causes apoptosis. Again, these results strongly suggest a role for an Nm23 protein in the regulation of cellular signalling processes, in a cell line that is growth factor-dependent for both proliferation and differentiation [9].

Nm23 in development and differentiation

Several biological processes have been proposed to be common to metastasis and normal tissue development. Thus both metastatic and embryonic cells proliferate, move and invade, suggesting that those processes that are naturally operative in embryogenesis are also turned on in malignant progression. Some suggestive evidence has led to the hypothesis that Nm23 proteins could play a role in the differentiation of normal tissues.

The identification of genes from other species as members of the *nm23* family provided support for this hypothesis. Thus *awd* (abnormal wing discs), an *nm23* homologue from *Drosophila melanogaster*, is required for normal fly development. Mutation or reduced expression of this gene cause alterations post-metamorphosis, leading to aberrant differentiation and necrosis of the imaginal discs, larval brain and proventriculus [13]. The involvement of *nm23*-homologue genes from *Myxococcus xanthus* (a soil bacterium) and *Dictyostelium discoideum* (a slime mould) in differentiation has also been proposed [3,15,47].

The *Drosophila awd* gene provides another biological system that is potentially useful for the elucidation of Nm23 function in the regulation of cellular signalling. A genetic analysis of this system has led to the identification of two loci that could interact with the *Drosophila nm23* homologue: *prune* (*pn*), a locus whose mutation causes an alteration in cyclohydrolase activity and results in an abnormal brown eye colour; and *tum-1*, an oncogenic version of the JAK (Janus kinase) family protein tyrosine kinase-encoding gene *hopscotch* (*hop*), which produces haematopoietic neoplasms resulting in lethality [48]. A Pro-97 to Ser mutation of *awd*, known as *killer of prune* (*awdK-pn*), causes the same developmental abnormalities as *awd* null mutants when co-expressed with mutations in the *pn* locus [13,14]. On the other hand, the *awdK-pn* mutation, in the absence of *pn* mutations, suppresses the phenotype produced by the *tum-1* oncogene. *Tum-1* lethality is also suppressed by *pn* mutations, suggesting the existence of a regulatory pathway involving the proteins encoded by these three genes [48].

Cloning of the *pn* gene has revealed limited sequence identity with the catalytic domain of mammalian GTPase-activating proteins (15–20% identity at the amino acid level) [49]. This identity was subject to considerable debate, however. A more recent database search has allowed us to identify another protein, yeast exopolyphosphatase 1 [50], which shows 25% identity at the amino acid level to the product of the *pn* locus. The potential significance of this similarity is highlighted by the recent description of a phosphatase for the Nm23 protein [51], and is under active investigation.

The first correlative evidence of a link between Nm23 and the differentiation of mammalian organisms came from the immunohistochemical analysis of mouse organogenesis through embryonic development. Nm23 expression was uniform and low during the first 10 days of embryogenesis. After day 10, increased Nm23 expression was observed, coincident with the functional development of different organs and tissues, such as brain, heart, kidney, skin, intestine and adrenals. This trend was not observed in all cases, and the lungs remained immunonegative during all developmental stages. In other tissues, such as the colonic epithelia and lactating mammary gland, Nm23 expression did not remain high in the adult [52].

A functional demonstration of a role for an *nm23* gene in cell differentiation was reported using MDA-MB-435 breast carcinoma cells. Upon transfection with *nm23-H1*, these cells acquired differentiated phenotypes, such as the ability to form duct-like structures, to produce and secrete basement membrane components and to produce milk glycoproteins when cultured in a three-dimensional system containing reconstituted basement membrane proteins [53]. None of the differentiated phenotypes were observed in two-dimensional culture on tissue culture plastic. These data reinforce the importance of tumour-cell–matrix interactions in *nm23* function.

Biochemical and structural features of Nm23 proteins

The genes of the *nm23* family encode polypeptides of 16–18 kDa that are highly conserved. Fig. 1 shows the amino acid sequences of the human and rodent proteins of this family. Three groups of conserved sequences can clearly be distinguished, with human DR-Nm23 the only known member of the third group. The differences between rodent and human sequences are less than 5% in each group, and the sequences of groups 1 and 2 are approx. 88% identical. DR-Nm23 is the least closely related member of this family, showing only 69 and 65% identity with Nm23-H1 and -H2 respectively. The fact that Nm23-H1 and -H2 proteins exhibit 77.5 and 77.7% sequence identity with *Drosophila* Awd, and approx. 60% identity with yeast nucleotide diphosphate kinase

```
           1                                                         60
Nm23-H1    .......... .......MAN CERTFIAIKP DGVQRGLVGE IIKRFEQKGF RLVGLKFMQA
Nm23-M1    .......... .......MAN SERTFIAIKP DGVQRGLVGE IIKRFEQKGF RLVGLKFLQA
Nm23-Rb    .......... .......MAN SERTFIAIKP DGVQRGLVGE IIKRFEQKGF RLVGLKFIQA

Nm23-H2    .......... .......MAN LERTFIAIKP DGVQRGLVGE IIKRFEQKGF RLVAMKFLRA
Nm23-M2    .......... .......MAN LERTFIAIKP DGVQRGLVGE IIKRFEQKGF RLVAMKFLRA
Nm23-Ra    .......... .......MAN LERTFIAIKP DGVQRGLVGE IIKRFEQKGF RLVAMKFLRA

DR-Nm23    MICLVLTIFA NLFPAACTGA HERTFLAVKP DGVQRRLVGE IVRRFERKGF KLVALKLVQS

consensus  .......... ........ .ERTF.A.KP DGVQR.LVGE I..RFE.KGF .LV..K....


           61                                                        120
Nm23-H1    SEDLLKEHYV DLKDRPFFAG LVKYMHSGPV VAMVWEGLNV VKTGRVMLGE TNPADSKPGT
Nm23-M1    SEDLLKEHYT DLKDRPFFTG LVKYMHSGPV VAMVWEGLNV VKTGRVMLGE TNPADSKPGT
Nm23-Rb    SEDLLKEHYI DLKDRPFFSG LVKYMHSGPV VAMVWEGLNV VKTGRVMLGE TNPADSKPGT

Nm23-H2    SEEHLKQHYI DLKDRPFFPG LVKYMNSGPV VAMVWEGLNV VKTGRVMLGE TNPADSKPGT
Nm23-M2    SEEHLKQHYI DLKDRPFFPG LVKYMNSGPV VAMVWEGLNV VKTGRVMLGE TNPADSKPGT
Nm23-Ra    SEEHLKQHYI DLKDRPFFPG LVKYMNSGPV VAMVWEGLNV VKTGRWMLGE TNPADSKPGT

DR-Nm23    SEELLREHYA ELRERPFYGR LVKYMASGPV VAMVWQGLDV VRTSRALIGA TNPADAPPGT

consensus  SE..L..HY. .L..RPF... LVKYM.SGPV VAMVW.GL.V V.T.R...G. TNPAD..PGT
                                                                        *

           121                                                       170
Nm23-H1    IRGDFCIQVG RNIIHGSDSV ESAEKEIGLW FHPEELVDYT SCAQNWIYE.
Nm23-M1    IRGDFCIQVG RNIIHGSDSV KSAEKEISLW FQPEELVEYK SCAQNWIYE.
Nm23-Rb    IRGDFCIQVG RNIIHGSDSV ESAEKEISLW FQPEELVDYK SCAQNWIYE.

Nm23-H2    IRGDFCIQVG RNIIHGSDSV KSAEKEISLW FKPEELVDYK SCAHDWVYE.
Nm23-M2    IRGDFCIQVG RNIIHGSDSV ESAEKEIHLW FKPEELIDYK SCAHDWVYE.
Nm23-Ra    IRGDFCIQVG RNIIHGSDSV ESAEKEIGLW FKPEELIDYK SCAHDWVYE*

DR-Nm23    IRGDFCIEVG .NLIHGSDSV ESARREIALW FRADELLCWE DSAGHWLYE*

consensus  IRGDFCI.VG .N.IHGSDSV .SA..EI.LW F...EL.... ..A..W.YE.
```

Fig. 1. Amino acid sequences of human and rodent Nm23 proteins. Amino acid residues common to all aligned sequences are shown. Phosphorylated serine and histidine residues are underlined. The Pro-96 residue, mutated in the *killer of prune* allele, is indicated with an asterisk.

(NDPK), tempts us to speculate that *DR-nm23* has diverged from the other *nm23* genes early in evolution, probably before the appearance of vertebrates. Confirmation of this hypothesis requires the identification of DR-Nm23 homologues in other species. The most notorious feature in the DR-Nm23 sequence is the presence of 17 extra residues in its N-terminus, which are not present in any other protein of this family. The regions of greatest variability between the sequences aligned in Fig. 1 are located between positions 37 and 50 and between positions 130 and 150, suggesting a possible role for these regions in the specificity of the different Nm23 molecules.

The best characterized property of Nm23 proteins is their capacity to use the terminal phosphate from a nucleoside triphosphate such as ATP to autophosphorylate a histidine residue, forming a high-energy intermediate from which the phosphate can be transferred to an acceptor molecule. When the acceptor molecule is a nucleoside diphosphate, the net result of the reaction is an NDPK activity, which has been described for more than 40 years [54–56]. The relevance of the NDPK activity for the biological effects of Nm23 in the modulation of tumour metastasis or differentiation has been subject to debate (reviewed in [7]). Evidence suggesting that the Nm23 NDPK activity is not directly responsible for its metastasis-suppressive or differentiation-inducing activities includes: (a) the lack of a correlation of total cellular or subcellular NDPK activity with Nm23 expression and metastasis-suppressive activity in transfection model systems [41,57]; and (b) the failure of human *nm23-H1* cDNA to abrogate all of the developmental defects upon its transformation of the null *awd* germ-line, despite a significant increase in NDPK activity [58].

The Nm23 phosphohistidine can also be transferred to histidine residues in other proteins, resulting in a protein-histidine kinase activity [59]. The significance of histidine protein kinases in mammalian cells is poorly understood [60], but similar enzymes in bacterial systems are part of a two-component system used to regulate signal transduction [61].

Besides this unstable phosphohistidine intermediate, low-energy phosphorylation of serine residues has been described for various Nm23 proteins [62–65]. We have demonstrated that this serine phosphorylation occurs both *in vivo* and *in vitro*, and that, in *nm23*-transfected melanoma cells, the level of autophosphorylation, but not of NDPK activity, correlates with the suppression of metastasis [62]. Two tryptic peptides from the human Nm23-H1 protein contained phosphorylated serine residues. The only serine residue in the first peptide was Ser-44. The second peptide, which exhibited 4-fold less autophosphorylation, contained three serine residues, at positions 120, 122 and 125, with Ser-120 the only strictly conserved residue among all described Nm23 homologues. Crystallographic data show that Ser-44 is located on the surface of the folded Nm23 proteins [66], and seems to be phosphorylated by intermolecular transfer (J.M.P. Freije, N.J. MacDonald and P.S. Steeg, unpublished work). On the other hand, Ser-120 has a buried position, and is probably phosphorylated by intramolecular transfer from the phosphohistidine intermediate.

Several other biochemical activities have been proposed for Nm23 proteins. Nm23-H2 was identified as a purine binding transcription factor for the c-*myc* promoter [67,68], but the specificity of the DNA binding has been questioned [69]. An extracellular role has also been proposed for Nm23, as a factor that inhibits the differentiation of myeloid leukaemia cells [70,71], and its presence on the cell surface of several cell lines has been reported [72]. However, the absence of a signal sequence from Nm23 proteins makes unclear the mechanisms by which these proteins could be secreted. A phosphatase specific for Nm23 proteins was recently purified [51]. This phosphatase has amino acid identity to Bax, an effector of mammalian programmed cell death, suggesting a connection of Nm23 proteins with signalling pathways involved in apoptosis, in good agreement with the biological effect described for human *DR-nm23* in the induction of apoptosis in myeloid cells [9].

Our recent studies have attempted to determine the relevance of several amino acids in Nm23-H1, implicated in the biochemical functions described above, for the *nm23-H1* metastasis-suppressive phenotype. We have performed site-directed mutagenesis of several amino acids in Nm23-H1, and are currently evaluating the biochemical properties of the mutant recombinant proteins. The biological effects of the site-directed mutants upon transfection into MDA-MB-435 human breast carcinoma cells were determined in an *in vitro* assay for one component of the metastatic process, tumour cell motility in Boyden chambers. We found that mutation of Pro-96 to serine (the *awd killer of prune* mutant in *Drosophila*) and of Ser-120 to glycine (the site of autophosphorylation, and a mutation found in human neuroblastomas) eliminated the motility-inhibitory activity of Nm23-H1, although the mutant recombinant proteins retained NDPK activity as well as the ability to autophosphorylate [39]. In comparison, mutation of Ser-44, another site of autophosphorylation, failed to affect significantly the motility-suppressive capacity of *nm23-H1*. These data suggest the importance of interactions of Nm23 with other cellular proteins, as opposed to general autophosphorylation or NDPK activities, as being relevant to its biological function.

Nm23 and translational research

We have used *nm23* expression as a marker in an attempt to identify chemotherapeutic agents that are preferentially inhibitory to highly aggressive tumour cells. To do this, the levels of Nm23 in a panel of breast carcinoma and melanoma cell lines were measured by Western blot, and correlated with the sensitivity of the cells to growth inhibition *in vitro* by various compounds, using the COMPARE computer algorithm [73]. The relationship of tumour cell sensitivity to chemotherapeutic compounds and Nm23 expression was calculated by Pearson correlation coefficients, where +1.0 signified that a compound was preferentially inhibitory to high-Nm23-expressing breast and melanoma cell lines, a correlation coefficient of −1.0 signified that the compound was preferentially inhibitory to low-Nm23-expressing cell lines, and a coefficient of 0 signified no relationship with Nm23 expression. Correlation coefficients were first obtained for 171 standard agents, i.e. drugs in clinical use, clinical trial or development. Correlation coefficients ranged from +0.845 to −0.631, which indicates a need for new agents active against the most aggressive tumour cells. Using the same approach, we identified 40 potential agents from the 30 000 available in the chemical repository of the Developmental Therapeutics Program of the National Cancer Institute whose activity against the tested cell lines was correlated inversely with their Nm23 expression levels, with a Pearson correlation coefficient of -0.64 or less. The preferential *in vitro* growth-inhibitory activity of four of these compounds against low-Nm23-expressing breast carcinoma cell lines was confirmed. Two of these agents have been found to exert an anti-motility effect *in vitro*, and both show weak inhibition of tubulin polymerization, suggestive of a common mechanism [74].

The COMPARE analysis also revealed an intriguing positive correlation between Nm23 expression levels and sensitivity to alkylating agents. When the standard agents were analysed, 21 out of the 30 agents with the highest correlation coefficients were alkylating agents. *In vitro* experiments using three panels of control- and *nm23*-transfected cell lines, of murine melanoma, human breast carcinoma and human ovarian carcinoma origin, determined that overexpression of Nm23 protein resulted in a quantitatively increased sensitivity to inhibition of growth by cisplatin [75]. For the murine melanoma cell lines, intravenous injection of tumour cells, followed by a single injection of cisplatin several days later, showed that cisplatin was preferentially inhibitory to pulmonary metastatic outgrowth of *nm23* transfectants *in vivo* as well. The mechanism of action for this intriguing observation is unknown, but we have found that *nm23-H1*-transfected breast carcinoma cells form greater numbers of interstrand cross-links upon exposure to cisplatin than do control transfectants, while DNA repair rates remain equivalent [75].

The significance of these data may lie in ongoing efforts to elevate tumour cell Nm23 expression *in vivo*. The promoter of *nm23-H1* is being intensively characterized in an attempt to identify the factors involved in its regulation. This promoter will be subject to cell-based drug screening efforts, in an effort to identify new compounds that will enter a tumour cell and turn on transcription of *nm23*. If such an agent can be identified, our data suggest that it may have improved clinical applicability in combination with cisplatin or other alkylating agent therapy.

References

1. Steeg, P.S., Bevilacqua, G., Kopper, L., Thorgeirsson, U.P., Talmadge, J.E., Liotta, L.A. and Sobel, M.E. (1988) J. Natl. Cancer Inst. **80**, 200–204

2. Rosengard, A.M., Krutzsch, H.C., Shearn, A., et al. (1989) Nature (London) **342**, 177–180

3. Caligo, M.A., Cipollini, G., Valromita, C.D., Bistocchi, M. and Bevilacqua, G. (1992) Anticancer Res. **12**, 969–973

4. Steeg, P.S., Bevilacqua, G., Pozzatti, R., Liotta, L.A. and Sobel, M.E. (1988) Cancer Res. **48**, 6550–6554

5. Su, Z.-Z., Austin, V.N., Zimmer, S.G. and Fisher, P.B. (1993) Oncogene **8**, 1211–1219

6. Lakshmi, M., Parker, C. and Sherbert, G. (1993) Anticancer Res. **13**, 299–304

7. DeLaRosa, A., Williams, R.L. and Steeg, P.S. (1995) Bioessays **17**, 53–62

8. Stahl, J.A., Leone, A., Rosengard, A.M., Porter, L., King, C.R. and Steeg, P.S. (1991) Cancer Res. **51**, 445–449

9. Venturelli, D., Martinez, R., Melotti, P., et al. (1995) Proc. Natl. Acad. Sci. U.S.A. **92**, 7435–7439

10. Urano, T., Takamiya, K., Furukawa, K. and Shiku, H. (1992) FEBS Lett. **309**, 358–362

11.   Kimura, N., Shimada, N., Nomura, K. and Watanabe, K. (1990) J. Biol. Chem. **265**, 15744–15749

12.   Shimada, N., Ishikawa, N., Munakata, Y., Toda, T., Watanabe, K. and Kimura, N. (1993) J. Biol. Chem. **268**, 2583–2589

13.   Dearolf, C., Hersperger, E. and Shearn, A. (1988) Dev. Biol. **129**, 159–168

14.   Dearolf, C., Tripoulas, N., Biggs, J. and Shearn, A. (1988) Dev. Biol. **129**, 169–178

15.   Muñoz-Dorado, J., Inoue, M. and Inoue, S. (1990) J. Biol. Chem. **265**, 2707–2712

16.   Hama, H., Almaula, N., Lerner, C.G., Inouye, S. and Inouye, M. (1991) Gene **105**, 31–36

17.   Troll, H., Winckler, T., Lascu, I., Muller, N., Saurin, W., Veron, M. and Mutzel, R. (1993) J. Biol. Chem. **268**, 25469–25475

18.   Wallet, V., Mutzel, R., Troll, H., Barzu, O., Wurster, B., Veron, M. and Lacombe, M.L. (1990) J. Natl. Cancer Inst. **82**, 1199–1202

19.   Bevilacqua, G., Sobel, M.E., Liotta, L.A. and Steeg, P.S. (1989) Cancer Res. **49**, 5185–5190

20.   Hennessy, C., Henry, J., May, F.E.B., Westly, B., Angus, B. and Lennard, T.W.J. (1991) J. Natl. Cancer Inst. **83**, 281–285

21.   Barnes, R., Masood, S., Barker, E., et al. (1991) Am. J. Pathol. **139**, 245–250

22.   Tokunaga, Y., Urano, T., Furakawa, K., Kondo, H., Kanematsu, T. and Shiku, H. (1993) Int. J. Cancer **55**, 66–71

23.   Cropp, C., Lidereau, R., Leone, A., et al. (1994) J. Natl. Cancer Inst. **86**, 1167–1169

24.   Hirayama, R., Sawai, S., Takagi, Y., et al. (1991) J. Natl. Cancer Inst. **83**, 1249–1250

25.   Royds, J.A., Stephenson, T.J., Rees, R.C., Shorthouse, A.J. and Silcocks, P.B. (1993) J. Natl. Cancer Inst. **85**, 727–731

26.   Kodera, Y., Isobe, K.-I., Yamauchi, M., et al. (1994) Cancer **73**, 259–265

27.   Ilijas, M., Pavelic, K., Sarcevic, B., et al. (1994) Int. J. Oncol. **5**, 1455–1457

28.   Mandai, M., Konishi, I., Koshiyama, M., et al. (1995) Cancer **75**, 2523–2529

29.   Kapitonovic, S., Spaventi, R., Vujsic, S., et al. (1995) Anticancer Res. **15**, 587–590

30.   Mandai, M., Konishi, I., Koshiyama, M., et al. (1994) Cancer Res. **54**, 1825–1830

31.   Boix, L., Bruix, J., Campo, E.,et al. (1994) Gastroenterology **107**, 486–491

32.   Yamaguchi, A., Urano, T., Goi, T., et al. (1994) Cancer **73**, 2280–2284

33.   Nakayama, T., Ohtsuru, A., Nakao, K., et al. (1992) J. Natl. Cancer Inst. **84**, 1349–1354

34.   Caligo, M.A., Grammatico, P., Cipollini, G., Vareso, L., Del Porto, G. and Bevilacqua, G. (1994) Melanoma Res. **4**, 179–184

35.   Hailat, N., Keim, D.R., Melhem, R.F., et al. (1991) J. Clin. Invest. **88**, 341–345

36.   Leone, A., Seeger, R.C., Hong, C.M., et al. (1993) Oncogene **8**, 855–865

37.   Nakamori, S., Ishikawa, O., Ohhigashi, H., et al. (1993) Clin. Exp. Metastasis **11**, 151–158

38.   Chang, C., Zhu, X.-x., Thoraval, D., et al. (1994) Nature (London) **370**, 335–336

39.   MacDonald, N.J., Freije, J.M.P., Stracke, M.L., Manrow, R.E. and Steeg, P.S. (1997) J. Biol. Chem., **271**, 25107–25116

40.   Leone, A., Flatow, U., King, C.R., Sandeen, M.A., Margulies, I.M.K., Liotta, L.A. and Steeg, P.S. (1991) Cell **65**, 25–35

41.   Leone, A., Flatow, U., VanHoutte, K. and Steeg, P.S. (1993) Oncogene **8**, 2325–2333

42.   Parhar, R.S., Shi, Y., Zou, M., Farid, N.R., Ernst, P. and Al-Sedairy, S. (1995) Int. J. Cancer **60**, 204–210

43.   Baba, H., Urano, T., Okada, K., et al. (1995) Cancer Res. **55**, 1977–1981

44.   Fukuda, M., Ishii, A., Yasutomo, Y., et al. (1997), Int. J. Cancer **65**, 531–537

45.   Kantor, J.D., McCormick, B., Steeg, P.S. and Zetter, B.R. (1993) Cancer Res. **53**, 1971–1973

46.   Freije, J.M.P., MacDonald, N.J. and Steeg, P.S. (1996) Curr. Top. Microbiol. Immunol. **213**, 215–232

47.   Muñoz-Dorado, J., Inoue, M. and Inoue, S. (1990) J. Biol. Chem. **265**, 2702–2706

48.   Zinyk, D.L., McGonnigal, B.G. and Dearolf, C. (1993) Nature Genet. **4**, 195–201

49.   Teng, D.H.F., Engele, C.M. and Venkatesh, T.R. (1991) Nature (London) **353**, 437–440

50.   Wurst, H., Shiba, T. and Kornberg, A. (1995) J. Bacteriol. **177**, 898–906

51. Shankar, S., Kavanaugh-Black, A., Kamath, S. and Chakabarty, A. (1995) J. Biol. Chem. **270**, 28246–28250

52. Lakso, M., Steeg, P.S. and Westphal, H. (1992) Cell. Growth Differ. **3**, 873–879

53. Howlett, A.R., Petersen, O.W., Steeg, P.S. and Bissell, M.J. (1994) J. Natl. Cancer Inst. **86**, 1838–1844

54. Berg, P. and Joklik, W.K. (1953) Nature (London) **172**, 1008–1009

55. Krebs, H.A. and Hems, R. (1953) Biochim. Biophys. Acta **12**, 172–180

56. Parks, R.E. and Agarwal, R.P. (1973) Enzymes 3rd Ed. **8**, 307–333

57. Golden, A., Benedict, M., Shearn, A., Kimura, N., Leone, A., Liotta, L.A. and Steeg, P.S. (1993) in Oncogenes and Tumor Suppressor Genes in Human Malignancies (Benz, C. and Liu, E., eds.), pp. 345–357, Kluwer Academic Publishers, Boston

58. Xu, J., Liu, L., Deng, F., Timmons, L., Hersperger, E., Steeg, P., Veron, M. and Shearn, A. (1997) Dev. Biol., **177**, 544–557

59. Wagner, P. and Vu, N.-D. (1995) J. Biol. Chem. **270**, 21758–21764

60. Crovello, C., Furie, B. and Furie, B. (1995) Cell **82**, 279–286

61. Hess, J., Bourret, R. and Simon, M. (1988) Nature (London) **336**, 139–143

62. MacDonald, N.J., DeLaRosa, A., Benedict, M.A., Freije, J.M.P., Krutsch, H. and Steeg, P.S. (1993) J. Biol. Chem. **269**, 25780–25789

63. Muñoz-Dorado, J., Almaula, N., Inouye, S. and Inouye, M. (1993) J. Bacteriol. **175**, 1176–1181

64. Hemmerich, S. and Pecht, I. (1992) Biochemistry **31**, 4580–4587

65. Bominaar, A., Tepper A. and Veron, M. (1994) FEBS Lett. **353**, 5–8

66. Webb, P., Perisic, O., Mendola, C., Backer, J. and Williams, R. (1995) J. Mol. Biol. **251**, 574–587

67. Postel, E.H., Berberich, S.J., Flint, S.J. and Ferrone, C.A. (1993) Science **261**, 478–480

68. Postel, E.H. and Ferrone, C.A. (1994) J. Biol. Chem. **269**, 8627–8630

69. Hildebrandt, M., Lacombe, M., Mesnildrey, S. and Veron, M. (1995) Nucleic Acids Res. **23**, 3858–3864

70. Okabe-Kado, J., Kasukabe, T., Honma, Y., Hayashi, M., Henzel, W.J. and Hozumi, M. (1992) Biochem. Biophys. Res. Commun. **182**, 987–994

71. Okabe-Kado, J., Kasukabe, T., Hozumi, M., et al. (1995) FEBS Lett. **363**, 311–315

72. Urano, T., Furukawa, K. and Shiku, H. (1993) Oncogene **8**, 1371–1376

73. Paull, K., Shoemaker, R., Hodes, L., et al. (1989) J. Natl. Cancer Inst. **81**, 1088–1092

74. Freije, J.M.P., Lawrence, J.A., Hollingshead, M.G. et al. (1997) Nature Med. **3**, 395–401

75. Ferguson, A.W., Flatow, U., MacDonald, N.J., Larminant, F., Bohr, V.A. and Steeg, P.S. (1997) Cancer Res., **56**, 2931–2935

Biochem. Soc. Symp. **63**, 273–294
Printed in Great Britain

24

Use of DNA transfer in the induction of metastasis in experimental mammary systems

**Roger Barraclough, Hai-juan Chen, Barry R. Davies,
Michael P.A. Davies, Youqiang Ke, Bryony H. Lloyd,
Adam Oates and Philip S. Rudland**

Department of Biochemistry, University of Liverpool, P.O. Box 147, Liverpool
L69 7ZB, U.K.

Abstract

The metastatic spread of cancer is a little understood process, in part because it is difficult to model the entire process using experimental approaches *in vitro*. The ability to transfer DNA into non-metastatic mammary cells and to observe the induction of metastasis *in vivo* provides a means for identifying DNA sequences that are associated with the development of metastatic capability. Using these techniques, a metastasis-associated cytoskeletal calcium binding protein, S100A4 (p9Ka), has been identified as an inducer of metastatic capability in benign rat mammary epithelial cells. Metastasis can also be induced in the rat mammary epithelial cells by fragments of DNA from metastatic, but not from benign, human breast tumour cells. These non-coding fragments of DNA act via the induction of osteopontin, an extracellular, integrin binding, calcium binding protein. Since both osteopontin and S100A4 are thought to be associated with malignancy in human breast cancer specimens, gene transfer techniques can identify genes for metastasis-inducing proteins that may play a role in breast cancer, and further suggest that cell migration/motility might be important in the metastatic process.

Introduction

Cancer is a process involving multiple steps that probably correspond to mutational events causing damage to somatic DNA [1]. Study of genes in which such damage occurs has led to the identification of a number of dominantly acting oncogenes and tumour suppressor genes [2] that contribute to the early development of a tumour. The protein products of these genes affect signal transduction and the cell cycle, and their oncogenic mechanisms are now well known at a molecular level [1]. However, for the more common solid cancers, the major clinical problem is the dissemination of the cancer, a little understood process, referred to as metastasis, whereby tumour cells spread from their site of origin to distant sites in the body. So far, few genes have been found that cause metastasis to occur. In view of the systemic nature of metastasis, it is not possible to study the entire process *in vitro*, although some individual steps of the process, such as the ability of cells to invade synthetic matrices or to adhere to particular substrata, can be studied in isolation using culture systems *in vitro* [3,4]. Techniques in which DNA is transferred into cultured cells and the cells subsequently tested for their metastatic capabilities *in vivo* provide an experimental approach for isolating and identifying DNA sequences, and their possible protein products, that confer the property of metastasis to non-metastatic tumour cells.

Early experiments in which DNA from metastatic cancer cells was transferred to non-metastatic tumour cells by transfection resulted in the transfected cells acquiring metastatic capabilities in syngeneic hosts or in nude mice. These experiments showed that the ability to metastasize *in vivo* can reside in changes in the genome of a metastatic cell [5–17]. Unfortunately, some of the early experiments utilized, as recipients, highly passaged, aneuploid, near-metastatic cell lines such as the NIH 3T3 fibroblast [14–17], in which an apparent metastatic phenotype could occur spontaneously prior to, or during, growth in the animal, as indicated by metastases occurring due to the transfection procedure or when a selectable plasmid DNA alone was transferred [14,16–19]. A further difficulty encountered in early experiments was the need to use the nude mouse as the recipient; many human carcinomas fail to grow and to metastasize in such immunodeficient mice unless additional genetic changes take place [20].

In our own laboratory, we have used as recipient a near-diploid, genetically stable, rat mammary epithelial cell line, Rama 37, of karyotype 42 ± 2.5 [21], derived from a benign 7,12-dimethylbenz-[a]-anthracene-induced mammary tumour [22]. This cell line produces relatively benign, non-metastatic, encapsulated tumours resembling human adenomas at about 50% of injection sites in the mammary fat pads of a syngeneic rat host [22]. These tumours fail to metastasize, and thus Rama 37 is a suitable mammary epithelial recipient cell line in which to test DNA for the ability to confer metastatic properties.

The experimental protocol employed is outlined in Fig. 1. Briefly, benign Rama 37 cells [22] as non-confluent monolayer cultures are transfected using the calcium phosphate procedure [23] with a plasmid containing a selectable marker, usually *neo* (which confers resistance to the antibiotic geneticin), but *gpt* has also been used [24]. The selectable marker is contained within plasmid DNA under the influence of the simian virus 40 (SV40) early promoter in pSV2*neo* [25] or pSV2*gpt* [26], or under the influence of the cytomegalovirus intermediate early promoter in pBKCMV (Stratagene). The test DNA is either

1
Insert the test DNA into a plasmid bearing a selectable marker gene,
pSV2*neo*, pSV2*gpt* or pCMV-1 (*neo*) and transfect the recombinant plasmid
into the benign rat tumour-derived epithelial cell line Rama 37*

2
Grow the cells in selective medium to kill any cells
that have not taken up the plasmid

3
Ring clone the surviving cells if required and inject 2×10^6 of the
surviving cells into the mammary fat pads of syngeneic rats

4
Examine the injected rats for primary tumours
in the mammary glands and for metastases in the lungs and
lymph nodes over a period of up to 16 weeks

Fig. I. Test system for metastasis-inducing DNA. *Alternatively, co-transfection of the test DNA and the plasmid bearing the selectable marker gene into the benign rat mammary-tumour-derived epithelial cell line Rama 37 produces transfectants that have taken up both the plasmid DNA and the test DNA.

co-transfected with, or inserted into, the cloning site of one of the above plasmids. After keeping the transfectants in a selective medium containing geneticin for a period of 2 weeks, the surviving geneticin-resistant cells are grown as pools of primary transfectants, or cells are ring cloned to provide transfected cell lines. The cells are subjected to a 'metastasis assay' in which 2×10^6 cells of the transfected cell lines or pools are injected subcutaneously into the mammary fat pads of 4–8-week-old female syngeneic rats; the rats are examined over a period of up to 16 weeks for the appearance of primary tumours in the mammary glands and for overt metastases; metastases to internal organs are detected at necropsy. While providing for the metastatic cells to leave the mammary gland, to survive in the circulation, and to adhere, invade and grow at the site of metastasis, the 'metastasis assay' must be well controlled. First, it is necessary to ensure that, during their transfer into the mammary glands, the cells are not injected into a blood vessel. This potential problem is overcome by isolating cells from any metastases and injecting them into the mammary fat pads of further rats. Secondly, it is necessary to ensure that the recipient cells do not exhibit metastatic activity, and that metastatic capability is not induced by transfection with plasmid DNA and by subsequent growth in selective medium. In several hundred individual metastasis assays, only one instance of a metastasis with Rama 37 cells with or without control plasmid has been observed.

Elevated levels of a metastasis-associated intracellular calcium binding protein can induce metastatic capability in benign rat mammary epithelial cells

S100A4 (p9Ka) is a member of the S100 family of proteins, a widely distributed family of calcium binding proteins of generally unknown function [27]. Although immunoreactive S100A4 displays a highly specific distribution within and among normal rat tissues [28], this distribution gives little help in understanding the role of this protein. Increased levels (about 16–20-fold) of S100A4 are present in the metastatic rat mammary epithelial cell line Rama 800 [29] relative to either a benign-tumour-derived epithelial counterpart or an epithelial cell line derived from normal rat mammary gland [30]. In mouse mammary epithelial cells, the level of the mRNA for murine S100A4 (*mts*1) is correlated quantitatively with the metastatic potential of the cells, measured by their ability to spread to the lungs within 4–5 weeks of intramuscular injection into recipient mice [31].

The normal gene for S100A4 has been cloned [32–34] and consists of a small untranslated 5′ non-coding exon and two coding exons, with the latter giving rise to the region of the protein which contains a calcium binding EF-hand domain [33]. The rat gene, contained in 10.3 kbp of cloned normal rat DNA [33], was inserted into the vector pSV2*neo* and the construct transfected into the benign non-metastatic rat mammary cell line Rama 37 using the calcium phosphate precipitation technique [23]. Geneticin-resistant transfected cells (*S100A4*/pSV2*neo*) arising from the expression of the *neo* gene contained 6–16-fold higher levels of mRNA for S100A4 and 8–14-fold higher levels of S100A4 protein than the recipient cells, and were subjected to the metastasis assay [35]. Parallel experiments were carried out using cells transfected with vector alone (pSV2*neo*) or vector containing control genes, either the activated c-Ha-*ras* oncogene (EJ*ras*/pSV2*neo*) or a growth factor gene, that for basic fibroblast growth factor (basic FGF/pSV2*neo*). The results (Table 1) showed that the *S100A4* gene, but not the oncogene or the growth factor gene, was able to induce metastatic capability in the Rama 37 cells [36].

The primary tumours produced by Rama 37 cells and by Rama 37 cells transfected with pSV2*neo* or EJ*ras*/pSV2*neo* produced adenomas with varying degrees of atypia and peripheral spindle cells. The tumours arising from Rama 37 cells transfected with 10–100 copies of *S100A4*/pSV2*neo* were histologically highly variable. The major component consisted of spindle cells of highly variable morphology, many with high nuclear/cytoplasmic ratios (Fig. 2). Some of these tumours had breached the surrounding connective tissue capsule and had invaded the adjacent host skeletal muscle [35]. Two *S100A4*/pSV2*neo* transfectant cell lines yielded metaplastic variants consisting of large mononuclear and giant multinucleated cells of malignant cytology as well as squamous elements [35]. The histology of metastatic lesions reflected that of the primary tumours (Fig. 2). Upon culture of cells from lung lesions and injection, these cells formed highly pleiomorphic spindle cell primary tumours and glandular tumours of a tubular, adenocarcinomatous appearance consisting of highly pleiomorphic, cuboidal epithelial-like cells lining duct-like structures, and sur-

Table I. Incidence of tumours and metastases produced by injection of primary transfectants and cultured tumours and metastases. Data from [36]. Rama 37 cells were transfected with pSV2neo containing the activated EJras cDNA, cDNA for basic fibroblast growth factor or the gene for S100A4 (p9Ka), and surviving transfectants were subjected to the metastasis assay. Cell lines from tumours or metastases (where present) were cultured and also subjected to the metastasis assay. Tumour incidence is defined as the number of tumours/number of sites injected. Latent periods are given as means, with ranges in parentheses. The incidence of metastases is defined as the number of animals with metastases/number of animals with tumours. Significantly more tumours than Rama 37 cells (Fisher exact test): *P<0.05; **P<0.01; ***P<0.002. †Significantly longer latent period than Rama 37 cells (P<0.001; Mann–Whitney U-test); ‡significantly shorter latent period than Rama 37 cells (P<0.001; Mann–Whitney U-test). Significantly more metastases than Rama 37 cells (Fisher exact test): §P<0.05; §§P<0.01.

Transfected DNA	Tumour incidence	Latent period in days (range)	Incidence of metastases
Primary transfectants			
None (Rama 37 cells)	22/46	33 (24–81)	0/20
pSV2neo	6/15	29 (14–33)	0/6
EJras/pSV2neo	20/40	23 (16–66)	0/20
Basic FGF/pSV2neo	9/41	71 (35–98)†	0/9
S100A4/pSV2neo	44/47***	11 (6–28)‡	16/29§§
Cultured tumours or metastases			
EJras/pSV2neo primary tumour	10/10**	7 (–)‡	0/10
Basic FGF/pSV2neo primary tumour	24/24**	10 (7–11)‡	0/24
S100A4/pSV2neo lung metastasis	42/52*	6 (4–7)‡	15/42§

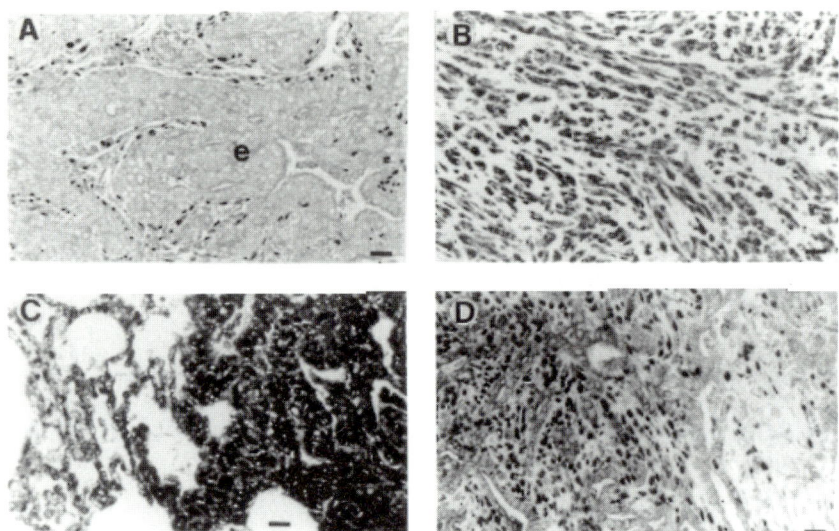

Fig. 2. Immunocytochemical staining for S100A4 (p9Ka) of tumours arising from Rama 37 cells and Rama 37 cells transfected with S100A4. (A) An adenomatous primary tumour arising from the injection of non-transfected Rama 37 cells into the mammary gland. There is virtually no staining of the epithelial cells (e) and moderate staining of the peripheral spindle cells. (B) Primary tumour of spindle cell type arising from the injection of Rama 37 cells that had been transfected with the *S100A4*/pSV2*neo* construct. The cytoplasm of the malignant spindle cells stains strongly for S100A4. (C) A lung metastasis produced by Rama 37 cells that had been transfected with *S100A4*/pSV2*neo*, showing uniform staining of the cells of the metastasis (on the right) and only slight staining of the adjacent lung tissue (on the left). (D) Adenomatous primary tumour produced by injection of a geneticin-resistant metastatic cell line isolated from a lung metastasis of *S100A4*/pSV2*neo*-transfected Rama 37 cells. There is strong staining of the elongated cells for S100A4. Bar = 17 μm. (Reproduced, with permission, from [35], ©1993, Macmillan Journals.)

rounding these, a minor component of more elongated cells. These tumours were highly invasive and invaded host skeletal muscle extensively [35].

Untransfected Rama 37 cells fluoresce only weakly with fluorescein-conjugated affinity-purified anti-S100A4 serum [35]. In contrast, the *S100A4/*pSV2*neo*-transfected cells contained abundant amounts of immunocytochemically detected S100A4 and possessed strongly immunofluorescing cytoplasmic filaments, particularly concentrated in the perinuclear region [35]. In dual-labelling experiments in which *S100A4*/pSV2*neo*-transfected cells were incubated simultaneously with tetramethylrhodamine isothiocyanate–phalloidin and fluorescein isothiocyanate-conjugated S100A4 antibodies, the staining patterns were virtually identical. The S100A4 immunofluorescence was completely abolished by preincubation of the antibodies with S100A4 protein [35]. These results strongly suggest that, in the transfected cells, the S100A4 is associating with the microfilamental cytoskeleton. Such results are consistent with experiments *in vitro* which suggest that S100A4 can bind to components of the cytoskeleton, i.e. actin [37], tropomyosin [38] and non-muscle myosin [39].

The human gene for S100A4 has been similarly transfected into benign Rama 37 cells, and has the same metastasis-inducing properties as rat *S100A4* in these cells. However, the metastases arising from transfection with the human *S100A4* gene, which occur predominantly in the lungs, tend to be slower-growing than those arising from transfer of the rat *S100A4* gene (B.H. Lloyd and R. Barraclough, unpublished work).

The rat *S100A4* gene induces metastasis in breast tumours when expressed in transgenic mice

Transgenic mice [40] containing 17 copies of the same rat *S100A4* gene construct that had induced metastasis in the benign rat mammary cell lines do not show any metastatic phenotype, despite rat S100A4 being expressed at a level greater than that which induces metastatic capability in the benign rat mammary tumour cells [35]. This result is consistent with S100A4 co-operating with other changes that have occurred in the immortal benign rat mammary cells but which are not present in the cells of the transgenic mouse. One such change concerns the c-*erbB-2* gene, the product of which is overexpressed on the cell membrane in 20–30% of human breast cancers, and is an indicator of a poor prognosis [41,42]. In order to find out whether such a change in benign mammary tumour cells might co-operate with the *S100A4* gene, the transgenic mice containing the additional *S100A4* genes have been mated with mice transgenic for the activated rodent c-*erbB-2* gene, *neu*, under the control of the mouse mammary tumour virus promoter to produce mouse strains that are bi-transgenic for *S100A4* and activated c-*erbB-2* (*neu*).

Of the mice transgenic for *neu*, 50% produced tumours by 14 months. Although some *neu*-positive cells were present in the lungs, these small clusters of cells were confined to the blood vessels. In contrast, bi-transgenic offspring containing both the *neu* and *S100A4* transgenes yielded tumours that formed metastases in the lungs of affected mice; these metastatic lesions were not surrounded by a complete basement membrane, indicating their invasive properties [43]. These experiments with transgenic mice are important because they show that *S100A4* induces metastatic capability in cells that are already tumorigenic, but not in normal cells.

S100A4 is elevated in malignant relative to benign human breast cancers, and is associated with distant metastasis and not with local recurrence

In order to find out whether the results with S100A4 in the model systems have identified a molecule that is relevant in human breast cancer, the levels of S100A4 were sought in a range of benign and malignant human mammary cell lines and tumour specimens. In order to quantify the levels more precisely, relative S100A4 mRNA levels were measured. A cloned DNA corresponding to exons 2 and 3 of the human *S100A4* gene [32] hybridized in Northern blotting experiments to a 760 bp mRNA corresponding to that for human S100A4. The results clearly showed that the mRNA for S100A4 is expressed at a 3–25-fold higher level in cultured invasive ductal carcinoma cell lines derived from pleural effusions than in SV40-immortalized normal human breast epithelial cell lines, or in cell lines derived from a benign human breast lesion (B.H. Lloyd and R. Barraclough, unpublished work). A similar result was found when human breast tumour specimens were examined (Fig. 3). For tumour specimens, relative levels of S100A4 mRNA were quantified and normalized using a previously described procedure [44]. In 144 breast lesions (113 invasive ductal carcinomas, 11 carcinomas *in situ*, five samples of fibrocystic disease and 15 samples of fibroadenoma), there was a statistically significantly higher mean level of S100A4 mRNA in the invasive carcinomas than in the benign lesions. In this regard, ductal carcinoma *in situ* resembled the invasive carcinomas. In a previous preliminary panel of 15 tumour specimens, high levels of S100A4 were correlated strongly with the level of urokinase-like plasminogen activator [45]. In the larger sample, there was an inverse correlation between S100A4 mRNA levels and the level of immunocytochemically detected oestrogen receptor, suggesting also a correlation between S100A4 levels and a more malignant tumour phenotype in human breast cancer. However, despite this correlation, when all 124 invasive carcinoma specimens were included, there was no significant correlation between the level of S100A4 mRNA and the number of affected lymph nodes, the most commonly used indicator of a poor prognosis in breast cancer. However, for patients who suffered early recurrence of their disease at a distant site, for example in lungs, bone or brain, the level of S100A4 was predictive of the time to the recurrence of the disease, whereas in those patients with local recurrence, for example in breast, skin or local lymph nodes, there was no relationship between S100A4 mRNA levels and the event-free interval. These results suggest that, as in the

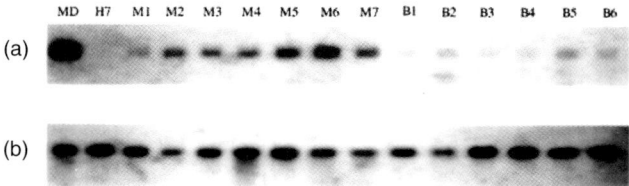

Fig. 3. mRNA for S100A4 in specimens of human breast tumours.
RNA, isolated from benign and malignant human tumour specimens, was subjected to agarose-gel electrophoresis and blotted on to Nylon filters. The filters were incubated with radioactively labelled probes corresponding to mRNAs for human S100A4 (a) and ribosomal protein 36B4 (b). Radioactive bands were visualized by autoradiography. The level of the ribosomal protein mRNA is similar in each sample, indicating equal loading. The level of the mRNA for S100A4 is markedly lower in the benign (B1–B6) than in the malignant (M1–M7) samples. MD and H7 refer to RNA from malignant MDA-MB-231 [72] and benign Huma7 [49] human mammary epithelial cells respectively.

rodent model systems, elevated levels of S100A4 mRNA in human cancers might be closely associated with dissemination to distant sites in the body. At the present time, the molecular basis underlying such a correlation is unknown.

Metastatic cells contain non-coding sequences in their DNA that can induce metastatic capability in non-metastatic benign rat mammary epithelial cells

In contrast to the recipient benign Rama 37 cells, the closely related malignant rat mammary cell line Rama 800 [46] forms primary tumours at a high incidence when injected into the mammary fat pads of syngeneic rats, and metastases appear in the lungs and lymph nodes of about 50% of tumour-bearing rats [46]. When Rama 37 cells were transfected with HindIII-cut genomic DNA from this metastatic cell line, there was a 90% incidence of primary tumours, and metastases occurred in a proportion of these animals (Table 2). In experiments under identical conditions in which pSV2neo alone or in which HindIII-cut salmon sperm DNA replaced the Rama 800 DNA, or in which a plasmid construct containing the polyoma large-T antigen gene was used, there were no metastases detectable [47]. The results of this experiment show that, in the Rama system, as in other systems [5–12,14], the ability to metastasize in vivo is transferable with the DNA of metastatic cells. The metastatic capability was maintained after culture and re-injection of cells from metastases and primary cultures (Fig. 4).

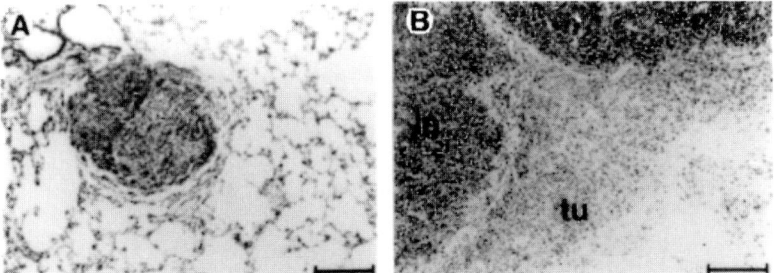

Fig. 4. Metastases produced by Rama 37 cells transfected with DNA from a metastatic rat mammary cell line. Rama 37 cells were transfected with DNA from the metastatic cell line Rama 800, and injected subcutaneously into the mammary glands. Tumours arose which metastasized to the lungs and/or lymph nodes. (A) Cells of a lymph node metastasis were cultured and injected subcutaneously into the mammary fat pad. A resulting metastasis in the lung is shown. (B) A cell line was obtained from a metastatic primary tumour in the mammary gland and injected subcutaneously into the mammary fat pad. A metastasis in a lymph node is shown in which tumour cells (tu) have breached the capsule and are beginning to invade from the edge of the lymph node (ln). Bar = 200 μm. (Reproduced, with permission, from [47], ©1990, Academic Press.)

Table 2. The metastatic phenotype can be induced by transfecting benign Rama 37 cells with DNA from malignant rat and human mammary tumours. Data are from [47][1], [24][2] and [21][3]. Tumour incidence is defined as the number of tumours/number of sites injected. Latent periods are given as means, with ranges in parentheses. The incidence of metastases is defined as the number of animals with metastases/number of animals with tumours. Significance of differences was as follows: [4]significantly more tumours than Rama 37 (P<0.001; Fisher exact test); [5]significantly less tumours than Rama 37 (P<0.05; Fisher exact test); [6]significantly shorter latent period than Rama 37 (P<0.05; Mann–Whitney U-test); [7]significantly more metastases than Rama 37 cells and HMT 3522/pSV2neo (Rama 37) (P<0.005) and Huma 7/neo (Rama 37) (P<0.01; Fisher exact test); [8]significantly more metastases than Rama 37 cells and HMT 3522/pSV2neo (Rama 37) (P<0.001) and Huma 7/neo (Rama 37) (P<0.01; Fisher exact test).

Transfecting DNA (cell line)	Phenotype of DNA source	Incidence of tumours	Latent period in days (range)	Incidence of metastasis
Experiment I				
None (Rama 37)[1]	—	36/74	44 (41–87)	0/36
None (Rama 800)[2]	—	12/12	55 (46–73)	5/12[9]
Salmon sperm/pSV2neo (Rama 37)[1]	Non-malignant	20/36	43 (25–62)	0/20
Rama 800/pSV2neo (Rama 37)[1]	Malignant	91/100[4]	19 (6–83)[6]	7/91
Experiment 2				
None (Rama 37)[3]	—	22/46	33 (24–81)	0/20
pSV2neo (Rama 37)[3]	Non-malignant	6/15	29 (14–43)	0/6
Salmon sperm/pSV2neo (Rama 37)[3]	Non-malignant	7/11	43 (25–62)	0/7
HMT 3522/pSV2neo (Rama 37)[3]	Non-malignant	28/85[5]	24 (20–31)	0/20
Huma 7/pSV2neo (Rama 37)[3]	Non-malignant	17/66[5]	22 (14–28)	0/10
Ca2-83/pSV2neo (Rama 37)[3]	Malignant	43/89	26 (12–68)	9/26[7]
MCF-7/pSV2neo (Rama 37)[3]	Malignant	32/82	27 (14–53)	8/16[8]
ZR-75-1/pSV2neo (Rama 37)[3]	Malignant	21/62	24 (20–43)	1/12

[9]Metastases in right axillary lymph node.

When *Hind*III-fragmented DNA from human breast cell lines of benign origin (HMT 3522 [48] or Huma 7 [49]) was transfected into Rama 37 cells and the transfectants tested in the metastasis assay, there was no evidence of metas-

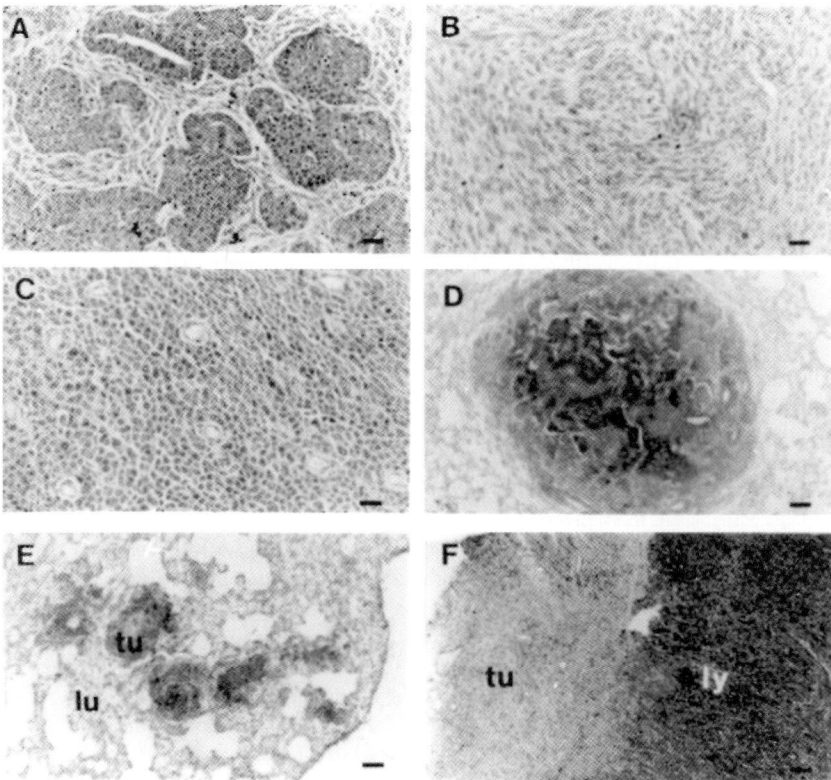

Fig. 5. Histology of tumours produced by untransfected Rama 37 cells and Rama 37 cells transfected with fragmented DNA from malignant human tumour cell lines. (A) Glandular primary tumour arising from the injection of untransfected Rama 37 cells into the mammary gland, consists of a mixture of epithelial cells often surrounding a central duct-like structure and spindle cells. (B) A primary tumour consisting of spindle cells produced by Rama 37 cells transfected with fragmented DNA from the malignant human breast tumour cell line Ca2-83. (C) A primary tumour consisting of cells intermediate in morphology between cuboidal and spindle cells produced by Rama 37 cells transfected with fragmented DNA from the malignant human breast tumour cell line MCF-7. (D) A cannon-ball metastasis in the lung of a rat injected with Rama 37 cells transfected with fragmented DNA from the malignant human breast tumour cell line Ca2-83. (E) Multiple micrometastases (tu) in the lung (lu) of a rat injected with Rama 37 cells transfected with fragmented DNA from the malignant human breast tumour cell line MCF-7. (F) Metastasis (tu) and lymphocytes (ly) in the lymph node of a rat injected with Rama 37 cells transfected with fragmented DNA from the malignant human breast tumour cell line Ca2-83. Scale bars: (A)–(C), 17 μm; (D)–(F), 70 μm. (Reproduced, with permission, from [21], ©1994, American Association for Cancer Research.)

tasis, despite primary tumours forming in 28/85 and17/66 injected sites respectively (Table 2). With DNA from one of two cell lines of malignant breast tumour origin (Ca2-83 [50] or MCF-7 [51]), the tumour incidence was similar to that with the benign cells, but metastases occurred in 9/26 and 8/16 tumour-bearing rats respectively, indicating that transfection of the human DNA has the metastasis-inducing effect observed with the DNA from metastatic rat cells. In these experiments, controls in which similarly fragmented salmon sperm DNA was co-transfected with pSV2neo failed to yield any metastases (Table 2). These experiments show that DNA from human malignant cells, but not from human benign cells, can induce metastatic capability in non-metastatic rat mammary cells.

The primary tumours produced by the DNA from the human malignant tumours were undifferentiated and anaplastic, consisting of spindle cells or cells intermediate in morphology between cuboidal, epithelial-like and spindle cells (Fig. 5). These were in marked contrast to the glandular elements of the

Table 3. The ability to induce metastatic capability is stable in cells cultured from primary tumours and metastases. Data are from [21]. DNA from the benign or malignant cell lines shown was co-transfected into Rama 37 cells with pSV2neo. The transfected cells were subjected to the metastasis assay. Cells from primary tumours and metastases were cultured and subjected to the metastasis assay. The results from this assay are shown. Tumour incidence is defined as the number of tumours/number of sites injected. Latent periods are given as means, with ranges in parentheses. The incidence of metastases is defined as the number of animals with metastases/ number of animals with tumours. Significantly more tumours than Rama 37 cells (Fisher exact test): *$P<0.05$; **$P<0.01$. †Significantly shorter latent period than Rama 37 and the original transfected cell pool from which the cells were derived ($P<0.001$; Mann–Whitney U test). Significantly more metastases than Rama 37 cells and benign HMT 3522 transfectants (Fisher exact test): ‡$P<0.05$; ‡‡$P<0.01$.

Transfecting DNA and source	Tumour incidence	Median latent period in days (range)	Incidence of metastasis
HMT-3522 (benign), primary tumour	18/18**	11 (9–12)†	0/18
Ca2-83 (malignant), lung metastasis	23/29*	5 (–)†	6/18‡
Ca2-83 (malignant), lung metastasis	28/28**	6 (4–8)†	3/24
Ca2-83 (malignant), lung metastasis	18/31	7 (4–9)†	4/13‡
Ca2-83 (malignant), lymph node metastasis	27/29**	7 (5–13)†	5/16‡
ZR-75 (malignant), lung metastasis	16/23	7 (5–7)†	7/12‡‡
MCF-7 (malignant), lung metastasis	24/24**	6 (–)†	3/20

tumours arising from the parental Rama 37 cells (Fig. 5A) or the elongated/spindle cells of benign morphology with occasional cords or nests of cuboidal epithelial cells reminiscent of the glandular structures that characterized the tumours produced by controls in which Rama 37 cells were transfected with salmon sperm DNA (results not shown).

Geneticin-resistant cell lines derived from primary tumours and from lung and lymph node metastases, when subjected to the metastasis assay, yielded primary tumours that had a somewhat shorter latent period than those that had arisen directly from the transfected cells. However, cell lines established from lung or lymph node metastases arising from Rama 37 cells transfected with Ca2-83 or MCF-7 DNA yielded metastases at about the same frequency as the primary transfectants, whereas cell lines isolated from the primary tumours that arose from injection of cells transfected with DNA from benign human tumours (e.g. HMT 3522) failed to yield any metastases after isolation and culture *in vitro* (Table 3). These results, taken together, suggest that the metastatic capability can be transferred in a dominant manner from the DNA of malignant human breast cancer cell lines to the benign Rama 37 cells, and that the DNA sequences responsible are maintained in an active form, at least in some of the cells, during the formation of metastases and cell culture.

The induction of the metastatic phenotype in the transfected Rama 37 cells might arise from the activity of a protein coding gene. However, this appears unlikely for two reasons. First, the DNA had been fragmented by digestion with *Hind*III prior to being transfected, and secondly, the frequency

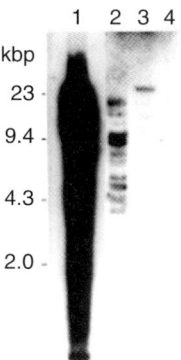

Fig. 6. Human DNA sequences are stably incorporated into the genomes of Rama 37 cells co-transfected with human DNA and pSV2neo. DNA isolated from cell lines was fragmented with the restriction enzyme *Hind*III and subjected to agarose-gel electrophoresis, Southern blotting and hybridization to an oligonucleotide probe corresponding to the primate-specific region of *alu* repetitive DNA. The probe hybridized strongly to DNA isolated from a human benign breast cell line (lane 1), and also to DNA from cell lines isolated from a lung metastasis arising from rat Rama 37 cells transfected with DNA from the human malignant mammary cell lines Ca2-83 (lane 2) or ZR-75 (lane 3). There was no hybridization to DNA from the recipient cell line Rama 37 (lane 4). (Reproduced, with permission, from [21], © 1994, American Association for Cancer Research.)

of occurrence of metastases in the Rama 37 cells caused by DNA from malignant rat or human breast cells occurs at too high a frequency (1–3%) to be due to the activity of a single-copy gene (estimated frequency 0.1%) [52]. Thus it is likely that it is non-coding human DNA that is involved. The presence of human DNA sequences within the genomic DNA of Geneticin-resistant cell lines isolated from metastases (Fig. 6) was shown by Southern blots using an oligonucleotide probe specific for the second monomer of primate *Alu* repeats, that does not cross-hybridize with any rat repetitive elements [21]. Rescue of the human sequences for possible identification was achieved by a novel tagging procedure.

Rescue and characterization of the metastasis-causing DNA sequences (MetDNA) from the genomes of transfected cells

DNA from a cell line (Ca2-LT1) isolated from a lung metastasis arising from Ca2-83-transfected Rama 37 cells was cut with the restriction enzyme *Hin*dIII, and double-stranded synthetic oligonucleotide 'tag' sequences (Fig. 7) were ligated to both ends of the DNA fragments. The tagged fragmented DNA was co-transfected into recipient Rama 37 cells. These tags (Fig. 7) provide restriction enzyme sites for the excision of transfected DNA fragments from the genome of the transfected cells, and specific primer sequences for amplification by PCR of sequences between the tags directly from DNA isolated from tumours and metastases. As a control, *Hin*dIII-fragmented DNA from a cell line isolated from a tumour originating from Rama 37 cells co-transfected with DNA from the benign human breast cell line HMT 3522 was also tagged. Tagged or untagged metastatic DNA, or tagged DNA from the benign cells, was transfected into Rama 37 cells and the resultant transfectants tested for metastatic capability (Table 4). The results clearly show that the tagging does not affect the ability of metastatic DNA to induce metastasis in the benign Rama 37 cells, and that the tagging process itself does not make the fragmented benign cell DNA metastatic (Table 4).

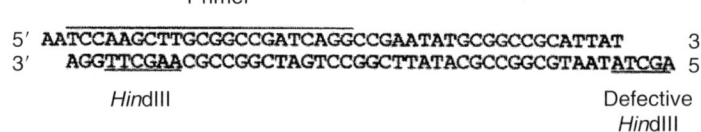

Primer

5′ AATCCAAGCTTGCGGCCGATCAGGCCGAATATGCGGCCGCATTAT   3′
3′   AGGTTCGAACGCCGGCTAGTCCGGCTTATACGCCGGCGTAATATCGA 5′

       *Hin*dIII   Defective
                                                               *Hin*dIII

Fig. 7. Double-stranded synthetic oligonucleotide sequences used to tag fragmented DNA prior to transfection into the Rama 37 cell line. The synthetic tag DNA contains a 3′ end consisting of the *Hin*dIII overhang for ligation to the *Hin*dIII-digested DNA, but without re-creating the *Hin*dIII site. An alternative *Hin*dIII site is provided near the 5′ end of the tag. The PCR primer used to amplify the tagged DNA from the genomes of transfected cells is overscored.

Table 4. Effect of tagging on the induction of metastases by DNA from benign and malignant cells, and rescue of metastasis-inducing DNA from transfected Rama 37 cells. To analyse the effect of tagging, DNA fragmented with *Hind*III from either a metastatic or a benign cell line, either with the synthetic DNA tag ligated to each end (tagged) or not (untagged), was transfected into benign Rama 37 cells and subjected to the metastasis assay. For rescue of tagged fragments, DNA from tagged metastatic transfectants was subjected to amplification by PCR using the primer shown in Fig. 7, and the PCR products were subjected to agarose-gel electrophoresis, purified and transfected into Rama 37 cells. *Significantly more metastases than Rama 37 cells ($P<0.05$; Fisher exact test).

Donor DNA	No. of rats	Tumours (%)	Metastases (%)
(a) Effect of tagging			
None	46	48	0
Untagged metastatic	31	77	17*
Tagged metastatic	37	78	21
Tagged benign	39	79	0
(b) Rescue of tagged fragments			
PCR fragment 1	30	93	43*
PCR fragment 2	40	90	25*

Cell lines were isolated from cultures of lung metastases arising from transfection of tagged and untagged DNA, and high-molecular-mass DNA was isolated. Amplification of the DNA between the tags by PCR was carried out using the primer contained in the tag sequence shown in Fig. 7. Two discrete but broad bands of approx. 1.0–1.4 kbp in size, termed F1 and F2, were obtained when the PCR products were subjected to agarose-gel electrophoresis. When these fragments were co-transfected with pSV2*neo* into Rama 37 cells and the transfectants introduced into mammary fat pads, significant metastasis was obtained (Table 4), strongly suggesting that these amplified bands contain DNA sequences that are active in the metastasis assay.

In order to find out whether the PCR fragments derived from F1 or F2 represented one or more sequences, the pooled PCR fragments were cloned into a plasmid vector and then the nucleotide sequences of individual cloned DNAs were determined. Only six different sequences were represented in the 30 clones examined. Co-transfection of representative samples of these six cloned sequences into Rama 37 cells with pSV2*neo* gave rise to transfected cells which produced mammary tumours with an incidence of 100% of the animals and metastases in the lungs with frequencies ranging from 12% to 50% of tumours. pSV2*neo* alone yielded tumours in only 50% of the animals, and there were no metastases.

Comparison of the six nucleotide sequences with entries in the GenBank nucleotide sequence database and with the eukaryotic promoter database yielded no exact matches with previously sequenced rat or human DNA. A comparison of the open reading frames over 50 amino acids in length occurring in the three forward and the three reverse translation frames from the six metastasis-inducing sequences failed to show any significant identity with existing proteins. This result is supported by Northern blotting experiments in which radioactive probes corresponding to the six MetDNA sequences failed to detect any mRNAs in the transfected metastatic cells. It is therefore unlikely that the MetDNAs are dominantly acting expressed genes that induce metastasis in a manner analogous to that of the dominantly acting oncogenes. More likely, MetDNAs act in the broadest sense in a regulatory capacity, albeit in an as yet unidentified manner. All six MetDNAs contain recognition sequences for transcription factors TCF-1 [53] and H1P1b [54], and all but one contain recognition sites for CTCF [55], H1P1a [54] and NF-IL6 [56]. All but one MetDNA sequence contain regions of Z-DNA [57]. One of the MetDNAs contains a sequence with 85–90% identity with a 102-nucleotide fragment of the rat whey acidic protein promoter [58], 30 nucleotides of which are duplicated in the MetDNA. Since the MetDNAs do not encode expressed mRNAs, it is possible that MetDNAs induce metastasis by affecting the level of the product of one or more critical metastasis-inducing genes.

MetDNA is associated with changes in the level of osteopontin and its mRNA, and osteopontin can induce the metastatic phenotype in Rama 37 cells

The technique of subtractive hybridization was employed [59–61] to identify cDNAs that are expressed at a markedly higher or lower level in Rama 37 cells than in a cell line (Ca2-LT1) isolated from a lung metastasis arising from Rama 37 cells transfected with DNA from the metastatic cell line Ca2-83 [50]. A cDNA library from the Ca2-LT1 cells subtracted with copy RNA corresponding to mRNA from the Rama 37 cells contained about 2000 cloned cDNAs [62]. Individual cloned cDNAs were screened on Northern blots to identify those that were differentially expressed. One particular clone, which was expressed at a 9 ± 1.2-fold higher level than in the Rama 37 cells, possessed over 99% identity with the mRNA for rat osteopontin [61]. Of the total number of cloned DNAs analysed in the subtracted library, 21% were cDNAs to rat osteopontin [61]. Using Northern blots, the level of the mRNA for osteopontin was found to be elevated 5.7–9-fold in three independent cell lines formed from the transfection of Rama 37 cells with DNA from the metastatic cell line Ca2-83 (Table 5). Furthermore, the spontaneously metastatic rat mammary cell line Rama 800 also exhibited an elevated level of osteopontin mRNA (Table 5). Immunocytochemical staining of tumours for osteopontin showed that osteopontin is expressed in primary mammary tumours and lung metastases arising from the transfection of Rama 37 cells with DNA from the malignant human tumour cell line Ca2-83, but that it is not detectable in mammary tumours arising from the recipient Rama 37 cell line (Fig. 8).

A full-length cloned cDNA for rat osteopontin mRNA obtained from the subtracted library (see above) was subcloned under the control of the cytomegalovirus intermediate early promoter into the *neo*-gene-containing phagemid expression vector pBKCMV [61]. Although the recipient Rama 37

Table 5. Levels of osteopontin mRNA in various malignant meta-static cell lines relative to that in the recipient Rama 37 cells. Levels of osteopontin mRNA were quantified by densitometry from hybridization signals on Northern blots relative to a constitutive non-muscle actin as a loading control. The corrected levels of osteopontin mRNA are expressed relative to the level in Rama 37 cells. Results are means ± S.E.M. of four determinations.

Source of cell line	Type of tumour	Relative level of osteopontin mRNA
Rama 37	Benign, non-metastatic	1.0
Lung metastasis arising from Rama 37 cells transfected with Ca2-83 DNA		
Line 1	Malignant, metastatic	9.0 ± 1.2
Line 2	Malignant, metastatic	7.6 ± 0.7
Lymph node metastasis arising from Rama 37 cells transfected with Ca2-83 DNA	Malignant, metastatic	5.7 ± 0.7
Rama 800 from a spontaneously metastatic rat mammary tumour	Malignant, metastatic	3.9 ± 0.6
Lymph node metastasis arising from Rama 37 cells transfected with the *S100A4* gene	Malignant, metastatic	0.9 ± 0.1

cells express mRNA for osteopontin, the geneticin-resistant transfectants expressed variable, but higher, levels of osteopontin mRNA, ranging from 1.4 to 6 times that in Rama 37 cells. Using Western blotting, it was shown that the levels of osteopontin reflected the levels of its mRNA. No metastases were obtained when Rama 37 cells were transfected with the pCMV-1 plasmid alone. However, when two of the pCMV.osteopontin transfectants, one expressing 6 times and one expressing 1.4 times the level of osteopontin mRNA in Rama 37 cells, were subjected to the metastasis assay, metastases were obtained with the former but not with the latter [61]. Primary tumours and metastases derived from the former transfectant expressed immunocytochemically detectable osteopontin (Fig. 8). These results strongly suggest that, in the present cell system, an elevation of the level of osteopontin of 4–6-fold is sufficient to induce metastasis. Cell lines isolated from a MetDNA-induced lung metastasis yielded metastases when injected into the mammary fat pads of syngeneic rats, showing stable induction of metastatic capability. These cell lines also possess elevated levels of osteopontin mRNA relative to the parental Rama

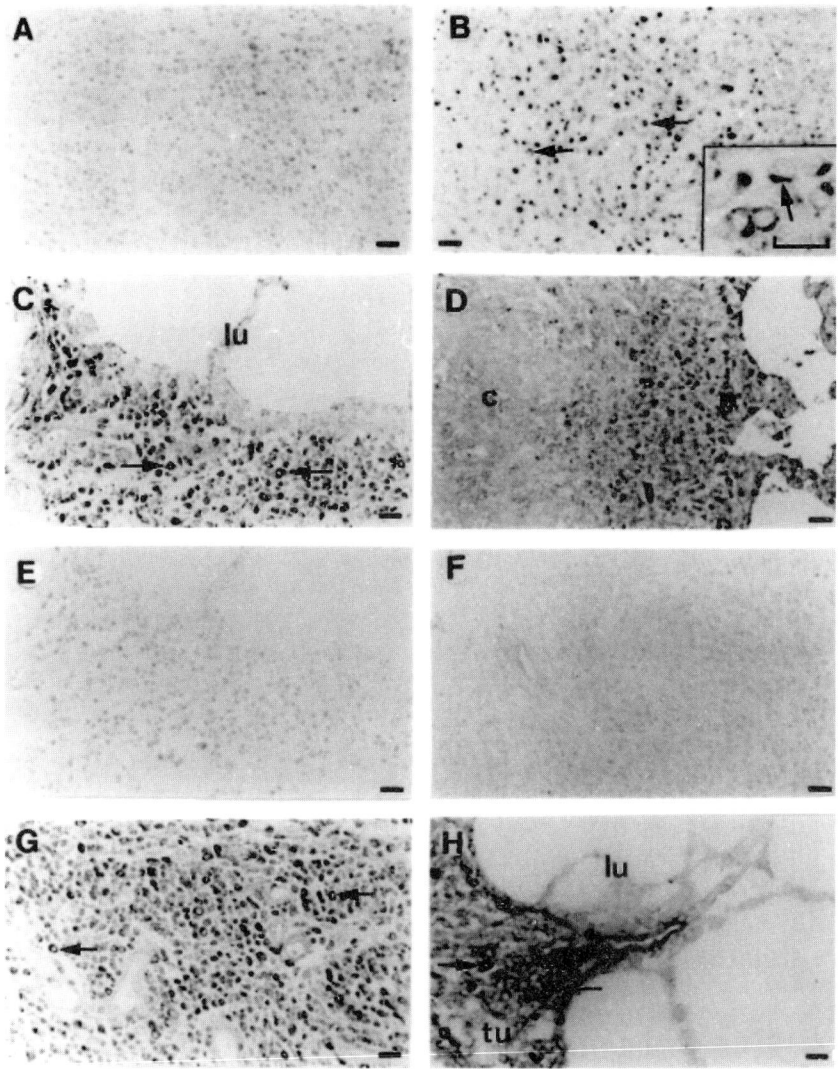

Fig. 8. Immunocytochemical staining of rat tumours and metastases for osteopontin. (A) A primary tumour arising from the injection of non-transfected Rama 37 cells into the mammary gland, showing no immunocytochemically detectable osteopontin. (B) Immunocytochemical staining of a primary tumour produced by Ca2-LT1 (the cell line used to construct the subtracted library that yielded osteopontin cDNA) confirms the presence of osteopontin (arrows). The inset shows the cytoplasmic and cell surface staining (arrow). (C) Virtually all the cells of a lung metastasis arising from injection of Ca2-LT1 stain for osteopontin (arrows), but there is little staining of the adjacent lung tissue. (D) In a lung metastasis there is an increasing gradient of staining ☞

37 cells, further strengthening the link between MetDNA and the elevation of osteopontin in the induction of metastasis in this system. The mechanism whereby non-coding MetDNAs raise osteopontin mRNA levels is at present unknown.

Osteopontin is an extracellularly located phosphoprotein with calcium binding properties [63]. In normal rat tissues, osteopontin is detected immuno-cytochemically in such tissues as lactating mammary gland, bladder and pancreas, as well as in bone [62]. Generally, staining is associated with the surfaces of epithelial cells and osteoblasts/osteoclasts [62], a distribution consistent with the proposed interaction of osteopontin with $\alpha v \beta 3$ integrin (vitronectin receptor) via a GRGDS binding site [64]. However, osteopontin has been associated previously with tumorigenesis and metastasis. In *ras*-transformed NIH 3T3 cells, the levels of osteopontin mRNA and protein correlate with the tumorigenic and metastatic potentials of the cells [65]. Although it is not known whether these correlations represent a causal relationship between osteopontin levels and metastasis *in vivo*, decreasing the levels of osteopontin using antisense technology has been reported to reduce the malignancy of these *ras*-transformed 3T3 cells *in vitro* [66], suggesting causality, at least in the culture situation.

Summary and conclusions

DNA transfer techniques have been employed to identify DNA sequences that can induce metastatic capability in benign mammary epithelial cells. The sequences isolated are not previously described oncogenes, but probably act by raising the level of an effector protein, a metastasis-associated extracellular calcium binding protein, osteopontin. Although there is a strong correlation between osteopontin levels and metastasis in model systems, it is not yet clear how osteopontin increases metastatic capability *in vivo*. It has been suggested that the correlation between osteopontin and metastatic potential in murine 3T3 fibroblasts arises from protection afforded to the cells by osteopontin against macrophage NO-mediated cytotoxicity [67]. However, osteopontin is associated with $\alpha v \beta 3$ integrin [64,68] and possibly with other integrins [69], and it is likely that the elevated levels of osteopontin might play a role in metastatic capability through an effect on cell adhesion [63] or cell motility/migration [63,70].

☞ **Fig. 8. (contd.)** from the centre (c) of the tumour to the periphery (p). (E) An adjacent section to (D) treated with osteopontin antibody blocked with antigen shows no staining. (F) A primary tumour arising from Rama 37 cells transfected with plasmid pBKCMV does not stain for osteopontin. (G) A primary tumour arising from injection of Rama 37 cells transfected with plasmid pBKCMV.osteopontin stains intensely for osteopontin. (H) A lung metastasis (tu) arising from injection of Rama 37 cells transfected with plasmid pBKCMV.osteopontin stains intensely for osteopontin (arrows), but there is little staining of adjacent lung tissue (lu). Scale bars = 18 μm (insert in B 19 μm). (Reproduced, with permission, from [61], © 1996, Macmillan Journals.)

Rama 37 cells can also acquire metastatic capability by expressing at an elevated level the gene for an intracellular cytoskeleton-associated calcium binding protein, S100A4 (p9Ka), which is probably involved in the regulation of cell motility [37–39]. Since cells transfected with the *S100A4* gene do not express increased levels of osteopontin, it is possible that S100A4 and osteopontin provide alternative routes towards metastatic capability in benign mammary cells. It is likely from the known properties of S100A4 and osteopontin that these routes affect cell motility/migration. That evidence is beginning to accumulate of an independent association between the levels of S100A4 (B.H. Lloyd and R. Barraclough, unpublished work) or of osteopontin [71] and human breast cancer suggests that both the S100A4 and osteopontin routes might be relevant to the development of breast cancers in humans.

We thank Glaxo Inc., the Ludwig Institute for Cancer Research and the North West Cancer Research Fund for past financial support, the Cancer and Polio Research Fund for past and present support, and the Medical Research Council for research studentships to B.R.D. and A.O.

References

1.   Cavenee, W. and White, R. (1995) Sci. Am. **March**, 50–57
2.   Weinberg, R. (1989) Cancer Res. **49**, 3713–3721
3.   Schor, S.L., Schor, A.M., Winn, B. and Rushton, G. (1982) Int. J. Cancer **29**, 57–62
4.   Isoai, A., Giga-Hama, Y., Shinkai, K., Mukai, M., Akedo, H. and Kumagai, H. (1992) Cancer Res. **52**, 1422–1426
5.   Gibbins, J., Nicholson, T. and Vozab, R. (1987) Proc. Aust. New Zeal. Soc. Cell Biol., L41
6.   Gibbins, J., Nicholson, T., Vozab, R., Ying, B. and Messerle, K. (1991) Anticancer Res. **11**, 129–138
7.   Glenn, J., McDonald, D., Horetsky, R. and Sexton, F. (1987) J. Surg. Res. **44**, 382–390
8.   Sorenson, G., Pettengill, O., Cate, C. and Pribish, D. (1988) Proc. Am. Assoc. Cancer Res. **29**, 61
9.   Ananthaswamy, H., Price, J., Goldberg, L. and Bales, E. (1988) J. Cell. Biochem. **36**, 137–146
10.   Radler-Pohl, A., Pohl, J. and Schirrmacher, V. (1988) Int. J. Cancer **41**, 840–846
11.   Tarin, D. (1988) Ciba Found. Symp. **141**, 149–169
12.   Thorgeirsson, U., Turpeenniemi-Hujanen, T., Williams, J., Westin, E., Heilman, C., Talmadge, J. and Liotta, L. (1985) Mol. Cell. Biol. **5**, 259–262
13.   Pickford, I. and Franks, L. (1988) Cancer Surv. **7**, 351–371
14.   Van Roy, F., Messiaen, L., Leibaut, G., Gao, J., Dragonetti, C., Fiers, W. and Marel, M. (1986) Cancer Res. **46**, 4787–4795
15.   Kasid, U., Weichselbaum, R., Brennan, T., Mark, G. and Dritschilo, A. (1989) Cancer Res. **49**, 3396–3400
16.   Kerbel, R., Waghorne, C., Man, H.S., Elliott, B. and Breitman, M. (1987) Proc. Natl. Acad. Sci. U.S.A. **84**, 1263–1267
17.   Verelle, P., Lescaut, V., Poupon, M. and Hillova, J. (1987) Anticancer Res. **7**, 181–186
18.   Vousden, K.H., Eccles, S.A., Purvies, H. and Marshall, C.J. (1986) Int. J. Cancer **37**, 425–433
19.   Waghorne, C., Kerbel, R. and Breitman, M. (1987) Oncogene **1**, 149–155
20.   Sharkey, F. and Fogh, J. (1979) Int. J. Cancer **24**, 733–738
21.   Davies, B.R., Barraclough, R. and Rudland, P.S. (1994) Cancer Res. **54**, 2785–2793

22. Dunnington, D.J., Monaghan, P., Hughes, C.M. and Rudland, P.S. (1983) J. Natl. Cancer Inst. **71**, 1227–1240

23. Graham, F.L. and van der Eb, E.S. (1973) Virology **52**, 456–467

24. Jamieson, S., Barraclough, B.R. and Rudland, P.S. (1990) Pathobiology **58**, 329–342

25. Southern, P.J. and Berg, P. (1982) J. Mol. Appl. Genet. **1**, 327–341

26. Mulligan, R.C. and Berg, P. (1980) Science **209**, 1422–1427

27. Hilt, D. and Kligman, D. (1991) in Novel Calcium-Binding Proteins: Fundamentals and Clinical Implications (Heizmann, C.W., ed.), pp. 65–103, Springer-Verlag, Berlin

28. Gibbs, F., Barraclough, R., Platt-Higgins, A., Rudland, P., Wilkinson, M. and Parry, E. (1995) J. Histochem. Cytochem. **43**, 169–180

29. Dunnington, D.J. (1984) Ph.D. Thesis, University of London

30. Barraclough, R., Dawson, K.J. and Rudland, P.S. (1984) Biochem. Biophys. Res. Commun. **120**, 351–358

31. Ebralidze, A., Tulchinsky, E., Grigorian, M., Afanayeva, A., Senin, V., Revazova, E. and Lukanidin, E. (1989) Genes Dev. **3**, l086–l093

32. Engelkamp, D., Schäfer, B.W., Mattei, M.G., Erne, P. and Heizmann, C.W. (1993) Proc. Natl. Acad. Sci. U.S.A. **90**, 6547–6551

33. Barraclough, R., Savin, J., Dube, S.K. and Rudland, P.S. (1987) J. Mol. Biol. **198**, 13–20

34. Tulchinsky, E.M., Grigorian, M.S., Ebralidze, A.K., Milshina, N.I. and Lukanidin, E.M. (1990) Gene **87**, 219–223

35. Davies, B.R., Davies, M.P.A., Gibbs, F.E.M., Barraclough, R. and Rudland, P.S. (1993) Oncogene **8**, 999–1008

36. Davies, B.R., Barraclough, R., Davies, M.P.A. and Rudland, P.S. (1993) Cell Biol. Int. **17**, 872–879

37. Watanabe, Y., Usada, N., Minami, H., et al. (1993) FEBS Lett. **324**, 51–55

38. Takenaga, K., Nakamura, Y., Sakiyama, S., Hasegawa, Y., Sato, K. and Endo, H. (1994) J. Cell Biol. **124**, 757–768

39. Ford, H. and Zain, S. (1995) Oncogene **10**, 1597–1605

40. Davies, M., Harris, S., Rudland, P. and Barraclough, R. (1995) DNA Cell Biol. **14**, 825–832

41. Slamon, D.J., Clark, G.M., Wong, S.G., Levin, W.J., Ullrich, A. and McGuire, W.L. (1987) Science **235**, 177–182

42. Winstanley, J., Cooke, T., Murray, G.D., et al. (1991) Br. J. Cancer **63**, 447–450

43. Davies, M.P.A., Rudland, P.S., Robertson, L., Parry, E.W., Jolicoeur, P. and Barraclough, R. (1996) Oncogene **13**, 1631–1637

44. Anandappa, S., Winstanley, J., Leinster, S., Green, B., Rudland, P. and Barraclough, R. (1994) Br. J. Cancer **69**, 772–776

45. Pedrocchi, M., Schäfer, B., Mueller, H., Eppenberger, U. and Heizmann, C. (1994) Int. J. Cancer **57**, 684–690

46. Dunnington, D.J., Kim, U., Hughes, C.M., Monaghan, P. and Rudland, P.S. (1984) Cancer Res. **44**, 5338–5346

47. Jamieson, S., Barraclough, R. and Rudland, P.S. (1990) Cell Biol. Int. Rep. **14**, 717–725

48. Briand, P., Petersen, O.W. and Van Deurs, B. (1987) In Vitro **23**, 181–188

49. Rudland, P.S., Ollerhead, G. and Barraclough, R. (1989) Dev. Biol. **136**, 167–180

50. Rudland, P.S., Hallowes, R.C., Cox, R.A., Ormerod, E.J. and Warburton, M.J. (1985) Cancer Res. **45**, 3864–3877

51. Soule, H., Vazquez, A., Long, A., Albert, S. and Brennan, M. (1973) J. Natl. Cancer Inst. **51**, 1409–1413

52. Bernstein, S. and Weinberg, R. (1985) Proc. Natl. Acad. Sci. U.S.A. **82**, 1726–1730

53. van de Wetering, M., Oosterwegel, M., Dooijes, D. and Clevers, H. (1991) EMBO J. **10**, 123–132

54. Means, A. and Farnham, P. (1990) Mol. Cell. Biol. **10**, 653–661

55.   Lobanenkov, V., Nicolas, R., Adler, V., Paterson, H., Klenova, E., Polotskaja, A. and Goodwin, G. (1990) Oncogene 5, 1743–1753

56.   Majello, B., Arcone, R., Toniatti, C. and Cilliberto, C. (1990) EMBO J. 9, 457–465

57.   Wang, A.-J., Quigley, G., Kolpak, F., Crawford, J., van Boom, J., van der Marel, G. and Rich, A. (1979) Nature (London) 282, 680–686

58.   Campbell, S. and Rosen, J. (1984) Nucleic Acids Res. 12, 8685–8697

59.   Rubenstein, L., Brice, A., Ciaranello, R., Denney, D., Porteus, M. and Usdin, T. (1990) Nucleic Acids Res. 18, 4833–4842

60.   Owens, G.P., Hahn, W.E. and Cohen, J.J. (1991) Mol. Cell. Biol. 11, 4177–4188

61.   Oates, A.J., Barraclough, R. and Rudland, P.S. (1996) Oncogene 13, 97–104

62.   Oates, A. (1995) Ph.D. Thesis, University of Liverpool

63.   Denhardt, D. and Guo, X. (1993) FASEB J. 7, 1475–1482

64.   Ross, F., Chappel, J., Alvarez, J.I., et al. (1993) J. Biol. Chem. 268, 9901–9907

65.   Craig, A., Bowden, G., Chambers, A., et al. (1990) Int. J. Cancer 46, 133–137

66.   Behrend, E.I., Craig, A.M., Wilson, S.M., Denhardt, D.T. and Chambers, A.F. (1994) Cancer Res. 54, 832–837

67.   Feng, B., Rollo, E. and Denhardt, D. (1995) Clin. Exp. Metastasis 13, 453–462

68.   Reinholt, F., Hultenby, K., Oldberg, A. and Heinegård, D. (1990) Proc. Natl. Acad. Sci. U.S.A. 87, 4473–4475

69.   Hu, D., Lin, E., Kovach, N., Hoyer, J. and Smith, J. (1995) J. Biol. Chem. 270, 26232–26238

70.   Liaw, L., Skinner, M., Raines, E., Ross, R., Cheresh, D., Schwartz, S. and Giachelli, C. (1995) J. Clin. Invest. 95, 713–724

71.   O'Malley, F., Harris, J., Doig, G., Kerkvliet, N., Saad, Z., Bautista, D., Tonkin, K. and Chambers, A. (1996) Lab. Invest. 74, 109

72.   Engel, L.W. and Young, N.A. (1978) Cancer Res. 38, 4327–4339

Biochem. Soc. Symp. **63**, 295–313
Printed in Great Britain

25

Matrix metalloproteinases and metastatic cancer

Mark I. Cockett[*]**, Gillian Murphy**[†]**, Mary L. Birch**[*]**,
James P. O'Connell**[*]**, Tom Crabbe**[*]**, Andy T. Millican**[*]**,
Ian R. Hart and Andrew J.P. Docherty**[*][‡]

[*]Celltech Research, Slough SL1 4EN, [†]Strangeways Research Laboratory,
Cambridge CB1 4RN, and [‡]Richard Dimbleby Department of Cancer Research,
St. Thomas's Hospital, London SE1 7EH, U.K.

Abstract

The rationale for matrix metalloproteinase (MMP) inhibition as a means to treat disease progression in breast cancer stems from the apparent involvement of MMPs in the hydrolysis of basement membranes during tumour cell invasion and subsequent metastasis. MMP-mediated matrix remodelling also appears to promote the growth of tumour cells, possibly by facilitating the proliferation and migration of endothelial cells and the neovascularization of tumour tissue. We found that transfection of the C127 breast cancer cell line by MMP-2 (gelatinase A), but not by MMP-1 or MMP-3 (collagenase and stromelysin respectively), gave rise to an invasive and metastatic phenotype. We were surprised to find that this phenotype depended not only on the catalytic properties of MMP-2 but also on properties associated with the MMP-2 non-catalytic C-terminal domain. Experiments with a synthetic gelatinase inhibitor revealed that a single dose could prevent the lungs of nude mice being colonized by the MMP-2 transfectants, and that the inhibitor had to be administered during or shortly after injection of the cells, indicating that an early event, such as the extravasation of the cells into the lung, is gelatinase-dependent in this system. In other studies employing long-term treatment with CT1746, an orally active gelatinase inhibitor, we have previously demonstrated a reduction in primary tumour growth rates, localized spread, and spontaneous metastasis, even when the treatment was commenced several days after tumour implantation. Furthermore, additive effects were recorded when gelatinase inhibitor therapy was combined with cytotoxic drug treatment. Since the gelatinase inhibitors can also inhibit bone resorption *in vitro*, these observations point to their potential for delaying disease recurrence and reducing rates of bone loss following conventional therapeutic strategies, in metastatic breast cancer.

Introduction

Tumour cell invasion and metastatic spread indicate a poor prognosis in cancer, and basement membrane hydrolysis is thought to be one of several events that occur during this process [1]. Several classes of proteinase are capable of such hydrolysis, but the matrix metalloproteinases (MMPs) have received particular attention [2], because their increased expression correlates with the invasiveness of several tumour types, including breast cancer [3–9]. More recently the manipulation of MMP expression by genetic means, or through the use of MMP inhibitors, has provided evidence in a variety of rodent models for a causal role for MMPs, not only in tumour cell invasion and metastasis but also in primary tumour growth [10–23]. The therapeutic potential of synthetic MMP inhibitors, some of which can be administered orally, is currently being evaluated in clinical trials involving a wide variety of cancer types [24,25].

The MMPs comprise a structurally related family of enzymes, of which 14 members have been identified in humans (Table 1 and Fig. 1) [26]. Although there is no evidence for what their true substrates are *in vivo*, it has been observed that, at physiological pH, these enzymes can degrade most of the extracellular proteins that support the structural integrity of connective tissue (Table 1). Stromelysins 1 and 2, matrilysin and gelatinases A and B are of potential interest in cancer because they can all cleave type IV collagen, a major component of basement membranes, although their precise cleavage positions do vary. More recent studies have localized gelatinase A and stromelysin 3 mRNA synthesis to the stromal cells surrounding tumours, whereas the protein was immunolocalized to the tumour [5–7,27–29]. This has led to speculation that malignant cells might switch on stromal cell synthesis of MMPs via tumour-cell-derived factors [30–32]. Whatever the cellular source, deregulated proteolytic activity within the matrix is likely to have profound local effects on the resident cell population through it leading to the loss of cell attachment sites or the localized release of sequestered growth factors and cytokines [32]. This view is supported by a number of elegant studies that have shown the importance of the co-ordinated expression of MMPs and tissue inhibitors of the MMPs (TIMPs) in the development and maintenance of normal breast morphology [33–36]. Finally, there is some evidence that the MMPs facilitate the migration of endothelial cells during the development of a tumour vasculature [37–41]. Such mechanisms may explain how the administration of an MMP inhibitor can delay the growth, or reduce the growth rate, of experimental tumours in rodent models.

Following secretion, the MMPs are controlled in part through their requirement for an activation event, which involves the autoproteolytic removal of the approx. 80-amino-acid propeptide (see Fig. 1). Once activated they are susceptible to inhibition by the tight non-covalently binding TIMPs, of which four have now been reported [42,43]. The propeptide does not appear

Table 1. The human MMP family. Molecular masses are for the human enzymes and are estimated by SDS/PAGE, or predicted without knowledge of their glycosylation status from the corresponding cDNAs (MT1–4-MMPs). Macrophage elastase is activated spontaneously in the absence of EDTA to a 22 kDa form which lacks the C-terminal domain [82].

Enzyme	MMP no.	Molecular mass (kDa)		Matrix substrates
		Latent	Active	
Interstitial collagenase	MMP-1	55	43	Collagen types I, II, III, VII and X, gelatin (limited), proteoglycan core protein
Neutrophil collagenase	MMP-8	75	58	Collagen types I, II and III, gelatin (limited), proteoglycan core protein
Collagenase 3	MMP-13	65	55	Collagen types I and IV, gelatin, proteoglycan, fibronectin, tenascin, and probably other extracellular matrix components
Gelatinase A	MMP-2	72	66	Gelatin, collagen types IV, V, VII and XI
Gelatinase B	MMP-9	92	86	Gelatin, collagen types IV and V, elastin
Stromelysin 1	MMP-3	57	46	Proteoglycan core protein, collagen types II, IV, IX, X and XI, procollagen, fibronectin, laminin, elastin (poor), gelatin (limited)
Stromelysin 2	MMP-10	57	46	As for stromelysin 1
Matrilysin	MMP-7	28	20	Proteoglycan, type IV collagen, elastin, fibronectin, gelatin
Macrophage elastase	MMP-12	54	45 (22)	Elastin
Stromelysin 3	MMP-11	51	44	α_1 Proteinase inhibitor
MT1-MMP	MMP-14	64	54	Progelatinase A, procollagenase 3, collagen, proteoglycan, fibronectin, tenascin
MT2-MMP	MMP-15	72	61	As for MT1-MMP
MT3-MMP	MMP-16	66	55	Progelatinase A
MT4-MMP	MMP-17	Unknown	54	Unknown

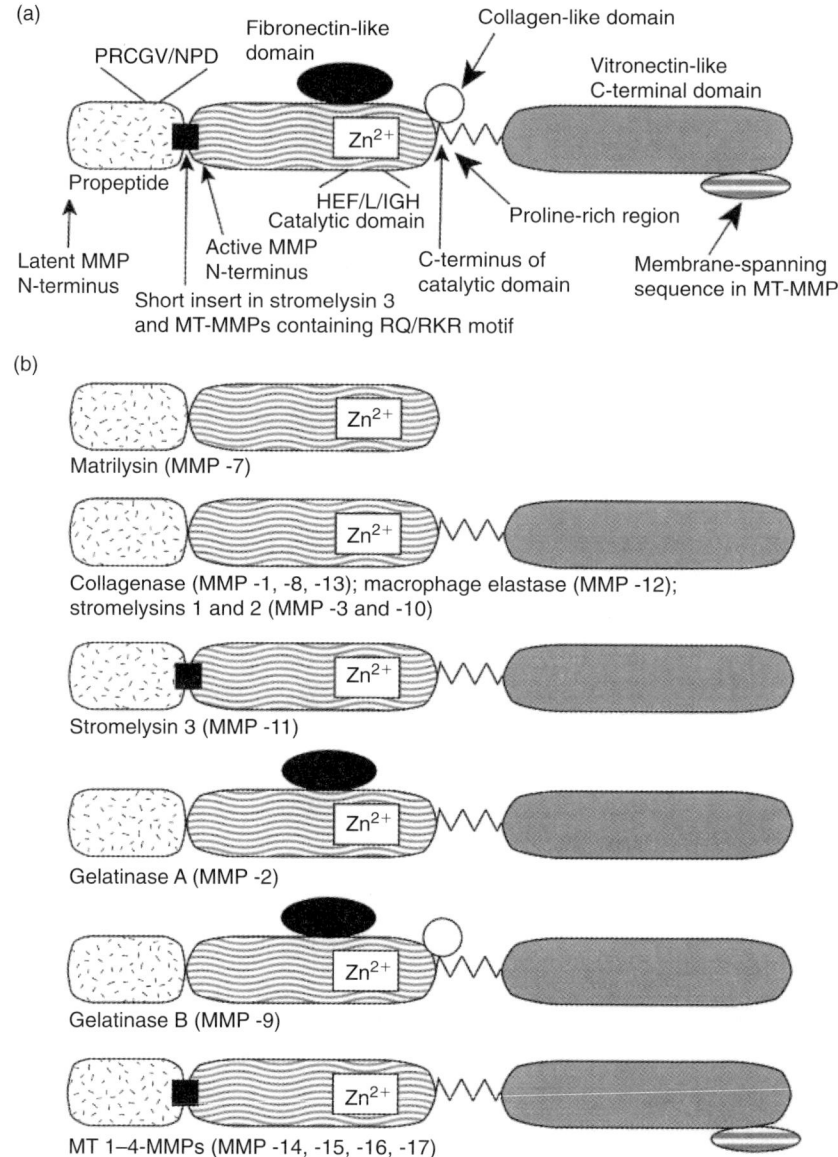

Fig. 1. (a) MMP domains, and (b) domain composition of each of the mammalian MMPs. The MMP family members share a high degree of amino acid sequence identity and, as shown, fall into classes depending on their domain composition. Matrilysin has the simplest domain arrangement, being composed of only a catalytic domain and propeptide. Within the propeptide the sequence motif PRCGV/NPD, which is found in all the MMPs, plays an important structural role in maintaining the latency of all MMP family members [83]. The amino acid sequence of all MMP catalytic domains is distinguished by containing the invariant motif HEXGHXXGXXH, where the three histidine residues co-ordinate the zinc atom at the active site and the glutamic acid ☞

to be susceptible to autoproteolytic cleavage unless its structure is perturbed, and *in vivo* it is thought that this may arise from propeptide clipping by proteinases such as plasmin [44,45]. Gelatinase A is unlike the other enzymes in that its activation cannot be initiated by such proteases [45,46]. Recent studies have, however, identified several membrane-type MMPs (MT-MMPs) that may act as gelatinase A activators on the cell surface [47–52]. In the case of MT1-MMP, increased expression correlates with increased processing of progelatinase A to active species [47,51–53]. Furthermore, progelatinase A can be isolated from cell membranes as a ternary complex with both MT1-MMP and TIMP-2 [54]. How these findings relate to reports of receptors for gelatinase A on the cell surface [55,56] is not yet clear, but they are consistent with the observation that gelatinase A can be activated by cell membranes following some sort of interaction that involves its C-terminal domain [57,58]. TIMP-2 also binds to the progelatinase A C-terminal domain [54,58–64], and at low concentrations appears to promote ternary complex formation, while at high concentrations it can block activation by cell membranes [57,61,63].

In this chapter we show that the expression of gelatinase A, but not of stromelysin-1 or interstitial collagenase, by transfected murine mammary tumour cells facilitates invasiveness into Matrigel, and promotes lung colonization upon tail vein injection. Furthermore, we demonstrate that this phenotype depends not only on the catalytic properties of gelatinase A, which can be reversed by the administration of a gelatinase inhibitor, but also on properties contributed by the non-catalytic C-terminal domain.

Exogeneously added gelatinase facilitates the *in vitro* invasion of a mammary tumour cell line

In an earlier attempt at determining which MMPs contribute most to invasive cancer, we employed *in situ* zymography to measure the relative levels

☞ **Fig. I (contd.)** residue is essential for catalysis. All MMPs except matrilysin possess an additional C-terminal domain, which in the case of gelatinase A confers cell binding properties on the enzyme [58,61,63], and in the case of the collagenases confers collagen specificity [84]. The MT-MMPs have in addition a C-terminally located transmembrane domain (and short cytoplasmic tail) that appear to locate these enzymes at the cell surface. Together with stromelysin 3 the MT-MMPs also have an approx. 10-amino-acid insertion between the propeptide and the catalytic domain that contains a sequence motif (RQ/RKR) which is recognized by members of the propeptide convertase family, such as furin. In the case of stromelysin 3, cleavage at this position leads to loss of the propeptide, and hence enzyme activation [85]. The gelatinases are somewhat different from all the other MMPs in that they both have three repeats of a fibronectin-like matrix binding domain located within their catalytic domains. Gelatinase B has an additional domain that has some identity with collagen, and which may simply act as an additional spacer, together with a proline-rich stretch of amino acids found in most of the MMPs between the catalytic and C-terminal domains.

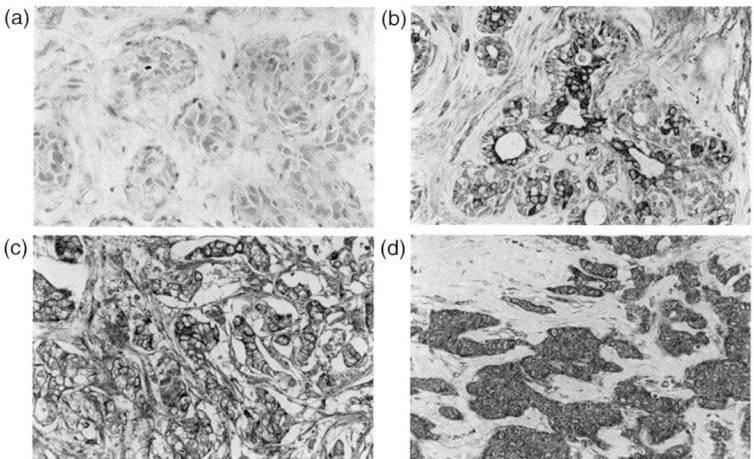

Fig. 2. Immunolocalization of gelatinase A in normal breast and in invasive carcinoma. (a) Normal breast lobule showing a low level of gelatinase A immunostaining, localized to the peripheral myoepithelial cells. The lobular epithelial component is unstained ($\times$ 150). (b) Grade I invasive carcinoma, no special type, showing well formed tubules and intense epithelial staining for gelatinase A, with preferential localization to the luminal surface ($\times$ 150). (c) Grade II invasive carcinoma, no special type, showing intense cytoplasmic staining of the malignant cells ($\times$ 200). (d) Grade III invasive carcinoma, no special type, showing complete absence of tubule formation, nuclear pleomorphism and mitotic activity. There is intense immunostaining for gelatinase A, which is restricted to the tumour cells ($\times$ 100). In some cases focal staining is observed on the epithelial cell surface (b and c). The immunostaining was undertaken by Dr Ken MacLennan at the ICRF Cancer Medicine Research Unit, St James's University Hospital, Leeds, U.K., using the monoclonal antibody (GL8) raised against human gelatinase, as described previously [86].

of gelatinase A, stromelysin 1 and interstitial collagenase mRNAs in breast cancer. Gelatinase A mRNA was found in higher abundance than those for stromelysin 1 or interstitial collagenase [4]. Immunostaining of breast cancer tissue sections, as shown in Fig. 2, also revealed increased levels of gelatinase A protein in the more invasive forms of this disease [3–5].

In order to explore whether the increased levels of gelatinase A might play a causal role in an invasive phenotype, we first measured the relative activities of interstitial collagenase, stromelysin 1, both full-length gelatinase A and a truncated version (Δ418–631) lacking the C-terminal domain (see Fig. 1), and gelatinase B to degrade a reconstituted basement membrane in the form of ^{14}C-labelled Matrigel (Fig. 3a). As previously demonstrated on gelatin and type IV collagen, the truncated version of gelatinase A was found to be equipotent with the full-length enzyme [58]. Stromelysin was found to be more active than gelatinase A when Matrigel was used as the substrate, and gelatinase B was less active. A low activity for interstitial collagenase on this substrate was observed, and this is probably explained by the low content of interstitial collagen in Matrigel.

We tested the ability of each of the enzymes, when added to tumour cells, to facilitate invasion through Matrigel-coated polycarbonate filters in a Transwell apparatus [65]. C127 cells were originally isolated from a murine mammary tumour [66], and although they synthesize low levels of TIMP-2, they do not synthesize detectable levels of TIMP-1 or any of the metalloproteinases described above. In each Transwell experiment we added the amount of enzyme that gave rise to 50% digestion of the Matrigel, as measured previously. Interstitial collagenase failed to achieve 50% digestion, and in this case we used 20 pmol of enzyme. With Matrigel-coated filters to which no enzyme had been added, we observed a decrease in the number of cells passing through the filter compared with non-coated filters (Figs. 3b and 1c). In the presence of gelatinase A, Δ418–631 gelatinase A or gelatinase B, significant invasion did occur if these enzymes were activated (Fig. 1b). Neither active nor latent interstitial collagenase nor stromelysin 1 gave rise to cell invasion (Fig. 1c). Therefore, even though stromelysin 1 is more capable of degrading Matrigel than either of the gelatinases, its activity on this substrate is apparently nonproductive for cell invasion *in vitro*.

In vitro invasion by cells expressing gelatinase A requires the enzyme to possess a C-terminal domain

We measured whether gelatinase expression by C127 cells could also facilitate cell invasion *in vitro* by transfecting the cells with a vector encoding progelatinase A, the truncated (Δ418–631) form or a catalytically inactive form of the enzyme, referred to as E375Q [67]. On submitting the three classes of transfectant to the Matrigel assay we found that they did not differ from the parent cell line in their ability to migrate through non-coated filters (Figs. 4a and 4b). However, in the presence of Matrigel the cell line secreting full-length enzyme achieved an enhanced level of invasion when compared with that obtained with the non-transfected cell line or with cells transfected with either the catalytically inactive E375Q gelatinase or the C-terminally truncated Δ418–631 form. This was despite the fact that both mutant gelatinase A cell lines secreted similar levels of gelatinase as the full-length gelatinase A cell line. We, and more recently others, have shown that gelatinase A activation by cells involves an interaction between the cell membrane and the gelatinase A C-terminal domain, and in the absence of this domain enzyme activation does not occur [58–63]. We showed above that when gelatinase A was added to Matrigel, it had to be activated for it to facilitate C127 cell invasion. Although we do not know the details of the activation mechanism employed by C127 cells, it seems likely that the failure of the Δ418–631 gelatinase transfectants to invade the Matrigel could arise from the inability of this form of the enzyme to become activated when expressed by C127 cells.

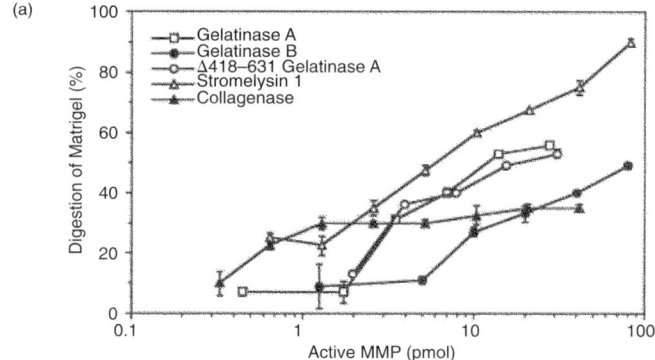

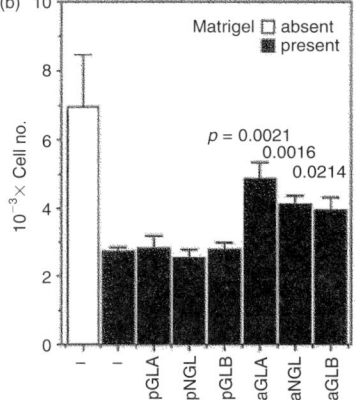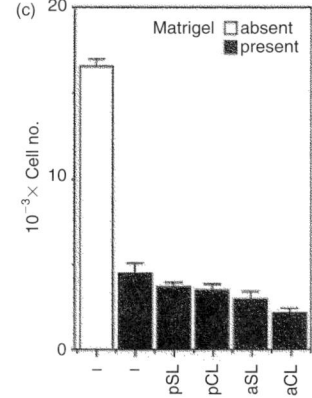

Fig. 3. Invasion of Matrigel by C127 cells in the presence of MMPs.
(a) Hydrolysis of Matrigel by the addition of MMPs. A 30 mg portion of Matrigel (Collaborative Research Inc.) labelled with [^{14}C]acetic anhydride dried on to the bottom of microtitre plate wells was incubated with activated preparations of each enzyme in 100 ml of 100 mM NaCl, 50 mM Tris/HCl, pH 7.4, 5 mM CaCl$_2$ and 0.5% Brij at 37 °C. After 24 h the amount of free ^{14}C was determined with a model 1500 Packard liquid scintillation analyser. The amount of Matrigel remaining was determined after further digestion with 1.00 ml of 0.5 mg/ml trypsin for 24 h at 37 °C. The digestion of the Matrigel by each metalloproteinase was calculated from the amount of ^{14}C present in the supernatant before and after trypsin digestion. A value of 100% digestion refers to the release of ^{14}C after trypsin alone, and 0% is the ^{14}C released after incubation with buffer alone. The molar quantities of each active enzyme were determined by active-site titration against a standard preparation of TIMP-1 [84]. (b, c) Matrigel invasion by C127 cells in the presence of: buffer without enzyme (−), gelatinase A (GLA), Δ418–631 gelatinase A (NGL), gelatinase B, (GLB), stromelysin (SL) or collagenase (CL). The prefixes 'a' and 'p' denote the presence of activated and latent enzyme respectively. Non-coated Transwells (Costar), or Transwells coated with 30 mg of Matrigel, were seeded with 5×10^5 C127 cells in serum-free Dulbecco's modified Eagle's medium. ☞

Expression of gelatinase A, but not stromelysin I or interstitial collagenase, by C127 cells conveys a metastatic phenotype that is dependent on both the gelatinase A catalytic domain and the non-catalytic C-terminal domain

We explored the behaviour of the MMP-secreting cells *in vivo* by examining the lung colonizing properties of human interstitial collagenase, stromelysin 1 and the gelatinase A-secreting C127 cell lines after their injection into the tail veins of Balb/c nu.nu mice. (Fig. 5a). Approx. 5×10^5 gelatinase A-secreting cells generated between 25 and 36 lung nodules after 4 weeks. Mice injected with the same number of untransfected cells or cells transfected with the vector alone or with collagenase or stromelysin gave rise to very low numbers of lung nodules (Fig. 5a). This is despite the stromelysin 1 and gelatinase A ($GL-A_1$) cell lines secreting equimolar amounts of enzyme (0.67 and 0.88 pg/24 h per cell respectively). The molar productivity of the interstitial collagenase cell line is twice that of the $GL-A_2$ cell line (0.36 and 0.21 pg/24 h per cell respectively) but, as shown in Fig. 5(a), the latter cell line generates significantly more lung nodules. The metastatic phenotype contributed by the gelatinase cDNA appeared to result from secretion of the enzyme, since other independently isolated gelatinase A transfectants showed a dose–response relationship between the amount of gelatinase A produced and the number of lung nodules (Fig. 5b).

Interestingly, mice injected with cells that secreted the truncated ($\Delta 418$–631) version of gelatinase A that lacks the C-terminal domain failed to develop lung nodules (Fig. 5a). This is despite the fact that, when activated, this form of the enzyme is catalytically competent with respect to its ability to cleave gelatin, type IV collagen or Matrigel (Fig. 3a), and is consistent with the finding that the cells secreting $\Delta 418$–631 gelatinase A were unable to invade Matrigel-coated filters *in vitro* (Fig. 4b).

The lung colonizing phenotype can be reversed by the administration of a synthetic gelatinase inhibitor

The metastatic phenotype appears to depend on the catalytic properties of gelatinase A or a closely related enzyme, because lung nodule formation

☞ **Fig. 3 (contd.)** The lower chamber contained the same medium with 10% foetal calf serum. Cells were seeded alone or in the presence of the amount of enzyme that gave 50% digestion of the Matrigel, except in the case of collagenase, where 20 pmol was used. The enzyme was added to the upper chamber of the Transwell apparatus and incubated at 37 °C for 60 min before addition of the cells. The total number of cells that traversed the filter was counted after incubation at 37 °C for 72 h, essentially as described in [65], except that the total number of cells passing through the filter was counted. The levels of significance (P) were calculated by two-tailed t test analysis using the StatView programme on an Apple Macintosh, comparing the numbers of cells in the lower chamber after incubation in the presence or absence of added enzyme.

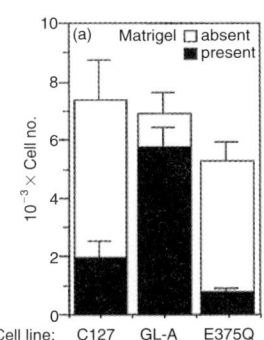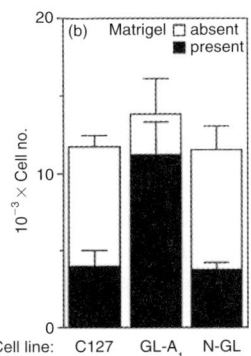

Fig. 4. Matrigel invasion by C127 cells expressing gelatinase A.
Invasion in the presence of Matrigel is increased in the gelatinase A-expressing
transfectants (GL-A) compared with the parental cell line (C127) or (a) C127
cells expressing the catalytically inactive form of gelatinase A (E375Q) or (b)
the C-terminally truncated Δ418–631 form of the enzyme (N-GL). The collage-
nase-expressing cell line (CL) was generated using a human collagenase-
encoding cDNA in a vector containing the murine metallothionein (mMT-1)
promoter, as previously described for the stromelysin-producing cell line (SL)
[87]. The control C127 cell line (CL/SL$_{con}$) was transfected with the same vector, except that it lacked a metalloproteinase coding sequence. The gelatinase
A-expressing C127 cell lines (GL-A$_1$ to GL-A$_6$) are independent isolates that
secrete different amounts of progelatinase A. They were established using the
vector pEE6hCMV.ne, as described previously [88], except that the hCMV promoter was replaced by the same mMT-1 promoter that was used to express
collagenase and stromelysin [87]. The C127 cell line expressing Δ418–631
gelatinase A (N-GL) was made using the pEE6hCMV.ne vector. The corresponding control cell lines (GL-A$_{con}$ and N-GL$_{con}$ respectively) were established
by transfecting C127 cells with the same vectors lacking gelatinase coding
sequences. Using ^{14}C-labelled casein or gelatin as substrate, no endogenous
murine metalloproteinase activity could be detected in serum-free C127 cell
conditioned media. This was confirmed by examining conditioned media on
casein and gelatin zymograms [58]. Using the collagenase diffuse fibril assay
[89], by comparison with standard human TIMP-2, 0.31 pg/24 h per cell murine
TIMP-2 was shown to be secreted. No murine TIMP-1 could be detected by
reverse zymography [58]. These estimates assume that the murine TIMPs have
specific activities that are similar to those of their human counterparts. The
specific production rates of the collagenase- and stromelysin-secreting transfectants grown for 24 h in serum-free Dulbecco's modified Eagle's medium was
determined by ELISA [91], and was 0.36 and 0.67 pg/24 h per cell respectively.
The productivity of each of the gelatinase A-secreting cell lines GL-A$_1$ to GL-A$_6$
was measured similarly [92], with values of 0.88, 0.21, 0.09, 0.02, <0.01 and
<0.01 pg/24 h per cell respectively. The truncated (Δ418–631) gelatinase A-
secreting cell line secreted approx. 0.5 pg/24 h per cell, as determined by
comparative zymography using purified preparations of the truncated enzyme
as a standard [58]. The relative productivity of all the gelatinase A-producing
cell lines was also confirmed by zymography and was found to parallel the
yields expected from the ELISA measurements.

could be reduced by the intravenous administration of CT543, a synthetic gelatinase inhibitor (Fig. 6). The effect appears to depend on the potency of the inhibitor, because the structurally related compound CT636, which has K_i values against gelatinase A and most of the other MMPs that are about 100-fold higher than those for CT543, had no effect in this model (Fig. 6). As previously shown by others [11,12], TIMP-1, the naturally occurring MMP inhibitor that has specificity for all of the MMPs, was also shown to reduce the number of lung nodules, but a direct comparison with the synthetic inhibitors is not possible because of differences in the molar amounts of each inhibitor used (Fig. 6).

Our results with the gelatinase inhibitor also indicate that the gelatinase must be activated for it to confer a metastatic phenotype. How this occurs in C127 cells is unknown, but examples where the focal activation of progelatinase A, sequestered on a cell surface, apparently confers directionality to an invading cell have been reported [68,69]. A scheme by which this may occur is depicted in Fig. 7. A key observation that supports the scheme is the finding

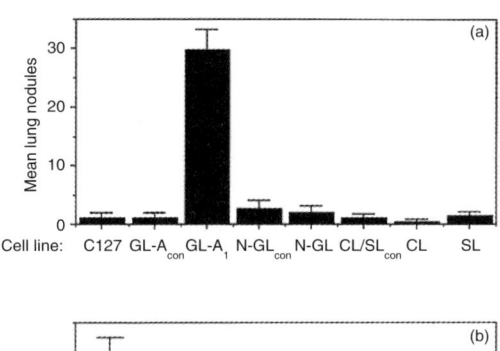

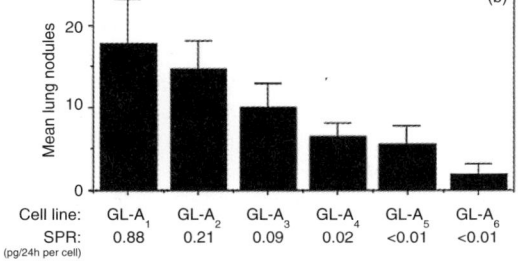

Fig. 5. Lung nodule formation in Balb/c nu.nu mice after tail vein injection of transfected C127 cell lines. (a) Lung nodules arising from the parental cell line or transfectants expressing gelatinase A (GL-A$_1$), truncated (Δ418–631) gelatinase A lacking the C-terminal domain (N-GL), collagenase (CL) or stromelysin (SL); GL-A$_{con}$, N-GL$_{con}$ and CL/SL$_{con}$ are the corresponding control cell lines lacking metalloproteinase coding sequences. (b) Lung nodule formation by independently isolated C127 clones possessing different specific production rates (SPR) for gelatinase A (GL-A$_1$ to GL-A$_6$). Approx. 5×10^5 C127 cells or C127 transfectants were injected into the tail veins of groups of 10 female Balb/c nu.nu mice. Lung nodules were scored 4 weeks after staining in Bouins fixative [90]. For details of the cell lines see Fig. 4.

that excess gelatinase A C-terminal domain, when added to cells *in vitro*, can block both cell binding and activation of gelatinase A on the cell surface [58,61,63]. We therefore conclude that our finding that the C-terminal domain is required for invasion *in vitro* and metastasis *in vivo* may result from it conferring cell binding properties on the enzyme that lead to its activation. The recent discovery of a family of MT-MMPs, and the localization of at least one of them (MT1-MMP) to the surface of invasive tumours cells, where it can be found associated with both TIMP-2 and progelatinase A, lends credence to this idea [45,54,63]. A prediction arising from the scheme shown in Fig. 7 is that an excess of progelatinase A, in a catalytically inactive form, might be able to compete with the endogenous wild-type enzyme for binding sites on either the cell surface or the extracellular matrix, or both. If so, we hypothesized that it could modify the invasive properties of the gelatinase A transfectants. As shown in Fig. 8, 1×10^6 GL-A$_1$ cells were incubated for 1 h with 25 μg of either a E375A catalytically inactive gelatinase A proenzyme or wild-type proenzyme, and then injected into the tail veins of Balb/c nu.nu mice. Cells that had been incubated with the catalytically inactive proenzyme generated significantly fewer lung nodules after 4 weeks compared with the number generated by untreated cells or cells that had been incubated with the wild-type proenzyme.

Conclusions

Spontaneous transformants of the murine mammary tumour C127 cell line, or variants that have been transformed by *ras*, have previously been shown to be tumorigenic but not metastatic [70]. From these data, Liotta and colleagues concluded that C127 cells, unlike NIH 3T3 cells, lack the genetic elements necessary for metastasis and that these elements are separate from those required for tumorigenicity [71,72]. Transfection of a rat bladder carcinoma cell line, that already expresses endogenous levels of interstitial collagenase and gelatinase B, with gelatinase A has also been reported to generate a more metastatic phenotype [21]. Our results go further, in that we show that expression of gelatinase A alone by C127 cells, which do not normally express MMPs, is sufficient to convert them into a more metastatic phenotype, and that this requires the enzyme to have an intact C-terminal domain. Transfection of cells with matrilysin [16] or gelatinase B [18] is also reported to give rise to a metastatic phenotype, but in both of these cases endogenous levels of gelatinase A were also synthesized by the recipient cells.

The inability of stromelysin or collagenase to confer the metastatic phenotype in our system may be due to these enzymes failing to become activated, or the activity of these enzymes simply being non-productive for invasion. Urokinase and plasmin are thought to be important stromelysin and collagenase activators *in vivo*, and both are present in our model (M.I. Crockett and G. Murphy, unpublished work). We therefore believe that it is unlikely that the stromelysin or collagenase failed to become active. The main collagenous component of basement membrane is type IV collagen, and therefore the explanation for interstitial collagenase failing to confer an invasive phenotype may be related to this enzyme having only poor activity on type IV collagen.

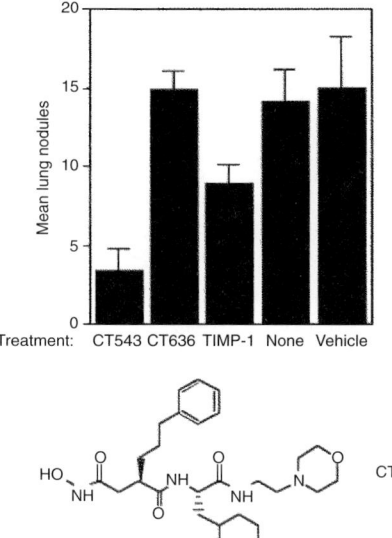

Fig. 6. Effects of metalloproteinase inhibitors on lung colony formation by the gelatinase A-secreting C127 GL-A1 cell line in Balb/c nu.nu mice. Metalloproteinase inhibitors were tested in mice injected with C127 GL-A$_1$ cells as described in the legend to Fig. 4, except that the cells were mixed with either 100 mg of CT543 or CT636 in 200 μl of PBS/ethanol (19:1, v/v), or 50 mg of TIMP-1 in 200 ml of PBS, prior to injection. Control groups received C127 GL-A$_1$ cells alone or cells mixed with 200 μl of PBS/ethanol (19:1, v/v). Inhibitor- or vehicle-treated groups received a second tail vein injection of drug or vehicle 24 h later. CT543 and CT636 are gelatinase substrate peptidomimetics which include a hydroxamic or carboxylic acid group respectively that acts as a zinc binding ligand [93]. The K_i values against gelatinase A, gelatinase B, stromelysin 1, collagenase and matrilysin are 0.1 nM, 1.53 nM, 24 nM, 210 nM and >10 mM respectively for CT543, and 10 nM, 67 nM, 1.47 mM, 57.8 mM and >10 mM respectively for CT636. The latter compound is therefore about 100-fold less potent than CT543, but they share a similar level of selectivity.

If cell mobility requires some degree of cell–matrix attachment, it could be that matrix degradation under some circumstances could be counter-productive for invasion, due to it leading to the loss of essential cell attachment sites. The details of the matrix loss will vary according to the precise substrate specificity of the particular enzyme involved. For example, it is known that stromelysin 1 cleaves within the globular N- and C-terminal non-helical regions of type IV collagen, whereas gelatinase A cleaves at a locus within the

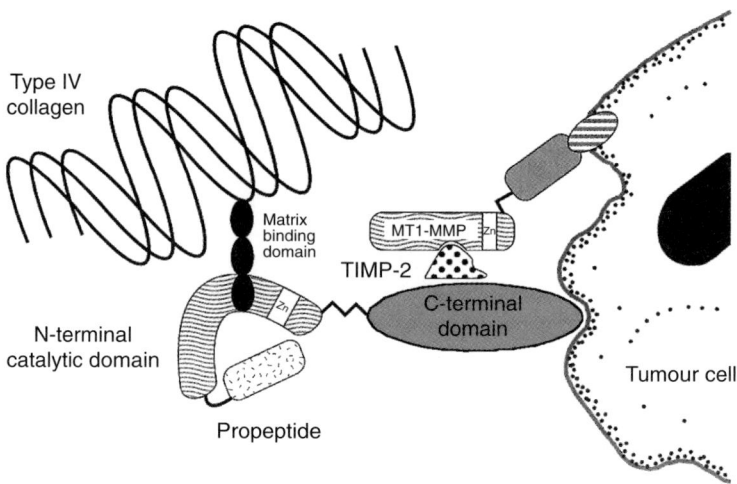

Fig. 7. Scheme showing the way in which gelatinase A may bind to both the cell surface and the extracellular matrix. Sequestration of progelatinase A on the cell surface by its C-terminal domain, possibly through interactions with cell-bound MT1-MMP and TIMP-2, integrin αvβ3 or other unknown receptors, is thought to give rise to its localized activation, at the motile front of invading cells [54–56,68,69]. The potential for gelatinase A to bind simultaneously to the extracellular cell matrix is also shown [94].

helical domain [73]. Indeed, it has been shown that, in the case of melanoma cells, gelatinase A activity directly modulates cell adhesion and spreading [69], whereas the overexpression of stromelysin 1 in transgenic mice is insufficient for progression of mammary adenocarcinomas to an invasive and metastatic phenotype [74].

Although there are several steps in the metastatic pathway that may be gelatinase A-dependent [1,38], it is most likely that the non-cytotoxic inhibitors used in this study reduce the number of lung colonies by preventing extravasation by the tumour cells, or their subsequent immediate invasion and establishment in the extravascular space. This is because the decrease in lung nodules observed at 4 weeks was accomplished by just two doses of an inhibitor, administered during the early part of the experiment: once at the time that the cells were injected, and again 24 h later. The clearance rate of the inhibitor is such that it is not expected to be present beyond the first 36 h.

Unfortunately, anti-metastasis therapy alone is unlikely to be of benefit to cancer patients with already disseminated disease. Furthermore, metastasis inhibition might be very hard to demonstrate in such patients. It is therefore encouraging that longer-term treatment with MMP inhibitors has been found to reduce primary tumour growth rates in a variety of cancer models, and this observation does not appear to be due to any cytotoxic effects of the MMP inhibitors on tumour cells ([13–15,17,19,20,22,23,95]. Although the mechanism by which they inhibit tumour growth is unknown, direct anti-angiogenic

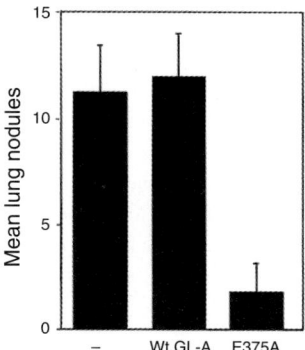

Fig. 8. Effect on lung nodule formation of mixing catalytically inactive gelatinase A with the C127 gelatinase A transfectants prior to tail vein injection. The tail veins of Balb/c nu.nu mice were injected with the GL-A$_1$ gelatinase A-secreting cell line after it had been incubated for 60 min in the absence ($-$) or in the presence of 25 mg of either wild-type (Wt.GL-A) or catalytically inactive (E375A) gelatinase A.

effects have been reported with MMP inhibitors ([40,41]; V. Mahaclevan, I.R. Hart and A.J.P. Docherty, unpublished work). In nearly all of these models, however, very high levels of inhibitor have been used. Furthermore, the inhibitors employed possess very broad enzyme specificity, being potent inhibitors of the entire MMP family. Since the plasma concentrations of inhibitor achieved in the animal models cited above are not usually reported, it is possible that the reduced rates of tumour growth arise from the inhibitors achieving concentrations at which they inhibit metalloproteinases other than the well characterized MMPs. Such a view is entirely plausible, given the avalanche of reports describing numerous physiological processing events mediated by as yet uncharacterized metalloproteinases ([75–78] and references therein). Nonetheless, these new enzymes are sufficiently related to the MMPs to be inhibited by the types of inhibitor currently used in cancer models [75,76].

The most promising setting in which MMP inhibitor therapy might be envisaged is following some kind of cytotoxic therapy to reduce the primary tumour burden. Recently we have successfully used such an approach in Lewis lung carcinoma-bearing mice [79]. Mice were treated continuously with an orally active gelatinase inhibitor starting several days after tumour implantation, in combination with either cisplatin (once on day 7) or cyclophosphamide (on days 5, 7, 9 and 11). For the optimal gelatinase inhibitor/cisplatin combination, a delay in tumour growth of 12.4 days was observed, compared with 4.5 days for cisplatin alone. For the cyclophosphamide/gelatinase inhibitor combination, the delay was increased from 19.5 to 30.9 days. The combination therapy also reduced the incidence of spontaneous pulmonary metastasis to 33% (gelatinase inhibitor/cisplatin) and 21% (gelatinase inhibitor/cyclophosphamide) of the vehicle-treated group, compared with 75% and 46% respectively for cisplatin and cyclophosphamide alone.

These findings, together with our observation that gelatinase inhibitors can block some kinds of bone resorption *in vitro* [80,81], indicate that chronically administered gelatinase inhibitors, in combination with established chemotherapies, might increase disease-free intervals in breast cancer patients, with a reduction in bone-metastasis-associated morbidity.

We gratefully acknowledge Simon Tickle and Terry Baker for monoclonal antibody GL8, Di Eaton for the K_i measurements and help with the active-site titrations, Mary Harrison for activity assays, Stan Zucker for construction of the gelatinase A active-site mutants and help with the ELISAs, and Geoff Yarranton for helpful comments on the manuscript. G.M. is supported by the Arthritis and Rheumatism Council, U.K.

References

1.   Hart, I.R. and Saini, A. (1992) Lancet **339**, 1453–1457
2.   MacDougall, J.R. and Matrisian, L.M. (1995) Cancer Metastasis Rev. **14**, 351–362
3.   Monteagudo, C., Merino, M.L., San, J.J., Liotta, L.A. and Stetler-Stevenson, W.G. (1990) Am. J. Pathol. **136**, 585–592
4.   Polette, M., Clavel, C., Cockett, M.I., Girod de Bentzmann, S., Murphy, G. and Birembaut, P. (1993) Invasion Metastasis **13**, 31–37
5.   Poulsom, R., Hanby, A.M., Pignatelli, M., Jeffery, R.E., Longcroft, J.M., Rogers, L. and Stamp, G.W.H. (1993) J. Clin. Pathol. **46**, 429–436
6.   Wolf, C., Rouyer, N., Lutz, Y., et al. (1993) Proc. Natl. Acad. Sci. U.S.A. **90**, 1843–1847
7.   Rouyer, N., Wolf, C., Chenard, M.P., Rio, M.C., Chambon, P., Bellocq, J.P. and Basset, P. (1995) Invasion Metastasis **14**, 269–275
8.   Onisto, M., Riccio, M.P., Scannapieco, P., et al. (1995) Int. J. Cancer **63**, 621–626
9.   Freiji, J.M., Diez-Itza, I., Balbin, M., Sanchez, R., Blasco, R., Tolivia, J. and Lopez-Otin, C. (1994) J. Biol. Chem. **269**, 16766–16773
10.   Frisch, S.M., Reich, R., Collier, I.E., Genrich, L.T., Martin, G. and Goldberg, G.I. (1990) Oncogene **5**, 75–83
11.   Schultz, R.M., Silberman, S., Persky, B., Bajkowski, A.S. and Carmichael, D.F. (1988) Cancer Res. **8**, 5539–5545
12.   Alvarez, O.A., Carmichael, D.F. and DeClerck, Y.A. (1990) J. Natl. Cancer Inst. **82**, 589–595
13.   Davies, B., Brown, P.D., East, N., Crimmin, M.J. and Balkwill, R. (1993) Cancer Res. **3**, 2087–2091
14.   Wang, X., Fu, X., Brown, P.D., Crimmin, M.J. and Hoffman, R.M. (1994) Cancer Res. **54**, 4726–4728
15.   Koop, S., Khokha, R., Schmidt, E.E., MacDonald, I.A., Morris, V.L. Chambers, A.F. and Groom, A.C. (1994) Cancer Res. **54**, 4791–4797
16.   Witty, J.P., McDonnell. S., Newell, K., Cannon, P., Navre, M., Tressler, R. and Matrisian, L.M. (1994) Cancer Res. **4**, 4805–4812
17.   Montgomery, A.M.P., Mueller, B.M., Reisfeld, R.A., Taylor, S.M. and DeClerck, Y.A. (1994) Cancer Res. **54**, 5467–5473
18.   Bernhard, E.J., Gruber, S.B. and Muschel, R.J. (1994) Proc. Natl. Acad. Sci. U.S.A. **91**, 4293–4297
19.   Chirivi, R.G., Garofalo, A., Crimmin, M.J., Bawden, L.J., Stoppacciaro, A., Brown, P.D. and Giavazzi, R. (1994) Int. J. Cancer **58**, 460–464

20. Naito, K., Kanbayashi, N., Nakajima, S., Murai, T., Arakawa, K., Nishimura, S. and Okuyama, A. (1994) Int. J. Cancer **58**, 730–735

21. Kawamata, H., Kameyama, S., Kawai, K., et al. (1995) Int. J. Cancer **63**, 568–575

22. Watson, S.A., Morris, T.M., Robinson, G., Crimmin, M.J., Brown, P.D. and Hardcastle, J.D. (1995) Cancer Res. **55**, 3629–3633

23. Low, J.A., Johnson, M.D., Bone, E.A. and Dickson, R.B. (1996) Clin. Cancer Res. **2**, 1207–1214

24 Brown, P.D. (1994) Ann. N.Y. Acad. Sci. **732**, 217–221

25. Beckett, R.P., Davidson, A.H., Drummond, A.H., Huxley, P. and Whittaker, M. (1996) Drug Discovery Today **1**, 16–26

26. Birkedal Hansen, H., Moore, W.G., Bodden, M.K., Windsor, L.J., Birkedal Hansen, B., DeCarlo, A. and Engler, J.A. (1993) Crit. Rev. Oral Biol. Med. **4**, 197–250

27. Pyke, C., Ralfkiaer, E., Huhtala, P., Hurskainen, T., Dano, K. and Tryggvason, K. (1992) Cancer Res. **52**, 1336–1341

28. Gray, S.T., Wilkins, R.J. and Yun, K. (1992) Am. J. Pathol. **141**, 301–306

29. Basset, P., Wolf, N., Rouyer, J.P., Bellocq, J.P., Rio, M.C. and Chambon, P. (1994) Cancer **74**, 1045–1049

30. Kataoka, H., DeCastro, R., Zucker, S. and Biswas, C. (1993) Cancer Res. **53**, 3154–3158

31. Noel, A.C., Polette, M., Lewalle, J.M., Munaut, C., Emonard, P., Birembaut, P. and Foidart, J.M. (1994) Int. J. Cancer **56**, 331–336

32. Crawford, H.C. and Matrisian, L.M. (1995) Invasion Metastasis **14**, 234–245

33. Talhouk, R.K., Bissel, M.J. and Werb, Z. (1992) J. Cell Biol. **118**, 1271–1282

34. Sympson, C.J., Talhouk, R.S., Alexander, C.M., Chin, J.R., Clift, S.M., Bissell, M.J. and Werb, Z. (1994) J. Cell Biol. **125**, 681–693

35. Witty, J.P., Wright, J.H. and Matrisian, L.M. (1995) Mol. Biol. Cell **6**, 1287–1303

36. Lund, L.R., Romer, J., Thomasset, N., et al. (1996) Development **122**, 181–193

37. Mignatti, P., Tsuboi, R., Robbins, E. and Rifkin, D.B. (1989) J. Cell Biol. **108**, 671–682

38. Liotta, L.A., Steeg, P.S. and Stetler-Stevenson, W.G. (1991) Cell **64**, 327–336

39. Schnaper, H.W., Grant, D.S., Stetler-Stevenson, W.G., et al. (1993) J. Cell. Physiol. **156**, 235–246

40. Galardy, R.E., Grobelny, D., Foellmer, H.G. and Fernandez, L.A. (1994) Cancer Res. **54**, 4715–4718

41. Taraboletti, G., Garofalo, A., Belotti, D., Drudis, T., Borsotti, P., Scanziani, E., Brown, P.D. and Giavazzi, R. (1995) J. Natl. Cancer Inst. **87**, 293–298

42. Docherty, A.J.P., O'Connell, J., Crabbe, T., Angal, S. and Murphy, G. (1992) Trends Biotechnol. **10**, 200–207

43. Apte, S.S., Olsen, B.R. and Murphy, G. (1995) J. Biol. Chem. **270**, 14313–14318

44. Murphy, G., Ward, R., Gavrilovic, J. and Atkinson, S. (1992) Matrix Suppl. **1**, 224–230

45. Atkinson, S.J., Ward, R.V., Reynolds, J.J. and Murphy, G. (1992) Biochem. J. **288**, 605–611

46. Hipps, D.S., Hembry, R.M., Docherty, A.J.P., Reynolds, J.J. and Murphy, G. (1991) Biol. Chem. Hoppe-Seyler **372**, 287–296

47. Sato, H., Takino, T., Okada, Y., Cao, J., Shinagawa, A., Yamamoto, E. and Seiki, M. (1994) Nature (London) **370**, 61–65

48. Will, H. and Hinzmann, B. (1995) Eur. J. Biochem. **231**, 602–608

49. Takino, T., Sato, H., Shinagawa, A. and Seiki, M. (1995) J. Biol. Chem. **270**, 23013–23020

50. Puente, X.S., Pendas, A.M., Llano, E., Velasco, G. and Lopez-Otin, C. (1996) Cancer Res. **56**, 944–949

51. Pei, D. and Weiss, S.J. (1996) J. Biol. Chem. **271**, 9135–9140

52. Will, H., Atkinson, S.J., Butler, G.S., Smith, B. and Murphy, G. (1996) J. Biol. Chem. **271**, 17119–17123

53. Atkinson, S.J., Crabbe, T., Cowell, S., et al. (1995) J. Biol. Chem. **270**, 30479–30485

54. Strongin, A.Y., Collier, I., Bannikov, G., Marmer, B.L., Grant, G.A. and Goldberg, G.I. (1995) J. Biol. Chem. **270**, 5331–5338

55. Emonard, H.P., Remacle, A.G., Noel, A.C., Grimaud, J.-A., Stetler-Stevenson, W.G. and Foidart, J.M. (1992) Cancer Res. **52**, 5845–5848

56. Brooks, P.C., Stromblad, S., Sanders, L.C., et al. (1996) Cell **85**, 683–693

57. Ward, R.V., Atkinson, S.J., Slocombe, P.M., Docherty, A.J.P., Reynolds, J.J. and Murphy, G. (1991) Biochim. Biophys. Acta **1079**, 242–246

58. Murphy, G., Willenbrock, F., Ward, R.V., Cockett, M.I., Eaton, D. and Docherty, A.J.P. (1992) Biochem. J. **283**, 637–641

59. Howard, E.W. and Banda, M.J. (1992) J. Biol. Chem. **266**, 17972–17977

60. Fridman, R., Fuerst, T.R., Bird, R.E., et al. (1992) J. Biol. Chem. **267**, 15398–15405

61. Strongin, A.Y., Marmer, B.L., Grant, G.A. and Goldberg, G.I. (1993) J. Biol. Chem. **268**, 14033–14039

62. Willenbrock, F., Crabbe, T., Slocombe, P.M., et al. (1993) Biochemistry **32**, 4330–4337

63. Ward, R.V., Atkinson, S.J., Reynolds, J.J. and Murphy, G. (1994) Biochem. J. **304**, 263–269

64. Imai, K., Ohuchi, E., Aoki, T., et al. (1996) Cancer Res. **56**, 2707–2710

65. Repesh, L.A. (1989) Invasion Metastasis **9**, 192–208

66. Lowy, D.R., Rands, E. and Scolnick, E.M. (1978) J. Virol. **26**, 291–298

67. Crabbe, T., Zucker, S., Cockett, M.I., et al. (1994) Biochemistry **33**, 6684–6690

68. Monsky, W.L., Kelly, T., Lin, C.-Y., Yeh, Y., Stetler-Stevenson, W.G., Mueller, S.C. and Chen, W.-T. (1993) Cancer Res. **53**, 3159–3164

69. Ray, J.M. and Stetler-Stevenson, W.G. (1995) EMBO J. **14**, 908–917

70. Muschel, R.J., Williams, J.E., Lowy, D.R. and Liotta, L.A. (1985) Am. J. Pathol. **121**, 1–8

71. Thorgeirsson, U.P., Turpeenniemi-Hujanen, T., Williams, J.E., Westin, E.H., Heilman, C.A., Talmadge, J.E. and Liotta, L.A. (1985) Mol. Cell. Biol. **5**, 259–262

72. Garbisa, S., Pozzatti, R., Muschel, R.J., et al. (1987) Cancer Res. **47**, 1523–1528

73. Eble, J., Ries, A., Lichy, A., et al. (1996) J. Biol. Chem., **271**, 30964–30970

74. Witty, J.P., Lempka, T., Coffey, Jr., R.J. and Matrisian, L.M. (1995) Cancer Res. **55**, 1401–1406

75. Mohler, K.M., Sleath, P.R., Fitzer, J.N., et al. (1994) Nature (London) **370**, 218–220

76. Walcheck, B., Kahn, J., Fisher, J.M., et al. (1996) Nature (London) **380**, 720–723

77. Goetzl, E.J., Banda, M.J. and Leppert, D. (1996) J. Immunol. **156**, 1–4

78. Arribas, J., Coodly, L., Vollmer, P., Kishimoto, T.K., Rose-John, S. and Massague, J. (1996) J. Biol. Chem. **271**, 11376–11382

79. Anderson, I.C., Shipp, M.A., Docherty, A.J.P. and Teicher, B.A. (1996) Cancer Res. **56**, 715–718

80. Hill, P.A., Murphy, G., Docherty, A.J.P., Hembry, R.M., Millican, T.A., Reynolds, J.J. and Meikle, M.C. (1994) J. Cell Sci. **107**, 3055–3064

81. Hill, P.A., Docherty, A.J.P., Bottomley, K.M.K., O'Connell, J.P., Morphy, J.R., Reynolds, J.J. and Meikle, M.C. (1995) Biochem. J. **308**, 167–175

82. Shapiro, S.D., Kobayashi, D.K. and Ley, T.J. (1993) J. Biol. Chem. **268**, 23824–23829

83. Springman, E., Angleton, E., Birkedal-Hansen, H. and Van Wart, H. (1990) Proc. Natl. Acad. Sci. U.S.A. **87**, 364–368

84. Murphy, G., Allan, J.A., Willenbrock, F., Cockett, M.I., O'Connell, J.P. and Docherty, A.J.P. (1992) J. Biol. Chem. **267**, 9612–9618

85. Pei, D. and Weiss, S.J. (1995) Nature (London) **375**, 244–247

86. Afzal, S., El-Nasir, L., Foulks, W.D., et al. (1996) Lab. Invest. **74**, 406–421

87. Docherty, A.J.P. and Murphy, G. (1990) Ann. Rheum. Dis. **49**, 469–479

88. Bebbington, C.R. (1991) Methods (San Diego) **2**, 136–145

89. Cawston, T.E. and Murphy, G. (1981) Methods Enzymol. **80**, 711–722

90. Cooksley, S., Hipkiss, J.B., Tickle, S.P., Holmes-Ievers, E., Docherty, A.J.P., Murphy, G. and Lawson, A.D.G. (1990) Matrix **10**, 285–291

91. Zucker, S., Lysik, R.M., Gurfinkel, M., et al. (1992) J. Immunol. Methods **148**, 189–198
92. Fidler, I.J. (1978) Methods Cancer Res. **15**, 399–439
93. Beeley, N.R.A., Ansell, P.R.J. and Docherty, A.J.P. (1994) Curr. Opin. Ther. Pat. **4**, 7–16
94. Allan, J.A., Docherty, A.J.P., Barker, P.J., Huskisson, N.S. and Reynolds, J.J. (1995) Biochem. J. **309**, 299–306
95. An, Z.L., Wang, X.E., Willmott, N., et al. (1997) Clin. Exp. Metastasis **15**, 184–195

Subject Index